PRINCIPLES *and* PRACTICE *of*

Interventional Cardiology

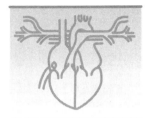

SUE APPLE, DNSc, RN, CCRN

Cardiology Clinical Nurse Specialist
Medical/Obstetrical/Ambulatory Clinical Nursing Division
The Washington Hospital Center
Washington, DC

JOSEPH LINDSAY, Jr., MD

Director, Section of Cardiology
The Washington Hospital Center
Washington, DC

Acquisitions Editor: Susan M. Glover, RN, MSN
Production Editor: Jennifer D. Weir
Coordinating Editorial Assistant: Hilarie M. Surrena

Copyright © 2000 Lippincott Williams & Wilkins

351 West Camden Street
Baltimore, Maryland 21201-2436 USA

227 East Washington Square
Philadelphia, PA 19106

Printed in the United States of America

Library of Congress Cataloging-in-Publication Data

Apple, Sue.
    Principles and practice of interventional cardiology / Sue Apple,
Joseph Lindsay, Jr.
        p.   cm.
    Includes index.
    ISBN 0-7817-1020-0
    1. Heart—Diseases—Treatment.   2. Heart—Surgery.   3. Coronary
heart disease—Surgery.   4. Myocardial revascularization.
    I. Lindsay, Joseph, 1932–   . II. Title.
    [DNLM: 1. Myocardial Revascularization—methods.   2. Myocardial
Revascularization—instrumentation.   WG 169 A648p 1999]
    RC683.8.A66   1999
    617.4'12—dc21
    DNLM/DLC   99-38188
    for Library of Congress   CIP

To purchase additional copies of this book, call our customer service department at **(800) 638-3030** or fax orders to **(301) 824-7390**. International customers should call **(301) 714-2324**.

99 00 01 02 03
1 2 3 4 5 6 7 8 9 10

*T*o the nurses, cardiovascular technicians, and all the other health care professionals at the Washington Hospital Center who deliver excellent care to patients undergoing percutaneous interventional procedures. Their avid interest in establishing the best practice area in this field inspired us to write this book.

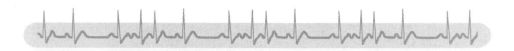

Contributors

Alexandre Abizaid, MD
Director, Intravascular Ultrasound
   Core Lab
Institute Dante Pazzanese of Cardiology
Brazil

Andrea S. Abizaid, MD
Director, Angiographic Core Lab
Interventional Cardiology
Institute Dante Pazzanese of Cardiology
Brazil

Sue Apple, RN, DNSc, CCRN
Medical/OB/Ambulatory Clinical
   Nursing Division
Washington Hospital Center
Washington, DC

George Dangas, MD
Director of Clinical Pharmacology &
   Endovascular Thrombosis
Cardiovascular Research Foundation
Cardiac Catheterization Laboratory
Washington Hospital Center
Washington, DC

Ann Greenberg, RN, MSN
Clinical Research Nurse Coordinator
Cardiovascular Research Foundation
Washington Hospital Center
Washington, DC

Rainer Hoffman, MD
Department of Internal Medicine
Section of Cardiology
Washington Hospital Center
Washington, DC

Mun K. Hong, MD
Cardiology Division (Interventional
   Cardiology)
Washington Hospital Center
Washington, DC

Katie Kehoe, RN, BSN, MS
Clinical Specialist, Cardiology
Washington Cardiology Center
Washington, DC

Kenneth M. Kent, MD
Director, Washington Hospital Center
Washington, DC

Ran Kornowski, MD
Director of Experimental Pharmacology
   and Myocardial Revascularization
Cardiovascular Research Foundation
Washington Hospital Center
Washington, DC

John R. Laird, MD, FACC, FACP
Director of Peripheral Vascular
   Interventions
Cardiology Research Foundation
Washington Hospital Center
Washington, DC

Alexandra J. Lansky, MD
Director, Angiographic Care Laboratory
   and Women's Cardiac Health Initiative
Cardiology Research Foundation
Washington Hospital Center
Washington, DC

Martin B. Leon, MD
Director and CEO, Cardiovascular
    Research Foundation
Washington Hospital Center
Washington, DC

Joseph Lindsay, Jr., MD
Director, Section of Cardiology
Washington Hospital Center
Washington, DC

Susan Marden, RN, MS
Clinical Nurse Specialist
Department of Nursing
National Institutes of Health
Bethesda, Maryland

Roxana Mehran, MD, FACC
Director of Clinical Research and
    Data Coordinating Center
Cardiovascular Research Foundation
Cardiac Catheterization Laboratory
Washington Hospital Center
Washington, DC

Gary S. Mintz, MD, FACC
Director, Coronary Ultrasound
Cardiovascular Research Foundation
Intravascular Ultrasound Imaging and
    Cardiac Catheterization Laboratories
Washington Hospital Center
Washington, DC

Nancy Morris, RN, BSN, RCVT
Cardiology Division
Cardiology Research Foundation
Washington Hospital Center
Washington, DC

Michael A. Peterson, MD
Cardiac Catheterization Laboratories
Cardiology Fellow
Washington Hospital Center
Washington, DC

Ellen E. Pinnow, RN, MS
Epidemiologist
Section of Cardiology
Washington Hospital Center
Washington, DC

Jorge F. Saucedo, MD
Assistant Professor of Internal Medicine
Director, Cardiac Catheterization
    Laboratories
John L. McClellan VA Hospital &
    UAMS Medical Center
Little Rock, Arkansas

Lucy Van Voorhees, MD
Director, Coronary Care Unit
Washington Hospital Center
Washington, DC

Ron Waksman, MD
Clinical Associate Professor of Medicine
    (Cardiology)
Georgetown University
Director of Experimental Angioplasty
    and Vascular Brachytherapy
Cardiovascular Research Foundation
Washington Hospital Center
Washington, DC

Carol Walsh, RCVT
Supervisor, IVUS Technical Services
Washington Hospital Center
Washington, DC

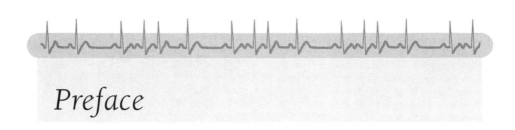

Preface

Percutaneous transluminal coronary angioplasty came to the Washington Hospital Center in the early 1980s, bringing to the cardiology nursing and technology staff a real sense of adventure and experimentation. Patient care in the catheterization laboratory and in the coronary care unit changed repeatedly as staff learned "on the job" the best way to care for patients undergoing these new procedures. The catheterization laboratory became more than a stop on the way to the operating room.

As the devices expanded from "plain old balloons" to include cutters, shavers, lasers, and stents, the catheterization laboratory also expanded to accommodate new interventionists and an exponential increase in patient volume. To handle this increase, nursing practice changed to provide care for these patients outside the intensive care unit. Lately, the catheterization laboratory has changed again to accommodate peripheral procedures, challenging the staff again to develop safe and effective ways to manage patients undergoing procedures in any part of the vascular tree, including the cerebral circulation.

With the growth of interventional procedures, there is a real need for a text to address the special needs of this population. This book is the outgrowth of years of experience with thousands of patients by many dedicated health care professionals, both in the catheterization laboratory and on the nursing units. It is intended to be a clinical reference for nurses, cardiovascular technicians, and other allied health care professionals who provide direct care for patients undergoing interventional procedures in the hospital setting.

The text is divided into four sections. Chapter 1 is a personal recounting of the development of interventional cardiology by Dr. Kent. The second section addresses the Basics—anatomy and physiology as well as coagulation. Percutaneous devices are covered in Section III. The last section addresses Clinical Issues, such as restenosis, management of the patients, and measurement of outcomes.

Our hope is that this book will become a valuable clinical resource for all practitioners in this exciting field.

Sue Apple
Joseph Lindsay, Jr.

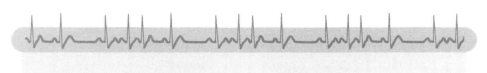

Acknowledgments

Special thanks to Dr. Kenneth Kent, who allowed extensive use of his personal archives, from which many of the angiographic cases in this book were taken.

To M. Katherine Kehoe, RN, MS, who spent hours helping to select and review catheterization films.

And finally to Brian K. Greer, Multimedia Coordinator, who provided essential computer and graphic skills.

Contents

Section III   Clinical Issues

CHAPTER 1

Development of Interventional Cardiology

KENNETH M. KENT, MD

Coronary heart disease (CHD) is the number one cause of death in the United States.[1] In addition to the 500,000 deaths each year, there is considerable morbidity associated with 500,000 nonfatal myocardial infarctions, as well as limitations of activity due to angina pectoris.

During each of the decades from 1960, mortality due to CHD has decreased. This phenomenon has resulted from many factors, including the Public Health initiatives from the National Heart Lung and Blood Institutes, which promoted control of major risk factors of CHD: systemic hypertension, cigarette smoking, and cholesterol.

Coronary revascularization procedures may now be having an impact on mortality from CHD. Evidence indicates that coronary revascularization through coronary artery bypass surgery (CABG) or percutaneous transluminal coronary angioplasty (PTCA) reduces morbidity, such as in those with angina associated with CHD.[2] Moreover, there are some subgroups in which revascularization definitely does prolong life.[3,4]

CABG procedures began in the 1960s, but it was Favalaro in 1968 who first described the modern technique of saphenous vein aortocoronary arterial grafting.[5] This operation revolutionized operative revascularization procedures. Although the saphenous veins used as conduits in such operations frequently degenerate and create late problems,[6] CABG has proved very effective in improving symptoms and increasing survival in certain groups of patients with CHD. New operative approaches attempt to use some, if not all, arterial conduits.

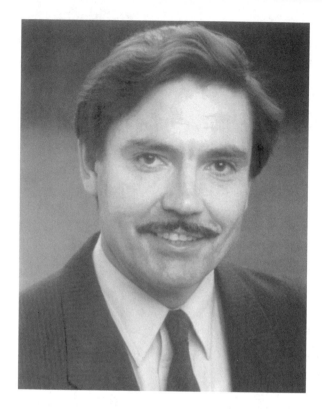

FIGURE 1-1 Andreas Gruentzig, the father of intervention cardiology. (Courtesy of Dr. Kenneth Kent.)

♥ Gruentzig and Percutaneous Transluminal Coronary Angioplasty

PTCA, the nonoperative approach to CHD, was introduced by Andreas Gruentzig (Fig. 1-1) working at University Hospital in Zurich. The first procedure was performed on September 16, 1977.[7] However, Gruentzig's interest in angioplasty began much earlier.

EARLY TRAINING

Gruentzig completed medical school at the University of Heidelberg and entered into the field of angiology. In this specialty, unique in Europe, physicians are trained to perform vascular imaging in all the various organ systems. Such physicians perform coronary, carotid, visceral, and peripheral angiography, whereas in the United States, coronary, carotid, and peripheral angiography were usually performed by cardiologists, neuroradiologists, and general radiologists, respectively.

PERIPHERAL ANGIOPLASTY—MID 1970S

Gruentzig's training led him to the work of Charles Dotter, who, in 1964, described a technique for enlarging the lumen of the superficial femoral arteries by catheters forced through arterial stenoses.[8] Dotter described the technique as first placing a very thin guidewire through the obstruction and then over the wire, passing a catheter through the obstruction. After the obstruction was enlarged, an even larger catheter was passed through it. With a series of catheters of increasing sizes, a much larger lumen was created. This rather crude approach was the first intravascular angioplasty procedure.

Dotter's technique required a large arteriotomy in the femoral vessel to create an adequate lumen. Furthermore, there were complications associated with trauma to the arterial plaque. Dotter's procedure gained little acceptance in the United States. However, Zeitler, working in Nuremberg, popularized the "Dottertechnique" and published a series of papers on both the initial and long-term results of the procedure in iliac and superficial femoral arteries of his patients.

Gruentzig learned of this technique and decided to improve it. He reasoned that a larger channel could be created more effectively by fashioning a balloon at the tip of a small catheter, which would then create a larger channel without increasing the size of the arteriotomy. He was still in training at the University Hospital in Zurich at that time. He located a chemist who assisted him in making a noncompliant balloon, which he affixed to the tip of a catheter. He tested this in animal experiments and proceeded to treat patients with obstructive peripheral arterial disease. This technique quickly proved to be an effective treatment.[9]

DEVELOPMENT OF CORONARY ANGIOPLASTY

Gruentzig had a keen interest in cardiology, his dream was to be able to treat obstructive coronary artery disease with nonoperative, percutaneous techniques. As his approach to treatment of peripheral vascular disease was gaining worldwide acceptance, he turned his attention to the coronary arteries. He created obstructions of the coronary arteries in dogs by placing ligatures around the vessels. He was then successful in dilating these obstructions with the homemade balloon dilatation catheters. He reported this work at the American Heart Association meeting in 1976.[10] Although there was much interest in this approach, a great deal of skepticism existed as to the applicability to human coronary atherosclerosis. Gruentzig continued developing his plan to use this transluminal dilatation approach in humans.

Gruentzig's plan met with even more skepticism in his own hospital environment; after all, he was still a fellow in training. He gained the cautious support of Senning, the Chief of Surgery, and Siegenthaler, the Chief of Medicine. He continued refining the balloon dilatation catheters. One of Gruentzig's greatest concerns was the time required to inflate the balloon. Dogs, which he used in the experiments, are very intolerant of ischemia. He had observed ventricular arrhythmia induced by ischemia associated with even brief balloon inflations. The obvious fear was that this would be a problem in humans. To help alleviate ischemia during balloon inflation, Gruentzig decided to use arterial blood from the contralateral femoral artery propelled through a rotary pump and perfused through the lumen of the balloon catheter through the tip beyond the inflated balloon. He prepared this perfusion system for the first cases but found that it was unnecessary.

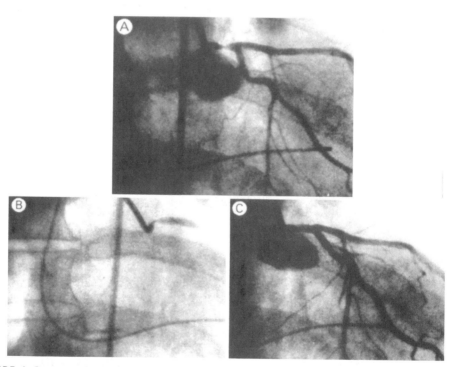

FIGURE 1-2 First PTCA in a human, Zurich, September 1977. Left anterior descending stenosis before **(A)** and after **(B)** balloon angioplasty by Dr. Gruentzig. **(C)** One month after the initial angioplasty. (From Topol EJ (ed): *Textbook of Interventional Cardiology.* Philadelphia, WB Saunders, 1990. Used with permission.)

FIRST HUMAN PTCA—1977

In September 1977, Gruentzig identified a suitable candidate for his first procedure, a young man with a single coronary stenosis of the proximal left anterior descending coronary artery. The patient was scheduled for surgery because of severe symptoms. Gruentzig met with him and discussed the possibility of avoiding an operation, the patient agreed. On September 16, 1977, with a number of skeptical surgeons as well as his own cardiology colleagues, but a very supportive catheterization laboratory staff, he successfully dilated this stenosis of the proximal left anterior descending coronary artery (Fig. 1-2). He documented a substantial reduction in the pressure gradient across the stenosis and a marked improvement in the angiographic appearance of the stenosis. His supporters cheered, his critics remained doubtful. He named the procedure "percutaneous transluminal coronary angioplasty" (PTCA).

Gruentzig was unable to find a second suitable candidate for this procedure at the University Hospital. He was invited by Kaltenbach to visit Frankfort, where they performed the second PTCA. In November 1977, at the American Heart Association meeting in Miami, he presented the results of PTCA in his first four patients. Again, the audience was divided, some were interested and enthusiastic; others remained skeptical.

DEMONSTRATION COURSES

Gruentzig was inundated with requests to visit his laboratory and observe the procedure. Once visitors arrived at the hospital, they were directed down a long hallway into the basement where Gruentzig frequently sat in his closet size office. So many visitors came that he decided to organize a demonstration course in which the attendees would sit in an auditorium and observe the PTCA procedures on television. Gruentzig was an enthusiastic and effective teacher, and these early courses in Zurich became the prototype for PTCA demonstration courses now performed around the world. With this format, observers would not only understand the fundamentals of the techniques but also see the failures and complications that occurred during the procedures. There was no way to hide the outcomes—both good and bad—during these live transmissions.

Proliferation of PTCA was hampered by the availability of the balloon dilatation catheters; each catheter was hand-made. Schneider, a catheter company located in Zurich decided to support Gruentzig. However, to purchase the catheters during 1978 to 1979, one had to travel to Zurich and pay cash in Swiss francs.

NATIONAL HEART, LUNG, AND BLOOD INSTITUTE, 1979

During 1979, the leadership of the National Heart Lung and Blood Institute (NHLBI) recognized the potential importance of PTCA and organized a conference in Bethesda, Maryland. Gruentzig and other physicians who had performed PTCA were invited; a cardiac surgeon, Vallee Willman, chaired the meeting. Physicians and statisticians who had participated in the Coronary Artery Surgery Study (CASS), the largest study at that time examining the effectiveness of bypass surgery, were in attendance. Data were presented on 205 patients who had undergone PTCA, the worldwide experience at the time. The outcome of that meeting was to establish a voluntary registry of patients undergoing PTCA.[11] The NHLBI agreed to provide administrative support as well as a data coordinating center. This became the basis for the NHLBI-PTCA Registry. Gruentzig's enthusiastic endorsement was instrumental in solidifying the support of the most physicians who were performing the procedure.

EARLY 1980s

In 1980, several important events occurred, Gruentzig moved to Emory University where he gained much greater support to advance this procedure. The demonstration courses moved to Emory, which increased the exposure of the procedure to American physicians. The United States Catheter Industries (USCI) obtained the rights from Schneider to manufacture and market the Gruentzig Dilica dilatation catheter, and the US Food and Drug Administration approved the catheter for sale in the United States.

A second workshop was held in Bethesda in 1981 during which the decision was made to cease enrollment of patients and concentrate on follow-up. A third workshop was held in 1983, initial and 1-year outcomes of PTCA procedures on 3070 patients were presented.[12] This was the first of many reports from this rich database.

During the mid 1980s, the demonstration courses for angioplasty flourished. Led by Gruentzig's model, initially at Zurich and later at Emory where he conducted courses twice a year, John Simpson conducted courses on the West Coast, and Hartzler conducted courses with live demonstrations in Kansas City and taped cases in Hawaii. Improvements in the angioplasty equipment continued as more manufacturers became interested in this rapidly expanding market. There was a great deal of enthusiasm for a second NHLBI sponsored PTCA registry to document that which seemed to be occurring, that is, improved success of the procedures. During 1985 to 1986, data were collected on 2060 patients undergoing PTCA at clinical sites, and improved outcome was established. Detre and associates[13] reported a comparison of the results of PTCA in the two registries, Registry I (1977–1981) and Registry II (1985–1986). Despite the fact that patients in Registry II were older, had more risk factors, and had more extensive coronary disease, the success rates for Registry II patients were greater and complications were less than those recorded in Registry I. This was undoubtedly due to improved catheters and guidewires, improved imaging equipment, a better understanding of the biologic responses, and management of complications.

A TRAGIC LOSS

In October 1985, the Interventional Cardiology community was shocked and saddened by the untimely death of Andreas Gruentzig. Most all physicians who were performing angioplasty at that time knew Andreas, had been impressed by his courage, conviction, and honesty, and had been moved by his compassion and love for life. In an interview conducted shortly before his death, he spoke of the future of angioplasty. He envisioned new balloons, lower in profile and made of stronger materials to withstand greater inflation pressures for hard plaque. He saw the need for different energy sources, such as lasers, to treat certain plaques. He saw the need for devices such as stents to scaffold or support arteries when uncontrolled dissections occurred. If he had lived, he would surely have embraced the new device angioplasty era.

❤ New Device Angioplasty—Late 1980s

Gruentzig's vision of the future of angioplasty began to develop shortly after his death, largely in response to the limitations inherent in balloon angioplasty.

DIRECTIONAL CORONARY ATHERECTOMY

John Simpson, who had introduced the first over-the-wire balloon approved in the United States, developed a microsurgical device placed at the tip of a catheter. This device could remove plaque from the wall of the artery. He began working with this Directional Atherectomy Catheter (DCA) in 1986 in peripheral arteries and subsequently in coronary arteries.[14] A multicenter clinical trial began in 1988, which demonstrated clinical successes and complications that were comparable to balloon angioplasty. Furthermore, investigators found that removing plaque resulted in substantial improvement in the angiographic appearance of the vessels.

Eccentric lesions, which were always a problem for balloon dilatation, could be effectively treated resulting in spectacular angiographic results. Ostial stenoses and bifurcation stenoses, which had remained challenges for balloon dilatation, were effectively treated with DCA.

The Interventional Cardiology community followed this investigation closely and was delighted with the FDA decision to approve this, the first non–balloon catheter, for angioplasty in 1990. Sales of this device soared. Although the second- and third-generation devices became available over the next few years, it remained a technical challenge. Guide catheters measuring 11 French (F) and subsequently 10F were necessary; the devices, 6F or 7F, were stiff and bulky and created marked ischemia during the procedure.   Despite these limitations, the angiographic appearances of the vessels were superior to that which could be achieved by balloons, and the enthusiasm continued. In the first comparative study of a new device to balloon dilatation, CAVEAT, a 1000-patient randomized study demonstrated no short- or long-term benefit in outcomes, success, complications, or restenosis in patients treated by DCA compared with those treated by balloon dilatation.[15] These results were at odds with many single-center experiences. In 1993, the Washington Cardiology Center (WCC) conducted a study with DCA combined with intravascular ultrasound the Optimal Atherectomy Restenosis Study (OARS) in which we hoped to achieve optimal atherectomy. We quickly learned that usual atherectomy, particularly as it was performed in CAVEAT with mostly 6F devices, resulted in very little plaque removal. Even using larger, 7F, atherectomy devices with iterative ultrasound guidance and aggressive postatherectomy dilatation, 60% of plaque remained after the procedure.[16]

A second 1000-patient multicenter study using different DCA strategies, 7F devices, and aggressive postatherectomy balloon dilatation, compared DCA with balloon angioplasty, Balloon vs Optimal Atherectomy Trial (BOAT).[17] This study demonstrated improved long-term outcome in patients undergoing DCA with decreased restenosis rates.

The results of this pivotal study became available as stents were approved for elective angioplasty in the United States (Johnson and Johnson Interventional Systems, August 1994). The ease of use of stents compared with DCA and efficacy studies that demonstrated the superiority of both stents and DCA compared with that of balloon angioplasty, resulted in a shift of usage from DCA to stents.

ROTATIONAL ATHERECTOMY

Two other mechanical atherectomy devices began clinical trials in the late 1980s: the rotation atherectomy device and transluminal extraction catheter. Rotational atherectomy is a conical device with industrial-grade diamond chips on the leading edge that rotated at 180,000 rpm and traveled over a guidewire.[18] This "drill" was effective in pulverizing plaque, particularly the hardened, fibrotic, and calcified elements of the plaque. The speed and the abrasive surface were effective in reducing the plaque to small particles, 95% were less than 5 microns—less than the size of a red blood cell. These small particles could pass through the microcirculation of the coronaries without causing damage.

For the first time, this device proved effective in treating calcified, undilatable stenoses, which accounted for 3% to 5% of PTCA failures in the previously published reports. Because this device was not in direct competition with stents and because it proved to be a valuable asset in treating rigid and undilatable stenoses, its use has continued until today. It is now frequently used to pretreat lesions that are subsequently treated with stents.

TRANSLUMINAL EXTRACTION CATHETER

The transluminal extraction catheter (TEC), another atherectomy device, was effective in removing soft plaque from the arterial wall. The entire catheter rotated, had cutting blades on the front end, and traveled over a guidewire. It also had a vacuum system to remove the plaque from the artery.[19]

This system had several deficiencies. It was large and required a 10F guidewire. The entire catheter rotated, which limited its use to the proximal portion of native arteries, and it was ineffective in fibrotic or calcified plaque. However, the TEC did prove effective in removing the soft obstructions in saphenous vein grafts.

EXCIMER LASER ANGIOPLASTY

Finally, excimer laser angioplasty started clinical trials in 1988.[20] This was perceived as an ideal solution for plaque removal. Unfortunately, although it seemed to remove plaque, a number of factors, including disruption of the arterial wall and dissections, limited its effectiveness in routine angioplasty. It may still have a role in treating long areas of stenoses or total occlusions; however, this has not been proved in clinical trials.

STENTS

Stents are metallic mesh-like structures, which are inserted and remain in the coronary arteries. Stents result in structural support of the vessel; this improves both the short- and long-term results.[21,22] Stents are currently used in at least 50% of angioplasty procedures in the United States.

The initial major deficiency of stents was the anticoagulant regimen. This was initiated because of the early thrombosis of the stent observed in animal trials and in some of the initial stent implants in humans. Patients were pretreated with aspirin, dipyridamole, and dextran for platelet inhibition. Immediately after the procedure, heparin was continued for 48 hours or until the patients became anticoagulated with coumadin. Groin hematomas and other bleeding problems were common, and length of hospital stay was 5 to 7 days.

Antonio Columbo was instrumental in documenting that if initial stent implantation was properly performed, this intense anticoagulation regimen was unnecessary.[23] The definitive study in the United States, the STARS trial proved that the antiplatelet regimen of aspirin and ticlopidine was superior to coumadin anticoagulation in preventing stent thrombosis.[24]

As stent designs improve, their usage will probably increase. Debulking before stent placement with rotational or directional atherectomy or with laser angioplasty has received a great deal of interest, and clinical trials to test this hypothesis are underway.

❤ Future Trends

During the past two decades, PTCA has been established as an effective treatment for obstructive coronary artery disease. In clinical trials, PTCA performed with balloon dilatation alone, has been compared with operative revascularization and proved to be just as effective in terms of death and myocardial infarction, but patients undergoing PTCA subsequently required more repeat revascularization procedures.[25] The deficiencies of balloon dilatation used in those trials have been addressed by new angioplasty devices. Endovascular stents have become the most popular new device. New frontiers include the exciting application of intravascular radiation therapy to limit restenosis after angioplasty, angiogenesis stimulated by controlled injury or gene therapy, and adjunctive pharmacology to improve the effectiveness of coronary angioplasty. As we enter the third decade of nonoperative coronary revascularization, we anticipate new solutions to the problems that have been identified during the past.

REFERENCES

1. Thom TJ, Kannel WB, Silbershatz H, D'Agonstine RB: Incidence, prevalence and mortality of cardiovascular diseases in the United States. In Alexander RW, et al: *The Heart*, pp. 3–18. New York, McGraw-Hill, 1998.
2. European Coronary Surgery Study Group: Long-term results of prospective randomized study of coronary artery bypass surgery in stable angina pectoris. *Lancet* 2:1173, 1982.

3. Myers WO, Schaff JV, Gersh BJ, et al: Improved survival of surgically treated patients with triple vessel coronary artery disease and severe angina pectoris: A report from the Coronary Artery Surgery Study (CASS) registry. *J Thorac Cardiovasc Surg* 97:487, 1989.

4. Frye RL, Gibbons RJ, Schaff HV, et al: Treatment of coronary artery disease. *J Am Coll Cardiol* 13:957, 1989.

5. Favalaro RG: Saphenous vein autograft replacement of severe segmental coronary artery occlusion: Operative technique. *Ann Thorac Surg* 5:334, 1968.

6. FitzGibbon GM, Kafka HP, Leach AJ, et al: Coronary bypass graft fate and patient outcome: Angiographic follow-up of 5,065 grafts related to survival and reoperation in 1388 patients during 25 years. *J Am Coll Cardiol* 28:616, 1996.

7. Gruentzig AR, Senning A, Siegenthaler WE: Non-operative dilatation of coronary artery stenosis: percutaneous transluminal coronary angioplasty. *N Engl J Med* 301:61,1979.

8. Dotter CT, Judkins MP: Transluminal treatment of arteriosclerotic obstructions: Description of a new technique and preliminary report of its application. *Circulation* 30:654, 1964.

9. Gruentzig AR: Die perkutane Rekanalisierung chronischer arterieller Verschlusse (Dotter-Prinzip) mit einem neuen doppellumigne Dilatationskatheter. *Fortschr Rontgenstr* 125:80, 1976.

10. Gruentzig AR, Turina MI, Schneider JA: Experimental percutaneous dilatation of coronary artery stenosis (abstr). *Circulation* 54:81, 1976.

11. Proceedings of the workshop on Percutaneous Transluminal Coronary Angioplasty, June 15–16, 1979. USDHEW NIH Publication no. 80-2030, March 1980.

12. Kent KM, Mullin SM, Passamani ER: Proceedings of the National Heart, Lung and Blood Institute on the Outcome of Percutaneous Transluminal Coronary Angioplasty. *Am J Cardiol* 53:1C–146C, 1984.

13. Detre KM, Holubkov R, Kelsey S, et al: Percutaneous transluminal coronary angioplasty in 1985–1986 and 1977–1981. The National Heart, Lung and Blood Registry. *N Engl J Med* 318:265, 1988.

14. Simpson JB, Johnson DE, Thapliyal HV: Transluminal atherectomy: A new approach to the treatment of atherosclerotic vascular disease (abstr). *Circulation* 72:III-146, 1985.

15. Topol EJ, Leya F, Pinkerton CA, et al: A comparison of directional atherectomy with coronary angioplasty in patients with coronary artery disease. *N Engl J Med* 329:221, 1993.

16. Simonton CA, Leon MB: Optimal directional coronary atherectomy: final results of the Optimal Atherectomy Restenosis Study (OARS). *Circulation* 97:332, 1998.

17. Baim DS, Cutlip DE, Sharma SK, et al: Final results of the balloon vs optimal atherectomy trial (BOAT). *Circulation* 97:309, 1998.

18. Ahn SS, Auth DC, Marcus DR, Moore WS: Removal of focal atheromatous lesions by angioscopically guided high speed rotary atherectomy. *J Vasc Surg* 7:292, 1988.

19. Stack RS, Perez JA, Newman GE, et al: Treatment of peripheral vascular disease with the Transluminal Extraction Catheter: Results of a multicenter study (abstr). *J Am Coll Cardiol* 13:227A, 1989.

20. Litvak F, Grundfest W, Eigler N, et al: Percutaneous excimer laser angioplasty. *Lancet* 2:102, 1989.
21. Serruys PW, de Jaigere P, Kiemeneij F, et al: A comparison of balloon-expandable-stent implantation with balloon angioplasty in patients with coronary artery disease. *N Engl J Med* 331:489, 1994.
22. Fischman DL, Leon MB, Baim DS, et al: A randomized comparison of coronary-stent placement and balloon angioplasty in the treatment of coronary artery disease. *N Engl J Med* 331:496, 1994.
23. Colombo A, Hall P, Nakamura S, et al: Intracoronary stenting without anticoagulation accomplished with intravascular ultrasound guidance. *Circulation* 91:1676, 1995.
24. Leon MB, Baim DS, Popma JJ, et al: A clinical trial comparing three antithrombotic-drug regimens after coronary-artery stenting (STARS). *N Engl J Med* 339:1665, 1998.
25. Writing group for the Bypass Angioplasty Revascularization Investigation (BARI) Investigators: Five-year clinical and functional outcome comparing bypass surgery and angioplasty in patients with multi-vessel coronary disease. A multicenter randomized trial. *JAMA* 277:715, 1997.

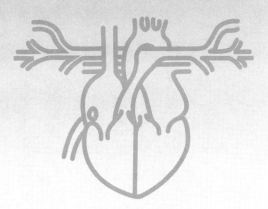

SECTION I

The Basics

CHAPTER 2

Coronary Anatomy and Physiology

SUSAN MARDEN, RN, MS

To understand coronary angiography and interventional procedures, it is necessary to have an understanding of the anatomy and physiology of the coronary vessels, first imaged in living humans by Sones in 1958.[1]

♥ Coronary Anatomy

The major coronary vessels, also referred to as the *epicardial arteries,* travel over the outer surface of the heart in grooved depressions or sulci (Fig. 2-1). Their ostia, or connections to the aorta, are located just beyond the cusps of the aortic valve (Fig. 2-2). The aortic cusps take their names from their association with the coronary arteries.

The left coronary artery originates from above the lateral or left coronary cusp of the aortic valve. The right coronary artery originates from above the anterior or right coronary cusp. The third cusp, referred to as the *noncoronary cusp,* is located posterior to the other cusps.

The sinuses of Valsalva, outpouchings of the aortic wall, lie behind each cusp. These sinuses enhance blood flow into the coronary arteries by allowing blood to pool around the openings and by preventing obstruction of the ostia by the valve cusps.

The coronary arteries lie in two orthogonal planes, the plane of the interventricular septum and the plane of the atrioventricular valves.

(text continues on page 20)

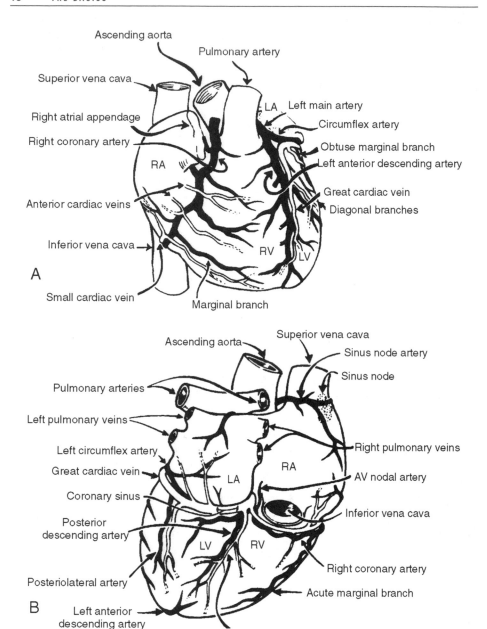

FIGURE 2−1 Diagram of the coronary arteries and veins of the heart. **(A)** Anterior view. **(B)** Posterior view. RA, right atrium; LA, left atrium; RV, right ventricle; LV, left ventricle. (Adapted from Walmsley R, Watson H: *Clinical Anatomy of the Heart*, pp. 203, 205. New York, Churchill Livingstone, 1978.)

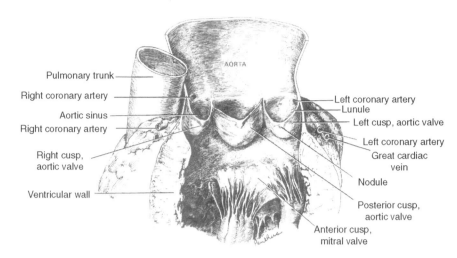

FIGURE 2–2 The aortic valve opened to reveal the ostia of the left and right coronary arteries. (From Clemente CD, Gray H [eds]: *Anatomy of the Human Body,* 13th ed. Philadelphia, Lea & Febiger, 1985. Adapted with permission.)

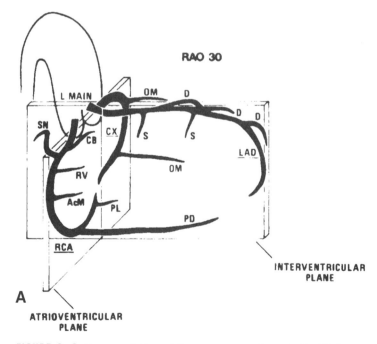

FIGURE 2–3 Representation of the coronary anatomy in the 30-degree right anterior oblique (RAO) projection **(A)** and cine views **(B** and **C)**.

(continued)

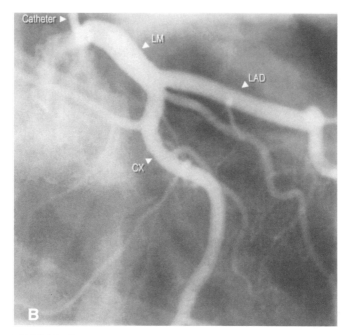

FIGURE 2–3 CONTINUED (**B**)

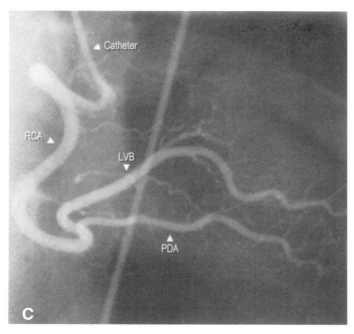

FIGURE 2–3 CONTINUED (**C**)

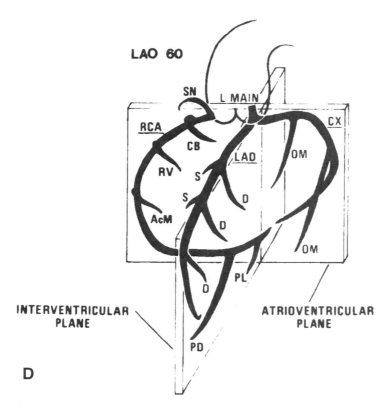

FIGURE 2–3 CONTINUED (D) Coronary anatomy in the 60-degree left anterior oblique (LAO) view is represented.

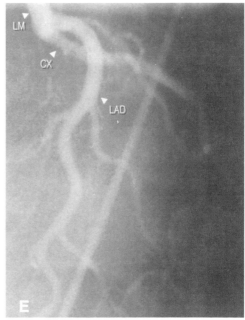

FIGURE 2–3 CONTINUED (E) Cine view from the LAO. Coronary branches are as indicated: L Main, left main); LAD, left anterior descending; D, diagonal); S, septal; CX, circumflex; OM, obtuse marginal; RCA, right coronary artery; CB, conus branch; SN, sinus node; AcM, acute marginal; PD, posterior descending; PL, posterolateral left ventricular. Figures in **A** and **D** adapted with permission from Baim DS, Grossman W: Coronary angiography. In Baim DS, Grossman W (eds): *Cardiac Catheterization, Angiography and Intervention,* 5th ed. Baltimore, Williams & Wilkins, 1995.)

Angiographic views of the coronary arteries include projections in these planes (Fig. 2-3).

♥ Coronary Arteries

The coronary arteries are medium-sized muscular vessels (Fig. 2-4). Their walls consist of three distinct layers of varying thickness. The intima is the inner most lining of the vessel. Its luminal surface consists of a single layer of endothelial cells that form a smooth, thrombus-resistant surface.[2] The highly selective permeability of the endothelial layer allows it to serve as a semipermeable barrier between the circulating blood and the arterial vessel wall.

Metabolically active, the endothelium produces highly potent substances that promote arterial vasodilation or vasoconstriction. These and other activities of the endothelium play a major role in maintaining vessel function. The internal elastic lamina forms the outer limit of the intima. It consists of a matrix of elastic fibers with multiple small openings, which permit cell movement between the intima and the media, the adjacent middle layer of the vessel. The media, the thickest portion of the normal coronary vessel, consists of multiple layers of smooth muscle cells

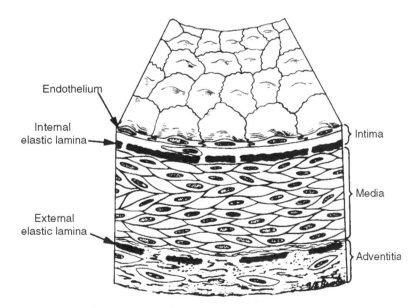

FIGURE 2–4 Structure of a normal muscular artery. (From Ross R, Glomset JA: The pathogenesis of atherosclerosis. *N Engl J Med* 295:369, 1976. Copyright 1976 Massachusetts Medical Society. All rights reserved.)

arranged in a spiraling pattern and surrounded by connective tissue. The internal and the external elastic laminae form the boundaries of the media, separating it from the intima and the outermost layer of the vessel, the adventitia. The smooth muscle cells within the media sustain the tone of the arterial wall allowing for a steady flow of blood through the vessel lumen. The size of the lumen of normal coronary arteries is regulated by the extent of contraction of the smooth muscle cells within the media. The adventitia is composed of an array of collagen fiber bundles, elastic fibers, numerous fibroblasts, and some smooth muscle cells. The adventitia contains a blood supply in the form of vasa vasorum or capillaries, venules, and arterioles. Nerve fibers and lymphatic channels are also distributed within this layer.

DISTRIBUTION OF THE CORONARY ARTERIES

Blood is supplied to the myocardium by the right and left coronary arteries and their branches. Smaller branches of the coronary arteries penetrate deep into the myocardial wall supplying blood directly to the pumping chambers and the conduction system. A network of very small branches interconnect the right and left coronary arteries. These arteries increase in size to provide collateral channels for blood flow if the major coronary

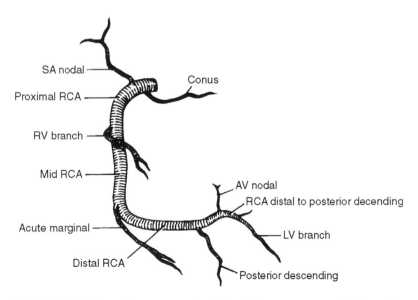

FIGURE 2–5 Schematic representation of the right coronary artery (RCA) and its branches. For anatomic reference, the RCA is divided into three regions: the proximal RCA, mid RCA, and distal RCA (From Hurst, JW, Schlant RC, Alexander WR [eds]: *The Heart: Arteries and Veins*, p. 2410. New York, McGraw-Hill, 1994. Reproduced with permission of the McGraw-Hill Company.)

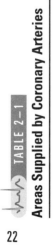 **TABLE 2–1**

Areas Supplied by Coronary Arteries

Structure	Usual Arterial Supply	Common Variants
Right atrium	Sinus node artery, branch of RCA (55%)*	Sinus node artery, branch of L circumflex (45%)
Left atrium	Major L circumflex†	Sinus node artery, branch of L circumflex (45%)
Right ventricle		
Anterior	Major RCA; minor LAD	
Posterior	Major RCA; posterior descending branch of RCA	Posterior descending may branch from L circumflex (10%)
	Minor LAD (ascending portion)	LAD terminates at apex (40%)
Left ventricle		
Posterior (diaphragmatic)	Major L circumflex, posterior descending branch of RCA; minor LAD (ascending portion)	Posterior descending may branch from L circumflex (10%)
		LAD terminates at apex (40%)
Anterior	LCA; L circumflex and LAD	
Apex	Major LAD	
Intraventricular septum	Major septal branches of LAD; minor posterior descending branch of RCA and AV nodal branch of RCA	Minor posterior descending may branch from L circumflex, and AV nodal may branch from L circumflex
LV papillary muscles		
Anterior	Diagonal branch of LAD; other branches of LAD, other branches of L circumflex	Diagonal may branch from circumflex
Posterior	RCA and L circumflex	RCA and LAD
Sinus node	Nodal artery from RCA (55%)	Nodal artery from L circumflex (45%)
AV node	RCA (90%)	L circumflex (10%)
Bundle of His	RCA (90%)	L circumflex (10%)
Right bundle	Major LAD septal branches; minor AV nodal artery	
Left anterior bundle	Major LAD septal branches; minor AV nodal artery	
Left posterior bundle	LAD septal branches and AV nodal artery	

RCA, right coronary artery; LAD, left anterior descending artery; L, left; LV, left ventricle; AV, atrioventricular.
*Percentages in parentheses denote frequency of occurrence in autopsy studies.
†Major and minor refer to degree of predominance of an artery in perfusing a structure.
From Boud EF, Halpenny CJ: Cardiac anatomy. In Woods SL, Froelicher ESS, Halpenny CJ, Motzer SH (eds): *Cardiac Nursing*, 3rd ed. Philadelphia, JB Lippincott, 1995.

arteries become obstructed. Table 2-1 summarizes the coronary vessels that supply the major cardiac structures and the common variations that may occur.

♥ Right Coronary Artery Anatomy

The right coronary artery originates from the right coronary sinus of Valsalva at the root of the aorta and travels toward the posterior wall of the left ventricle around the right atrioventricular groove (Fig. 2-5;see also Fig. 2-1). It branches as it proceeds along the atrioventricular groove to form the conus artery, the sinus node artery, and acute marginal branches. The conus artery travels across the right ventricular outflow tract toward the left anterior descending artery (LAD), providing a collateral blood supply if LAD occlusion occurs. The sinus node artery branches to supply the right atrium and the sinus node in approximately 50% to 60% of the population.[3,4] The acute marginal branches supply the right ventricle.

After the right coronary artery has circled the atrioventricular groove to the posterior side of the heart, the right coronary artery commonly gives rise to the posterior descending artery (PDA) in 85% to 90% of the population. The point at which the branch takes off at right angles into the posteriointerventricular groove has been called the "crux" of the heart (see Fig. 2-1).[3,4] The right coronary artery is considered the dominant artery if it provides the PDA. This important branch supplies blood to the posterior interventricular septum and the diaphragmatic portion of the left ventricle. After branching to form the PDA, the right coronary artery continues beyond the crux and terminates as one or more posterior ventricular branches. The posterior ventricular branches supply the inferior surface of the left ventricle. The AV nodal artery originating from the distal portion of the right coronary artery commonly supplies the atrioventricular bundle.

The anatomy of the right coronary artery is shown depicted in Figure 2-5. The posterior descending artery follows along the posteriointerventricular groove toward the apex of the heart (see Fig. 2-1). Branches arising from the PDA supply the posterior apical portion of the interventricular septum and the posterior-inferior surface of the left ventricle.

♥ Left Coronary Artery Anatomy

The left coronary artery originates from the left coronary sinus of Valsalva at the root of the aorta. Its initial 1 or 2 centimeters are termed the

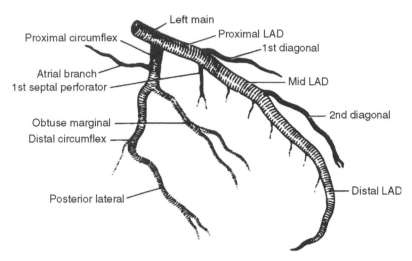

FIGURE 2–6 The left coronary artery and its branches. For anatomic reference, the left descending coronary artery (LAD) is divided into three regions: proximal LAD, mid LAD, and distal LAD. The left circumflex (LCX) is divided into two regions: the proximal LCX and the distal LCX. (From Hurst JW, Schlant RC, Alexander WR [eds]: *The Heart: Arteries and Veins,* p. 2408. New York, McGraw-Hill, 1994. Reproduced with permission of the McGraw-Hill Company.)

left main coronary artery. After this short course, it divides into two branches, the LAD and the left circumflex artery (LCX) (Fig. 2-6; see also Fig. 2-1).

The LAD continues in the direction of the left main artery along the anterior interventricular groove toward the apex of the heart (see Fig. 2-1), often extending around the apex of the heart to join the PDA. If the LAD is short, the PDA extends around the apex to join the LAD anteriorly. The LAD gives rise to diagonal and septal branches. The diagonal branches of the LAD course leftward along the anterior lateral surface of the left ventricle (see Fig. 2-1). The septal branches originate at a right angle from the LAD to perforate the ventricular septum. The major branches of the LAD in the order that they originate include the first diagonal branch, the first septal perforator, and the second diagonal branch (see Fig. 2-6).

The LCX emerges from the left coronary artery at a right angle and traverses the atrioventricular groove toward the left lateral wall of the heart (see Fig. 2-1). One to several obtuse marginal branches commonly originate from the LCX and traverse the lateral and posterolateral free right atrium near the tricuspid valve. This extensive coronary sinus system drains the right and left atrium, the interventricular septum, the left ventricle and a portion of the right ventricle. A second venous system in the heart, comprised of several anterior veins (see Fig. 2-1), drains venous blood from the anterior portion of the right ventricle directly into the right atrium at multiple sites. The third venous drainage system in the heart consists of tiny venous outlets in the myocardium known as thebesian veins. These allow a small portion of coronary venous drainage to return directly into the cardiac chambers.

❤ Physiology of the Coronary Circulation

The heart requires an abundant blood supply to perform the continuous work demanded of it. Paradoxically, it must generate sufficient pressure and flow in the aorta for perfusion of its own muscle in addition to providing blood flow to other body organs.

The rate of blood flow through the coronary arteries is dictated by myocardial oxygen need.[6,7] The major determinants of myocardial oxygen consumption include heart rate, ventricular wall tension (related to pressure and radius), and contractility. Coronary blood flow increases when myocardial oxygen needs rise and decreases as myocardial oxygen demands decline. Because heart muscle extracts initially all the oxygen from the blood delivered to it at rest, increased demands for oxygen can be met only by augmenting the rate of coronary blood flow. A low oxygen content in myocardial tissue induces vasodilation of the coronary arterioles, thereby increasing coronary blood flow. This ability of the coronary vasculature to modulate blood flow in response to increases in myocardial oxygen demand is referred to as *autoregulation*. Coronary blood flow is regulated to a lesser extent by other factors to include autonomic nervous system stimulation, circulating catecholamines, and pharmacologic agents.

Total coronary blood flow is greatest during relaxation of the heart muscle and diminishes abruptly during left ventricular contraction. The smaller intramural coronary vessels are compressed during ventricular contraction, causing a reduction in blood flow particularly to the inner most (subendocardial) layer of the heart. The subepicardial layer of the heart is adequately perfused during relaxation and contraction of the heart muscle. Ventricular contraction does not compromise the larger coronary vessels. The blood supply to the muscular myocardial layer is reduced during ventricular contraction to an intermediate degree when compared with blood supply to the other heart layers (Fig. 2-7).

wall of the left ventricle (see Fig. 2-6). The LCX supplies the sinus n
in approximately 40% to 50% of the population.[3,4] The LCX provid
the PDA in a small portion of the population (10% to 15%), and when
does, the heart is said to be "left dominant."[3,4] The entire inferior wall
the left ventricle and the septum is supplied by the left coronary syste
when the LCX is dominant.

In summary, the relative lengths of the RCA and the LCX vary sub
stantially with regard to the share of the posterior coronary circulatio
they provide.

♥ The Coronary Veins

Three separate coronary venous systems drain deoxygenated blood
returned from the myocardium.[5] The major venous drainage system, the
coronary sinus and its three branches, the great, middle, and small veins
(see Fig. 2-1), travel along side the epicardial coronary arteries. The great
vein parallels the LAD, while the middle and small vein travel along the
right coronary artery. All three join posteriorly to form the coronary
sinus.

The coronary sinus, beginning at the crux of the heart, is approximately 2 to 3 cm in length, and drains the coronary venous blood into the

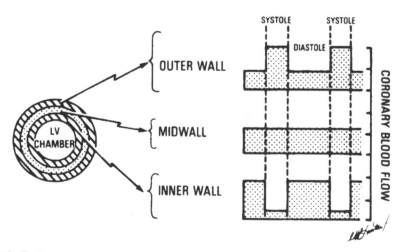

FIGURE 2–7 Diagram of coronary blood flow in systole and diastole in the layers of the heart.
Note that systolic flow predominates in the outer wall, whereas diastolic flow with minimal sys-
tolic flow is present in the inner wall. (Adapted with permission from West JB: *Best and Taylor's
Physiological Basis of Medical Practice,* 12th ed, p. 270. Baltimore, Williams & Wilkins, 1991.)

♥ Conclusion

This chapter has provided a brief overview of coronary anatomy and physiology. Familiarity with these topics is the essential first step in understanding the field of interventional cardiology.

REFERENCES

1. Hurst JW: History of cardiac catheterization. In King SB III, Douglas JS Jr (eds): *Coronary Arteriography and Angioplasty*, pp. 1–9. New York, McGraw-Hill, 1985.
2. Ross R: The pathogenesis of atherosclerosis. In Braunwald E (ed): *Heart Disease: A Textbook of Cardiovascular Medicine*, pp. 1105–1111. Philadelphia, WB Saunders, 1997.
3. Waller BF, Schlant RC: Anatomy of the heart. In Hurst JW, Schlant RC, Alexander WR (eds): *The Heart: Arteries and Veins*, pp. 59–112. New York, McGraw-Hill, 1994.
4. Bittl J, Levin D: Coronary arteriography. In Braunwald E (ed): *Heart Disease: A Textbook of Cardiovascular Medicine*, pp. 240–272. Philadelphia, WB Saunders, 1997.
5. James TN: *Anatomy of the Coronary Arteries*. New York, Paul B Hoeber, 1961.
6. Guyton AC: *Textbook of Medical Physiology*, pp. 221–341. Philadelphia, WB Saunders, 1991.
7. West JB: *Best and Taylor's Physiological Basis of Medical Practice*, pp. 222–290. Baltimore, Williams & Wilkins, 1991.

BIBLIOGRAPHY

Berne RM, Levy MN: *Cardiovascular Physiology*. St. Louis, Mosby-Year Book, 1992.

Bond EF, Halpenny CJ: Cardiac anatomy. In Woods S, Sivaragjan E, Halpenny J, Underhill Motzer S (eds): *Cardiac Nursing*, pp. 11–25. Philadelphia, JB Lippincott, 1995.

Bond EF, Halpenny CJ: Physiology of the heart. In Woods S, Sivaragjan E, Halpenny J, Underhill Motzer S (eds): *Cardiac Nursing*, pp. 26–57. Philadelphia, JB Lippincott, 1995.

Franch RH, King SB, Douglas JS: Techniques of cardiac catheterization including coronary arteriography. In Hurst JW, Schlant RC, Alexander WR (eds): *The Heart: Arteries and Veins*, pp. 2381–2420. New York, McGraw-Hill, 1994.

Ford P: Physiology of the cardiovascular system. In Price SA, Wilson LM (eds): *Pathophysiology: Clinical Concepts of Disease Processes*, pp. 304–314. New York, McGraw-Hill, 1978.

Gauthier DK: Anatomy and physiology of the heart. In Kinney MR, Packa DR (eds): *Anderoli's Comprehensive Cardiac Care*. St. Louis, Mosby, 1996.

Gray H, Clemente CD: *Anatomy of the Human Body*, pp. 620–665. Philadelphia, Lea & Febiger, 1985.

Levick JR: *An Introduction to Cardiovascular Physiology*, pp. 1–24. Oxford, Butterworth-Heinemann Ltd, 1995.

Ross R, Glomset JA: The pathogenesis of atherosclerosis (part 1 of 2). *N Engl J Med* 295:369, 1976.

Ross R: The vessel wall. In Fozzard HA, Jennings RB, Haber E, et al (eds): *The Heart and Cardiovascular System-Scientific Foundations*, pp. 163–170. New York, Raven Press, 1991.

Schlant RC, Sonnenblick EH: Normal physiology of the cardiovascular system. In Hurst JW, Schlant RC, Alexander WR (eds): *The Heart: Arteries and Veins*, pp. 113–152. New York, McGraw-Hill, 1994.

Thebodeau GA, Patton KT: *Anatomy and Physiology*, pp. 614–681. St. Louis, Mosby, 1996.

Van DeGraff KM: *Human Anatomy*, pp. 486–495. Dubuque, IA, Wm C. Brown Publishers, 1992.

Van DeGraff KM, Fox SI: *Concepts of Human Anatomy and Physiology*, pp. 621–680. Dubuque, IA, Wm C. Brown Publishers, 1995.

Vaska PL: Cardiovascular anatomy and physiology. In Clochesy J, Breu C, Cardin S, et al (eds): *Critical Care Nursing*, pp. 311–334. Philadelphia, WB Saunders, 1996.

CHAPTER 3

Coronary Artery Disease

ROXANA MEHRAN, MD, FACC, GEORGE DANGAS, MD, MICHAEL A. PETERSON, MD, AND MARTIN B. LEON, MD

The clinical presentation of coronary atherosclerotic heart disease (CAD) has changed little since the description of angina by Heberden 200 years ago.[1] However, current research into the atherosclerotic process and the physiology of the coronary circulation has produced an understanding of CAD that allows a more therapeutic focus on its prevention and treatment.

This chapter provides a brief overview of the pathophysiology and clinical manifestations of CAD.

❤ Pathophysiology

Atherosclerosis results from the interplay between multiple components of the blood vessel wall and molecules in the circulating blood. As early as 1851, von Rokitansky[2] suggested that intimal thickening resulted from fibrin deposition with subsequent organization by fibroblast and lipid accumulation. Virchow, in 1856,[3] proposed that blood lipids enter the arterial wall and interact with proteoglycans and promote intimal proliferation. Some years later, Ross integrated both theories into a more complex "response to injury" hypothesis.[4] His theory focuses on endothelial cell injury leading to monocyte adhesion and progression, followed by a complex chain of events culminating in the formation of the atheromatous plaque.

THE ENDOTHELIUM

The pathogenesis of atherosclerosis cannot be understood without an understanding of the function of the vascular endothelium. Not merely a passive barrier to diffusion, it performs a number of functions, including maintenance of a nonthrombogenic surface, control of vascular smooth muscle cell proliferation, and control of smooth muscle tone.

The endothelium modulates vascular tone by elaborating several vasoactive substances. Endothelium relaxing factor (EDRF), now known to be nitrous oxide (NO), is synthesized in intact endothelium from l-arginine.[5] NO stimulates guanylate cyclase to produce cyclic guanosine monophosphate (cGMP), which in turn produces vascular smooth muscle relaxation by decreasing cytosolic free Ca^{++}. The endothelium also forms prostacyclin (PGI_2) from arachidonic acid. This substance produces smooth muscle relaxation, but inhibits platelet adherence to the endothelium.[6] Another vasoactive peptide secreted by the endothelium is endothelin.[7] This substance, or more accurately family of substances, is a powerful vasoconstrictor. Thus, endothelial-mediated vascular tone is determined by a balance between vasodilator and vasoconstrictor activity. An abnormal endothelium has reduced or absent responses to the usual stimulants of endothelial vasodilation (e.g., acetylcholine, shear stress). Vasoconstriction rather than the physiologic vasodilator response may be produced.

As stated earlier, it is plausible that endothelial dysfunction is one of the earliest manifestations of atherogenesis. A study by Nabel and associates[8] found that angiographically normal segments of mildly atherosclerotic coronary arteries fail to dilate when exposed to increased flow (i.e., sheer stress). Most of these vessels not only failed to dilate, but in fact constricted. These observations provide support to the idea that endothelial dysfunction precedes grossly visible atherosclerosis. As a consequence, whether because of decreased production or increased inactivation, normal concentrations of NO do not reach the vascular smooth muscle cells to modulate vasoconstrictor substances.

There are data to support the concept that endothelial dysfunction may extend into the coronary microcirculation (i.e., microvascular endothelial dysfunction[9,10]). Patients with atherosclerosis have an impaired capacity to increase blood flow in response to endothelium-mediated agonists independent of any effect of endothelial dysfunction in epicardial coronary arteries.

Even in patients with no overt coronary disease, major risk factors for atherosclerosis appear to be associated with endothelial dysfunction. These include hypertension,[11] diabetes mellitus,[12] smoking,[13] and hypercholesterolemia.[14]

PHASE 1: INJURY

Initial injury may be the result of physical, chemical, or perhaps infectious processes. With respect to physical injury, shear stress plays an important role.[15] The preferred sites of atherogenesis are regions of low shear stress with complex secondary flow patterns, zones of standing recirculation, and regions of oscillatory hemodynamic changes occurring mostly at bending points and bifurcations.

In streams and rivers, silting or sedimentation occurs at points of branching. This effect is exaggerated as the angle of the branches becomes more obtuse. In bends, particularly sharp bends, silting occurs on the inner curvature, whereas "scouring" or erosion takes place on the outer curve of a flowing stream. In arteries, these outer curves are usually the sites of intimal injury. In similar fashion, the contraction of the heart, by tugging on portions of vessel that are partly anchored or tethered by a perforating branch artery, can make the artery unusually subject to intimal tears.

Therefore, several "hydraulic" forces are at work. Bifurcations, bends, and other curves create points of high- and low-shear force or drag. High shear tends to move or slide the intima across the medial and adventitial layers, leading to lifting, disruption, and thickening.[16] Caro,[17] on the other hand, alludes to zones of very low shear on the inside of curves and near bifurcations as problem areas. He suggested that low shear leads to a thick boundary layer, sequestration of platelets and macromolecules, and, in some manner, increased transmural permeability.

These processes are further affected by the level of arterial pressure. Increased arterial pressure accelerates atherosclerosis, not only in the systemic but also in the pulmonary circuit. Hypertension and hyperlipidemia increase the permeability of the arterial endothelium to the passage of macromolecules.

Circulating chemical factors also contribute to early endothelial injury. For example, advanced glycosylated end products in diabetes (type I), chemical irritants in tobacco smoke, circulating vasoactive amines, immune complexes, infections, and x-radiation can cause intimal injury. Homocystinuria in man denudes the endothelium and induces a massive platelet reaction, muscular hyperplasia, and eventually thromboatherosclerosis.[18]

Several infectious agents have been indicated as possible contributors to coronary arterial injury.[19] Fabricant and associates[20] found lesions in chickens infected with avian herpes virus that resemble the lesions found in human atherosclerosis. *Chlamydia pneumoniae*, a bacterial pathogen, causes upper respiratory infections in humans. When exposed to cultures of human vascular endothelial cells, it produces an increase in tissue factor as well as an increase in platelet adhesion. This process links *C. pneumoniae* infection and coagulation.

Muhlestein and colleagues[21] studied specimens of human coronary arteries obtained during atherectomy procedures. More than 75% were positive by immunofluorescence techniques for *C. pneumoniae*. Infection with cytomegalovirus has been cited as a risk factor for the rapid development of atherosclerosis in the coronary arteries of cardiac transplant patients. Epidemiologic studies have demonstrated an elevation in serum antibodies to cytomegalovirus in patients with documented CAD when compared with antibodies found in control subjects.

PHASE 2: RESPONSE TO INJURY

Endothelial injury allows circulating lipid particles to enter the subintimal layers of the artery. There they are engulfed by macrophages, forming *foam cells*. The internalization and accumulation of lipid particles occur by two mechanisms. One is active and depends on specific cell wall receptors. The other is passive entry, independent of receptors.

Endothelial cells and macrophages have a distinct high-affinity receptor that binds avidly to low-density lipoprotein particles (LDL) that have been oxidatively modified by endothelial cells.[22] Oxidized LDL particles are toxic to proliferating cells and may create a vicious cycle of injury and inflammation.[23]

Macrophages play a significant, but incompletely understood role in plaque formation. In a recent study Moreno and colleagues[24] looked at macrophage content of plaques removed from patients with acute coronary syndromes compared with that of patients with chronic stable angina. Macrophage-rich areas were more common in plaques from patients with acute coronary syndromes, but were also present in patients with stable symptoms. Macrophages may act as antigen-presenting cells for T lymphocytes, scavenger cells to remove noxious substances, and a source of growth-regulatory molecules and cytokines.

Vascular smooth muscle cells migrate from the media and proliferate in the intima, a process called *neointimal hyperplasia*. Some of these imbibe lipid particles and become foam cells. The stimulus for smooth muscle cell proliferation in atherogenesis is not completely understood. Experimental data have shown that after endothelial injury, growth factors and other mitogens are released. After the integrity of the endothelial layer has been restored, smooth muscle cells no longer proliferate.

In response to these complex processes, a visible atherosclerotic plaque is formed. The lipid-rich interior is separated from the lumen by a thin fibromuscular cap covered with endothelial cells. A tear in this cap exposes the interior contents to blood leading to thrombosis and the potential for an acute event.

♥ Physiology of the Coronary Circulation

To understand fully the concept of myocardial ischemia, attention must first be paid to the normal physiology of the coronary vascular bed. The existence of a critical balance between myocardial blood supply and oxygen need has long been appreciated. Stated simply, ischemia results when myocardial oxygen need outstrips the capacity of the coronary circulation to provide oxygen.

Unlike other muscular tissue, the myocardium extracts nearly all the oxygen presented to it. Thus, the arteriovenous oxygen difference is wide, and coronary venous blood has a very low oxygen content. It follows that the only way an increase in oxygen demand can be met is by increasing coronary blood flow. The critical impact of restriction of flow in this vascular bed can be appreciated.

The coronary bed is a low-flow, high-resistance system at rest. When myocardial oxygen demand increases, local factors (including adenosine) produce vasodilatation of the arteriolar bed, lowering resistance and increasing flow. When organ flow is regulated in this way by tissue demand, *autoregulation* is said to exist.

Coronary blood flow takes place principally in diastole. Compression of the intramuscular vessels during left ventricular systole limits flow during systole. Recognition of this unusual characteristic is important because tachycardia may reduce coronary flow because diastole is shortened.

Ischemia in a patient with stable coronary atherosclerosis results largely from an increase in oxygen need dictated by activity or emotion. Resting flow is not affected until the stenosis reaches about 90%; microvascular tone may also influence the degree of stenosis, and the pressure in the arterial bed distal to the stenosis may decline. Moreover, coronary "steal" may result when the arterioles in an ischemic vascular bed reach maximal vasodilatation at a time when further dilatation and decline in resistance in adjacent beds can occur. This sets the stage for shunting toward the lesser resistance and away from ischemic areas in which no further decline in resistance is possible.

Most acute coronary syndromes result from abrupt reduction of the lumen of a coronary artery by spasm or, far more often, thrombosis. The process by which rupture of an atherosclerotic plaque leads to thrombosis has already been addressed. An active (recently ruptured) atherosclerotic plaque often has identifiable angiographic features. Ambrose and associates[25] found that patients with stable angina had smooth, usually concentric borders. Eccentric stenoses with irregular edges are character-istically found in patients with unstable syndromes.

This brief description of the physiology of the coronary circulation is intended to provide a basis for understanding the descriptions of the clinical syndromes that follow.

❤ Clinical Manifestations of Coronary Atherosclerosis

When an atherosclerotic plaque narrows a coronary artery by ±50% of its luminal diameter, myocardial blood flow remains adequate to maintain myocyte metabolism at rest but can not rise to meet an increase in myocardial oxygen, for example, during increased physical activity. In that circumstance, chest discomfort appears during exertion, emotional upset, or other stimuli.

EXERTIONAL ANGINA

More than 200 years ago, Heberden described the features of that dis-comfort and named it "angina pectoris."[1]

There is disorder of the breast, marked with strong and peculiar symp-toms, considerable for the kind of danger belonging to it, and not extremely rare. . . . The seat of it, and sense of strangling and anxiety with which it is attended, may make it not improperly be called angina pectoris.

Those who are afflicted with it are seized, while they are walking, and more particularly when they walk soon after eating, with a painful and most disagreeable sensation in the breast, which seems as if it would

---

DISPLAY 3–1　Canadian Cardiac Society Classification of Angina

Class I. No discomfort from ordinary physical activity (walking or climbing stairs). Discom-fort is produced by more strenuous physical activity such as walking rapidly or uphill, or walking after a meal or in the cold

Class II. Slight limitation of normal activity

Class III. Marked limitation of normal activity

Class IV. Inability to carry on normal activity without symptoms often associated with angina at rest

Adapted from Campeau L: Grading of angina pectoris (Letter). *Circulation* 54:522, 1976.

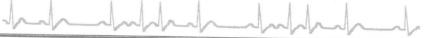

take their life away, if it were to increase or to continue: the moment they stand still, all this uneasiness vanishes_ and it will come on, not only when the persons are walking, but when they are lying down, and oblige them to rise up out of their beds every night for many months together . . . this complaint was greatest in winter; another, that it was aggravated by warm weather. . . .

Descriptors used by patients to describe angina include pressure, tightness, burning, choking, aching, and constricting. Visceral in origin, the pain is unlikely to be described as sticking, stabbing, cutting, shooting, or jabbing—adjectives more characteristically used for musculoskeletal pain. Once initiated, the discomfort persists for several minutes after the stimulus has been terminated but rarely for more than 10 to 15 minutes. Nitroglycerin administration often shortens the duration of symptoms. Fleeting, sharp pain lasting only a few seconds is virtually never a manifestation of myocardial ischemia, and a chest ache lasting for hours at a time is also uncharacteristic. Typically located behind the sternum, angina often radiates to the neck, jaw, or arms. It may be centered over the precordium and more unusually over the right chest, mid-back, or epigastrium.[26]

The threshold for discomfort may vary. This is true because variations in vasomotor tone in the affected artery alter the degree of the narrowing. Increased tone during exposure to cold is believed to partly account for the lower threshold of pain experienced by some patients in cold weather. Some patients experience angina only in the early morning hours when vasomotor tone is greatest. Alterations in vasomotor tone may also account for nocturnal angina in patients with otherwise stable exertional symptoms.[27]

Several factors may combine to provoke angina. For example, exercise capacity may not be as great after a meal when cardiac output is increased because of the need for greater splanchnic flow. Severe anemia, as in gas-

---

DISPLAY 3-2 Braunwald's Classification of Unstable Angina

Class I. New-onset (<2 months in duration), severe (three or more times per day), or accelerated angina (more frequent and precipitated by less exertion than formerly)

Class II. Angina at rest, but none within 48 hours

Class III. One or more episodes of angina at rest within 48 hours

Adapted from Braunwald E: Unstable angina: A classification. *Circulation* 80:410, 1989.

trointestinal bleeding, or hypoxemia from pulmonary disease may also produce reduced effort capacity or even discomfort at rest.

When the angina patient's effort capacity has been consistent for several weeks or months, he or she is said to have "stable angina." The Canadian Cardiac Society's Classification (CCSC) of angina is widely used to describe the degree of incapacity produced (Display 3-1). The degree of disability often corresponds to the level of exercise the patient is able to attain on treadmill testing. Although far from perfect correlates, both CCSC class and level of treadmill exercise are good predictors of the risk of future myocardial infarction or death.

ACUTE ISCHEMIC SYNDROMES

Acute events punctuate the clinical course of many patients with CAD. In most instances, these events are triggered by rupture of a plaque, exposing the blood to the lipid and collagen materials that had been contained by the endothelium-covered fibrous cap.[19,27] The ensuing thrombus abruptly increases the severity of the narrowing at the site of plaque rupture. Depending on the degree and location of the new obstruction and on the amount of available collateral circulation, one of several clinical syndromes result. When the obstruction is severe enough to reduce resting coronary flow below that required to maintain viability of the myocytes, myocardial infarction occurs. When the new obstruction provides barely enough flow to maintain myocyte viability, recurring rest angina may appear. When the new obstruction is less severe or the collateral circulation more adequate, effort angina may appear for the first time or, in a patient who already has angina, the level of effort required to produce symptoms may be diminished.[28]

The classification of unstable angina by Braunwald is extremely useful in understanding this clinical syndrome and its prognostic importance (Display 3-2). The likelihood of a fatal or nonfatal infarction in the short and intermediate term is increased as the symptom complex descends the classification scale. Ischemic electrocardiographic changes or elevated serum indices of myocardial injury may accompany this syndrome, especially in patients with class III symptoms. In the presence of a rise in cardiac enzymes a diagnosis of non–Q-wave myocardial infarction is appropriate, but does not fundamentally change the treatment strategy.

VASOSPASTIC (PRINZMETAL'S) ANGINA

In the late 1950s, Prinzmetal[29] described a series of patients with angina that, instead of occurring with effort, occurred at rest, and instead of

ST-segment depression on the electrocardiogram during pain, patients manifest ST-segment elevation. This syndrome is now attributed to focal coronary vasospasm.[30] That is, a segment with little or no fixed obstruction might, in response to vasoconstrictor stimuli, completely or nearly completely close the artery. Thus, symptoms would not occur during activity when vasodilator stimuli predominate but rather at rest when vasomotor tone is increased, as in the early morning hours.

It is likely that atherosclerosis is the fundamental vascular abnormality. Even though it may not be apparent from angiography, it sets the stage for abnormal vascular reactivity. Many patients have effort angina as well as vasospastic symptoms, and coronary arteriograms may show atherosclerotic narrowing in arteries other than those responsible for the ST elevation.

SYNDROME X

Typical effort angina is infrequently encountered in patients with normal coronary arteries and no other basis for the symptom (e.g., aortic stenosis, pulmonary hypertension). Some evidence ischemic patterns on stress testing. The pathophysiologic basis for syndrome X has not been entirely elucidated. Structural or functional abnormalities in arteries or arterioles too small to be visible on angiography have been suggested as being the basis for it. Other observers consider it to be related to hypersensitivity of the cardiac sensory fibers.[31,32]

♥ Conclusion

Diagnosis and management of patients with CAD continue to present a clinical challenge to health care providers. Future research will help to clarify the basic mechanisms of this complicated disease.

REFERENCES

1. Heberden W: Some account of a disorder of the breast. *Med Trans Coll Phys* 2:59, 1772.
2. von Rokitansky C: *A Manual of Pathological Anatomy*, vol 4, p. 261. Day GE, transl. London, Sydenham Society, 1852.
3. Virchow R: *Phlogose und thrombose in gefassystem, gesammelte abhandlungen zur wissenschaftlichen medicin*, p. 458. Frankfurt-am-Main, Germany, Meidinger Sohn, 1856.
4. Ross R: The pathogenesis of atherosclerosis: An update. *N Engl J Med* 314:488, 1986.

5. Furchgott RF, Zawadski JV: The obligatory role of endothelial cells in the relaxation of arterial smooth muscle by acetylcholine. *Nature* 288:373, 1980.

6. Vanhoutte PM: Endothelium-dependent contractions in arteries and veins. *Blood Vessels* 24:141, 1987.

7. Griffith TM, Edwards DH, Lewis MJ, et al: The nature of endothelium-derived vascular relaxing factor. *Nature* 308:645, 1984.

8. Nabel EG, Selwyn AP, Ganz P: Large coronary arteries in humans are responsive to changing blood flow: An endothelium-dependent mechanism that fails in patients with atherosclerosis. *J Am Coll Cardiol* 16:349, 1990.

9. Sellke FW, Armstrong ML, Harrison DG: Endothelium-dependent vascular relaxation is abnormal in the coronary microcirculation of atherosclerotic primate. *Circulation* 81:1586, 1990.

10. Zeiher AM, Drexler H, Willschlager H, Just H: Endothelial dysfunction of the coronary microvasculature is associated with impaired coronary blood flow regulation in patients with early artherosclerosis. *Circulation* 84:1984, 1991.

11. Panza JA, Quyyumi AA, Epstein SE: Abnormal endothelium-dependent vascular relaxation in patients with essential hypertension. *N Engl J Med* 323:22, 1990.

12. Nitenberg A, Valensi P, Sachs R, et al: Impairment of coronary vascular reserve and ACh-induced coronary vasodilation in diabetic patients with angiographically normal coronary arteries and normal left ventricular systolic function. *Diabetes* 42:1017, 1993.

13. Celemajer DS, Sorensen KE, Georgadopoulos D, et al: Cigarette smoking is associated with dose-related and potentially reversible impairment of endothelium-dependent dilation in healthy young adults. *Circulation* 88:2149, 1993.

14. Levine GN, Keaney JF, Vita JA: Cholesterol reduction in cardiovascular diseases. Clinical benefits and possible mechanisms. *N Engl J Med* 332:512, 1995.

15. Fuster V, Badimon L, Badimon JJ, Chesebro JH: The pathogenesis of coronary artery disease and the acute coronary syndromes. *N Engl J Med* 326:242, 1992.

16. Fry DL: Response of the arterial wall to certain physical factors. In *Atherogenesis: Initiating Factors*, p. 121. Amsterdam, NY, Ciba Foundation Symposium 12. Associated Scientific Publishers, 1973.

17. Caro CG: Transport of material between blood and wall in arteries. In *Atherogenesis: Initiating Factors*, p. 127. Amsterdam, NY, Ciba Foundation Symposium 12. Associated Scientific Publishers, 1973.

18. Harker LA, Slichter SJ, Scott CR, Ross R: Homocystinemia. Vascular injury and thrombosis. *N Engl J Med* 291:537, 1974.

19. Ross R: Atherosclerosis: An inflammatory disease. *Circulation* 340:115, 1999.

20. Fabricant CG, Fabricant J, Litrenta MM, Minick CR: Virus-induced atherosclerosis. *J Exp Med* 148:335, 1978.

21. Muhlestein JB, Hammond EH, Carlquist JF, et al: Increased incidence of *Chlamydia* species within the coronary arteries of patients with symptomatic

atherosclerosis versus other forms of cardiovascular disease. *J Am Coll Cardiol* 27:1555, 1996.

22. Parthasarathy S, Steinbrecher UP, Barnett J, et al: Essential role of phospholipase A2 activity in endothelial cell-induced modification of low density lipoprotein. *Proc Natl Acad Sci* 76:333, 1979.

23. Shaikh M, Marini S, Quincy JR, et al: Modified plasma-derived lipoproteins in human atherosclerotic plaques. *Atherosclerosis* 69:165, 1988.

24. Moreno P, Falk E, Palacios I, et al: Macrophage infiltration in acute coronary syndromes: Implications for plaque rupture. *Circulation* 90:775, 1994.

25. Ambrose JA, Winters SL, Stern A, et al: Angiographic morphology and the pathogenesis of unstable angina. *J Am Coll Cardiol* 5:609, 1985.

26. Braunwald B: The history. In Braunwald B (ed): *Heart Disease: A Textbook of Cardiovascular Medicine,* 5th ed. Philadelphia, WB Saunders, 1997.

27. Fuster V: Mechanisms leading to myocardial infarction: Insights from studies of vascular biology. *N Engl J Med* 90:2126, 1994.

28. Yun DD, Alpert JS: Acute coronary syndromes. *Cardiology* 88:223, 1997.

29. Prinzmetal M, Kennamer R, Masori, et al: A variant form of angina pectoris. *Am J Med* 27:375, 1959.

30. Mayer S, Hillis LD: Prinzmetal's variant angina. *Clin Cardiol* 21:243, 1998.

31. Kaski JC, Elliott PM: Angina pectoris and normal coronary arteriograms: Clinical presentation and hemodynamic characteristics. *Am J Cardiol* 76:35D, 1995.

32. Buus NH, Bottcher M, Botker HE, et al: Reduced vasodilator capacity in Syndrome X related to structure and function of resistance arteries. *Am J Cardiol* 83:149, 1999.

CHAPTER 4

Peripheral Vascular Disease

JORGE F. SAUCEDO, MD, AND JOHN R. LAIRD, MD, FACC, FACP

The 1990s have witnessed a trend toward the treatment of all forms of vascular disease in the cardiac catheterization laboratory. In effect, this trend is combining Andreas Gruentzig's original work in peripheral arteries with his later developments in the coronary circulation.[1]

To address this most recent development in the field of interventional cardiology, this chapter provides an overview of the clinical assessment and diagnosis of atherosclerosis in the peripheral and cerebral circulation.

♥ Peripheral Arterial Disease

Assessment of the peripheral circulation can be performed objectively and in a reproducible fashion with a good history, complete physical examination, and a few simple noninvasive studies. Although the diagnosis of peripheral arterial disease (PAD) is often delayed until the patient is symptomatic, PAD, even when asymptomatic, is an important marker for the presence of cardiovascular or other systemic illness.[2] Occlusive arterial disease can present acutely or chronically and is most often due to atherosclerosis. Features that suggest a nonatherosclerotic cause for PAD include the onset of symptoms in patients less than 40 years of age, involvement of the upper extremity, and the development of acute vessel occlusion without antecedent symptoms in the involved extremity.[3]

Peripheral arterial atherosclerotic obstructions are commonly seen at branch points and bifurcations (Fig. 4-1). Upper extremity involvement is less common than lower extremity involvement. Upper extremity arteries distal to the origin of the subclavian artery are rarely affected. Patients with diabetes mellitus have a different pattern and distribution of atherosclerosis. They tend to have more extensive disease of the tibial and peroneal arteries and less involvement of the aortoiliac segment.

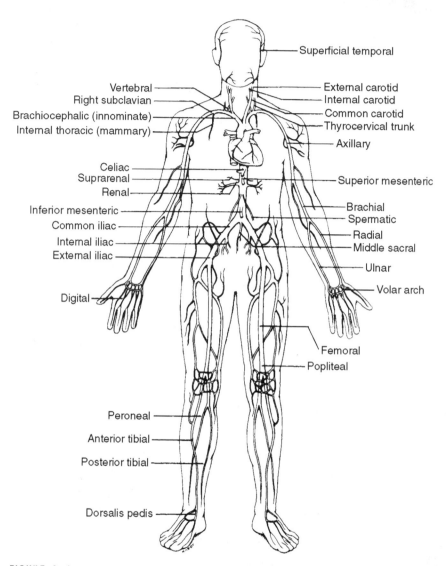

FIGURE 4–1 Distribution of the major peripheral arteries. (From Chaffee EE, Lytle IM [eds]: *Basic Physiology and Anatomy.* Philadelphia, JB Lippincott, 1980. Used with permission.)

CLINICAL MANIFESTATIONS AND DIAGNOSIS

The hallmark symptom of PAD is intermittent claudication. This is most often described as a discomfort or cramping of the lower extremity, which occurs with walking and is relieved within 2 to 3 minutes with rest. This discomfort is reproducible and constant in its occurrence with walking. The distance the patient can walk without symptoms may decrease slowly over time as the severity of the PAD progresses. The location of the claudication symptoms can be of some value in localizing the site of occlusive arterial disease. Generally, the level of claudication discomfort is distal to the obstruction site. For example, a hemodynamically significant obstruction of the iliac artery most often causes thigh or buttock claudication, whereas an obstruction in the superficial femoral artery most commonly produces calf claudication.

A number of disorders may produce symptoms that mimic intermittent claudication, including osteoarthritis of the hip or knee, sciatica, muscle strain, osteoporosis, plantar neuroma, or foot strain. One important disorder that mimics intermittent claudication is lumbar spinal stenosis. Lumbar spinal stenosis produces a symptom complex referred to as *pseudoclaudication.* This is a discomfort in the lower extremities, which occurs with weight bearing and walking and is relieved by sitting down or flexing the lumbar spine. This can be differentiated from true claudication by the fact that it occurs with standing alone as well as walking.

If the PAD is extensive and multilevel, the patient may present with the symptom complex known as "rest pain." Ischemic rest pain is typically described as a severe burning discomfort in the foot and toes, which is worse at night or when the extremity is exposed to a cool environment. This can sometimes be confused with the pain of peripheral neuropathy. Patients with ischemic rest pain often get some relief with dependency of the limb and describe having to hang their foot off the side of the bed during the night. When PAD has progressed to this extent, there is often other evidence of severe ischemia, including pallor on elevation of the legs, dependent rubor, and delayed venous filling time. In contrast to patients with peripheral neuropathy, patients with ischemic rest pain usually do not have symmetric symptoms and do not have signs of associated neuropathy such as absent or diminished deep tendon reflexes or loss of touch or vibratory sensation.[4]

Another manifestation of progressive and severe arterial insufficiency is major or minor tissue loss including ischemic ulceration or gangrene or both. Ischemic ulcers can be confused with other types of ulcers, including those associated with chronic venous insufficiency and various neuropathic diseases. Ischemic ulcers are often very painful and typically have an ischemic base with a discrete border. They are most often found distally on the toes or heels and may occur after some type of trauma.

The clinical presentation of an arterial embolism is often dramatic, with the development of an acutely ischemic limb. The clinical syndrome of acute limb ischemia is defined by the five P's Pain, Pallor, Paresthesia, Paralysis, and Pulselessness. Most embolic episodes to the lower extremities originate in the heart. Less often, an abdominal aortic aneurysm or diseased proximal artery may serve as the source of embolism. The findings with an acute arterial occlusion vary, depending on the size of the artery occluded and the extent of collateral circulation.

Microembolization of cholesterol crystals and fibrin platelet aggregates (atheromatous embolization syndrome) can occur in the setting of severe atherosclerosis. Atheromatous embolization often affects the dermal arterioles and digital arteries. Clinical manifestations of atheromatous embolization include purple or blue toes, gangrene, livedo reticularis,

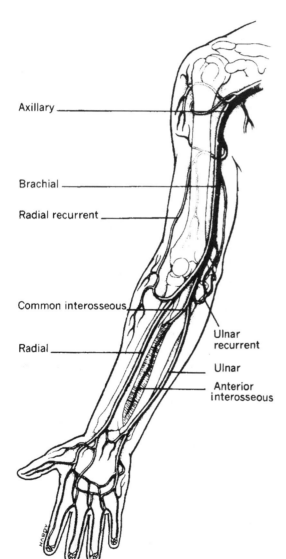

FIGURE 4–2 Distribution of major arteries of the arm. (From Chaffee EE, Lytle IM [eds]: *Basic Physiology and Anatomy.* Philadelphia, JB Lippincott, 1980. Used with permission.)

abdominal pain, ischemic bowel, and a variety of constitutional symptoms. If renal insufficiency and hypertension develop, atheroembolization to the renal arteries should be suspected.

Thromboangiitis obliterans (Buerger's disease) usually occurs in men younger than 40 years who have a long smoking history. These patients most commonly present with ulceration and gangrenous changes of the digits. The upper extremity is involved in at least 40% of patients with thromboangiitis obliterans.

PHYSICAL EXAMINATION

Complete evaluation of the peripheral arterial circulation should be included in the physical examination of every patient, particularly those with suspected coronary artery disease. Examination of the upper extremities should include measurement of the blood pressure in both arms. A difference of more than 10 mm Hg between the arms suggests the presence of an obstructing lesion in the subclavian or innominate artery. The brachial, radial, and ulnar pulses should be carefully examined (Fig. 4-2), and the intensity of the pulse noted. On auscultation, a systolic bruit may indicate turbulence caused by stenosis. If there is concern about possible occlusion of either the ulnar or radial artery, an Allen's test should be performed. The patient is asked to make a tight fist, and the examiner then occludes both the ulnar and radial arteries. The patient is instructed to open the hand, and the pressure applied to one of the two arteries is released. Prompt return of color to the hand determines patency of that artery. The maneuver is then repeated, releasing the pressure on the other artery to evaluate its patency.

Examination of the lower extremity should include careful palpation of the femoral, popliteal, and distal pulses. In examining the lower extremities, keep in mind that one or both pedal pulses are absent in about 12% of healthy persons.[5] The absence of the posterior tibial artery pulse is reported to be the best single criterion for the presence of occlusive arterial disease of the lower extremities.[6] Auscultation over the femoral and popliteal arteries should be performed to evaluate for the presence of a bruit. The development of pallor of the limb on elevation provides information regarding the degree of ischemia. Significant obstructive arterial disease may be present if pallor occurs after elevation of an extremity at 60 degrees for 1 minute.

The presence of tendinous and tuberous xanthomas and xanthelasma may be a clue to the presence of a severe lipid abnormality, associated with an increased risk of premature atherosclerosis and PAD. Also, arcus senilis in a young patient may be a sign of premature atherosclerosis. Fun-

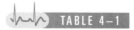 **TABLE 4–1**

Interpretation of Ankle Brachial Index

ABI	Symptoms	Severity
0.9–1.3	Asymptomatic	No significant lesions
0.6–0.9	Claudication	Single stenosis or occlusion
0.4–0.6	Claudication	Multilevel disease
0.2–0.4	Rest pain	Multilevel occlusions
<0.2	Impending tissue loss	Multilevel occlusions

The ankle brachial index (ABI) is determined by dividing the ankle systolic pressure by the brachial systolic pressure.

doscopic examination of a patient with PAD may demonstrate findings of hypertension, diabetes mellitus, or atheromatous embolization.

NONINVASIVE AND INVASIVE ASSESSMENT

Assessment of the patient with PAD includes measurement of the ankle brachial index, Doppler arterial waveform measurements, duplex scanning, and arteriography.

ANKLE BRACHIAL INDEX

One of the most widely used noninvasive tests to evaluate the degree of arterial obstruction is the measurement of the systolic blood pressure at the brachial and ankle levels using a Doppler device. If the patient has a significant obstruction of the lower extremities, the systolic pressure at the ankle level will be lower than the brachial systolic pressure. The normal ankle brachial index should be greater than 0.95. In general, patients with chronic occlusive arterial disease and an ankle brachial index of greater than 0.6 have a single-segment occlusion or stenosis and suffer from mild to moderate claudication. If lower values are measured, multiple levels of involvement and more severe symptoms are usually present (Table 4-1).

More precise localization of the level of obstruction can be obtained from segmental pressures. This involves performing serial measurements of the ankle pressure with blood pressure cuffs inflated at the level of the upper thigh, lower thigh, calf, and ankle (Fig.4-3). Additional information regarding the severity of PAD and the degree of functional impairment can be obtained by performing ankle brachial indices before and after exercise on a treadmill.

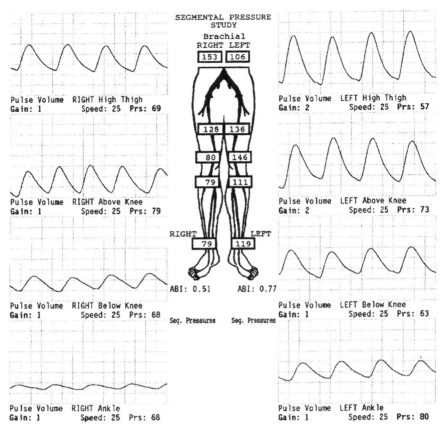

FIGURE 4–3 Segmental pressures and ankle brachial indices (ABIs) indicating bilateral lower extremity occlusive disease with more severe involvement of the right lower extremity. In addition, there is a probable significant stenosis or occlusion of the left subclavian artery (asymmetry between right and left brachial pressures). Prs, pressure.

DOPPLER WAVEFORM ASSESSMENT

The normal arterial velocity waveform has three separate and distinct phases. These phases include the forward-flow velocity associated with systole, the reverse-flow component that occurs in late systole and early diastole, and a secondary-forward flow component that is seen in late diastole. If this triphasic waveform is noted, the likelihood of significant disease proximal to the recording site is low. If there is arterial stenosis that exceeds 50%, the characteristics of this waveform are altered.[7] Blunting of the systolic peak occurs with loss of the reverse-flow component, resulting in a monophasic waveform[8] (see Fig. 4-3). Of note, the normal waveform from the brachial, radial, and ulnar arteries may not show the reverse-flow component in as many as 50% of person.

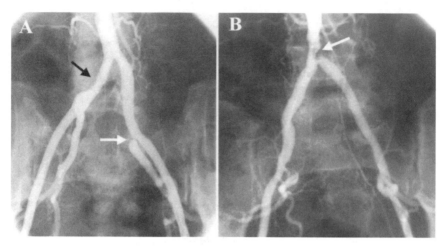

FIGURE 4–4 Distal aortography demonstrating the iliac vasculature in two patients. **(A)** Mild narrowing of the right common iliac artery (*black arrow*) and a significant stenosis at the origin of the left internal iliac artery (*white arrow*). **(B)** Severe atherosclerotic narrowing of the distal abdominal aorta involving the aortoiliac bifurcation is present (*white arrow*).

DUPLEX SCANNING

Ultrasonic duplex scanners combine B-mode imaging of the vessel with Doppler color and spectral waveform analysis. Changes in the Doppler-derived blood flow velocities can be used to estimate the severity and the location of stenoses. Identifying the location and extent of the disease with duplex scanning may permit therapeutic decisions before angiography. This technique is particularly important for the noninvasive evaluation of the patients with suspected disease of the extracranial carotid arteries. It is also an important modality to evaluate the results of percutaneous transluminal angioplasty (PTA) and document patency of distal bypass grafts (graft surveillance). Duplex scanning also allows for the evaluation of suspected aortic or peripheral aneurysms and groin masses after percutaneous coronary angiography and angioplasty. The transducer used in duplex scanning can be used to compress femoral pseudoaneurysms, thus allowing thrombosis and healing to occur.[9]

ARTERIOGRAPHY

Arteriography remains the "gold standard" for determination of the location and severity of occlusive arterial disease. It is best reserved for patients in whom revascularization is planned. Indications for arteriography include exertional and resting ischemia, vasculitis, embolus, thrombotic disease, vascular tumors and arterial aneurysms. Femoral catheterization can be performed by puncturing the common femoral artery on the same side of the affected leg or by puncturing the contralateral femoral artery. Contrast injection for peripheral arteriography of the legs can be performed with nonselective aortic injection by positioning the catheter at the infrarenal aortic level (Fig. 4-4). Imaging is performed by filming from the aorta to the feet. Many laboratories have now abandoned the traditional "cut-film" techniques for digital acquisition and digital subtraction angiography.

TREATMENT

Risk factor modification is the cornerstone of care for the patient with atherosclerotic peripheral vascular disease. The patient should be strongly advised to quit smoking. Continued tobacco use has been shown to be a risk factor for the progression of ischemia and decreases the likelihood of limb salvage in the setting of acute limb ischemia.[10,11]

Different approaches are available for the management of intermittent claudication. A walking program should be advised for all patients. Regular walking for periods up to 30 minutes per day with rest as needed to relieve claudication may increase the patient's walking distance significantly.[12] A variety of pharmacologic agents have been tried with limited success. Pentoxifylline is reported to promote blood flow owing to its effect on blood viscosity, erythrocyte deformability, platelet aggregation, and plasma fibrinogen concentration.[13] Several studies have reported modest improvement in walking distance in 50% to 60% of patients when 400 mg of pentoxifylline is taken three times per day. The full benefit of this drug may not be noted until after 12 weeks of treatment. Revascularization can be considered when symptoms persist despite the above measures and are lifestyle limiting or limb threatening. Percutaneous endovascular approaches to revascularization may include balloon angioplasty, atherectomy, laser-assisted angioplasty, stenting, or pharmacologic/mechanical thrombectomy.[14-16] Surgical techniques may include endarterectomy, embolectomy, or bypass surgery using autologous vein or synthetic graft material.[17]

❤ Extracranial Cerebrovascular Disease

Strokes account for 10% to 12% of all deaths in industrialized countries and are the third leading cause of death in the United States. The cause of stroke is multifactorial and includes ischemic stroke in 80%,

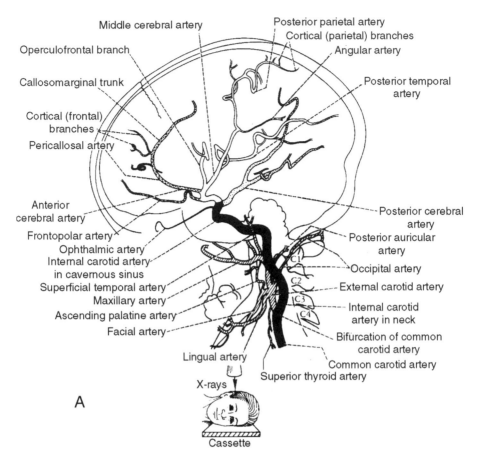

FIGURE 4-5 Major arteries of the cerebral circulation from three different radiographic views. **A**, lateral view; **B**, anteroposterior (angled) view; **C**, anteroposterior view. (From Snell RS: *Clinical Neuroanatomy for Medical Students.* Boston, Little, Brown, 1980. Used with permission.)

intracerebral hemorrhage in 10%, and subarachnoid hemorrhage in 5% of cases.

Atherosclerotic plaque is the underlying cause of most ischemic strokes. The plaque is most frequently found at the carotid bifurcation and is subject to ulceration, thrombosis, and embolization to the distal cerebral arteries. Hemodynamic forces are believed to play a role in the development of atherosclerosis at this level because the carotid artery bulb is exposed to low and oscillating shear stress. Distal embolism is the most common mechanism by which atherosclerotic plaque causes ischemic stroke. In addition, the heart is responsible for 20% of ischemic strokes in adults aged 45 to 60. The cardiac risk factors that favor embolism

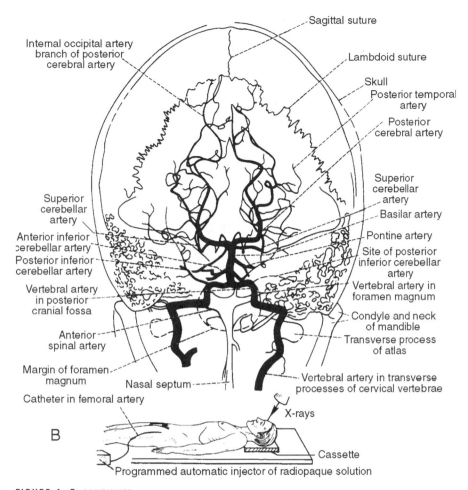

FIGURE 4-5 CONTINUED

include prosthetic heart valves, valvular heart disease, atrial fibrillation, recent myocardial infarction, endocarditis, and cardiomyopathy.[18]

CLINICAL MANIFESTATIONS AND DIAGNOSIS

The brain receives 15% of the total cardiac output via the carotid and vertebral arteries (Fig. 4-5). The clinical manifestations of cerebrovascular disease depend on the artery affected. The carotid arteries supply blood to the anterior and middle portion of the brain, whereas the vertebral arteries supply the posterior aspect of the brain. These vessels coalesce at the circle of Willis and are connected via the anterior and posterior commu-

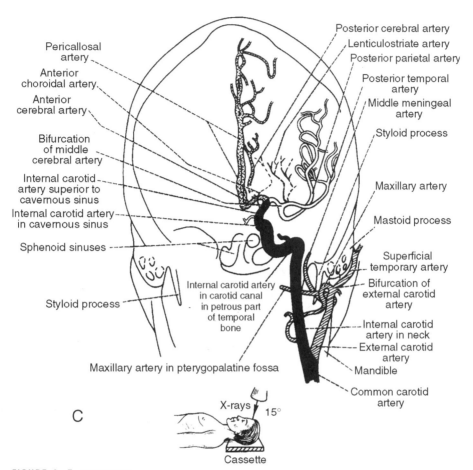

Pericallosal artery

Anterior choroidal artery

Anterior cerebral artery

Bifurcation of middle cerebral artery

Internal carotid artery superior to cavernous sinus

Internal carotid artery in cavernous sinus

Sphenoid sinuses

Styloid process

Internal carotid artery in carotid canal in petrous part of temporal bone

Maxillary artery in pterygopalatine fossa

Posterior cerebral artery

Lenticulostriate artery

Posterior parietal artery

Posterior temporal artery

Middle meningeal artery

Styloid process

Maxillary artery

Mastoid process

Superficial temporary artery

Bifurcation of external carotid artery

Internal carotid artery in neck

External carotid artery

Mandible

Common carotid artery

C

X-rays   15°

Cassette

FIGURE 4–5 CONTINUED

nicating arteries.[19] Autopsy studies have shown that the circle of Willis is incomplete in up to 50% of humans.

Transient ischemic attack (TIA) is defined as an episode of temporary cerebral dysfunction that resolves within 24 hours. Most TIAs last only a few minutes. These events are usually secondary to embolization of small amounts of atheroma, platelets, or fibrin.

Reversible ischemic neurologic deficit (RIND) is a reversible neurologic event that lasts more than 24 hours, but generally less than 1 week; it may represent a small cerebral infarct.

A *completed stroke* is a nonreversible neurologic deterioration, which generally has stabilized after 24 hours for the carotid circulation and after 72 hours for the vertebrobasilar circulation. The differentiation between ischemic and hemorrhagic stroke must be made by computerized tomography (CT) scan or by magnetic resonance imaging before definitive therapy is initiated. When the stroke is secondary to embolism from the internal carotid artery, the territory of the middle cerebral artery is the most commonly affected. This results in contralateral hemiplegia or hemiparesis with hemihypesthesia. Ischemia of the dominant hemisphere results in aphasia whereas ischemia of the nondominant hemisphere causes apraxia (defects in body image and the inability to perform specific tasks). When embolization to the ophthalmic artery occurs (first major branch of the internal carotid artery), amaurosis fugax or monocular blindness may be seen. Amaurosis fugax occurs in 30% of symptomatic cases of total internal carotid artery occlusion.

Another important clinical manifestation of cerebrovascular disease is the *lacunar stroke*. This usually affects the internal capsule and thalamus and is secondary to occlusion of penetrating end-arterial branches of the anterior, middle, posterior, and basilar arteries. A person usually with a lacunar stroke presents with a pure motor deficit, but pure sensory loss is also commonly seen. These strokes most commonly occur in diabetic and hypertensive patients.[20]

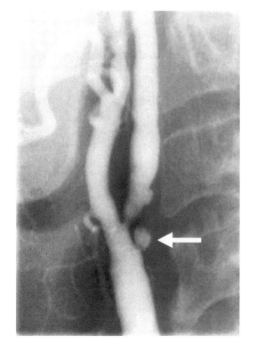

FIGURE 4–6 Carotid angiography demonstrating carotid bifurcation atherosclerotic disease with a severe stenosis at the origin of the internal carotid artery with ulcerated plaque in the distal common carotid artery (*arrow*).

PHYSICAL EXAMINATION

The physical examination of the vascular system of patients with cerebrovascular disease should include those maneuvers performed in patients with arterial vascular disease. Special attention should be placed on the examination of the vessels of the cervical region.

Auscultation over the vessels of the neck and head should be performed very carefully. Examination of the carotid artery with the stethoscope should begin as high as the level of the mandible. This auscultation continues slowly down the course of the common carotid artery to the base of the neck. After noting the presence and intensity of bruits, the subclavian artery can be examined over the supraclavicular area. The presence of vertebral artery bruits is best heard in the area posterior to the sternocleidomastoid muscles. Auscultation of the aortic and pulmonic valves must be performed to determine whether or not the neck bruits originate from the heart. A bruit that is heard during both systole and diastole may indicate a severe arterial stenosis, an arteriovenous malformation, an arteriovenous fistula, or a venous hum.[4] Although the presence of a cervical bruit is a helpful diagnostic sign, the absence of a bruit does not exclude significant arterial disease. Only 40% of patients with significant internal carotid artery stenosis have an audible bruit; of those patients with a bruit, only 20% will have a hemodynamically significant stenosis of the internal carotid artery.[21,22]

NONINVASIVE AND INVASIVE EVALUATION

Evaluation of the patient with cerebrovascular disease includes carotid duplex measurements, magnetic resonance angiography, and arteriography.

DUPLEX ULTRASOUND

Duplex ultrasound is the initial study performed in most patients with suspected extracranial cerebrovascular disease. Carotid duplex combines B-mode ultrasound and Doppler color and spectral waveform analysis to evaluate the degree of narrowing in the carotid arteries. Classification schemes have been developed to characterize the severity of stenosis based on the peak systolic and diastolic flow velocities in the internal carotid artery. Many studies have documented the reproducibility of this technique and have demonstrated the safety of performing carotid endarterectomy based solely on the results of duplex ultrasound without carotid angiography.[23,24]

MAGNETIC RESONANCE ANGIOGRAPHY

Magnetic resonance angiography (MRA) offers some advantages over duplex ultrasound, including less operator variability and the ability to visualize areas not well seen by duplex ultrasound, such as the proximal common carotid artery, distal extracranial internal carotid artery, and the intracranial vessels. MRA is an expensive technique, however, and is limited in defining certain types of vascular anatomy as well as plaque characteristics, including the presence of plaque ulceration. In addition, MRA may overestimate the severity of stenosis, particularly in the setting of subtotal occlusion.

ARTERIOGRAPHY

Intra-arterial digital subtraction angiography is presently the "gold standard" for the evaluation of cerebrovascular disease. Supra-aortic vessel assessment can be performed from aortic arch injections. Selective catheterization of the carotid arteries is then performed to further evaluate the carotid bifurcation (Fig. 4-6). Selective angiography can also provide information regarding intracranial collateral flow from the vertebrobasilar system and the contralateral carotid artery.

Selective carotid catheterization is performed with preshaped catheters including various "head hunters" and a variety of hockey-stick curves.[25] The volume and rate of contrast injection during selective carotid arteriography are variable. The two views most frequently obtained are the anteroposterior and the lateral projections, but oblique views may be needed to visualize a stenosis at the origin of the internal carotid artery. The projection that reveals the highest degree of stenosis is used to calculate the percentage of the diameter of stenosis. The minimal lumen diameter in the region of the stenosis is compared with the diameter of the more distal, nontapering segment of the internal carotid artery during these calculations.

TREATMENT

Aspirin and ticlopidine have an important role in reducing the incidence of stroke and death from cerebrovascular causes. Ticlopidine should be considered for the treatment of the patient who is unable to tolerate aspirin or with recurrent symptoms on aspirin therapy (American Heart Association guidelines, 1994).[26]

For the treatment of evolving or progressing stroke, anticoagulation and fibrinolytic agents can be used after a mandatory CT scan is performed to exclude cerebral hemorrhage.

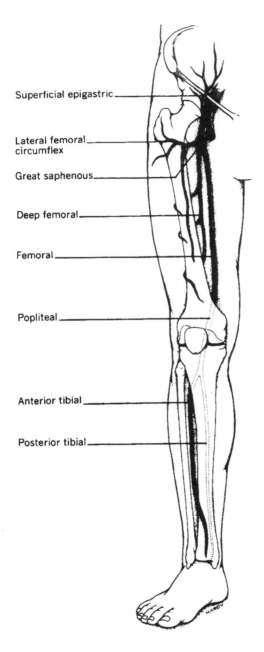

Superficial epigastric

Lateral femoral circumflex

Great saphenous

Deep femoral

Femoral

Popliteal

Anterior tibial

Posterior tibial

FIGURE 4–7 Major veins of the lower extremities. (From Chaffee EE, Lytle IM [eds]: *Basic Physiology and Anatomy.* Philadelphia, JB Lippincott, 1980. Used with permission.)

CAROTID ENDARTERECTOMY

Data from randomized trials of patients with symptomatic or asymptomatic extracranial cerebrovascular disease are now available. The North American Symptomatic Carotid Endarterectomy Trial (NASCET)[27] and the Asymptomatic Carotid Atherosclerosis Study (ACAS)[28] have shown carotid endarterectomy to be superior to medical therapy for the prevention of stroke or death in the setting of high-grade symptomatic and asymptomatic lesions of the carotid bifurcation.

PERCUTANEOUS CEREBROVASCULAR INTERVENTIONS

The use of percutaneous transluminal angioplasty (PTA) or primary stenting of stenotic lesions of the internal and common carotid arteries has generated significant interest in recent years, particularly for the treatment of patients at high risk for complications from standard carotid endarterectomy. Initial reports have showed that carotid PTA for symptomatic disease has a high initial technical success rate and a complication rate near 4%.

Carotid stenting is currently favored over balloon angioplasty because of improved angiographic results and reduced complications with this technique. Although the initial results with carotid stenting appear promising, long-term follow-up is not available. Randomized trials comparing carotid stenting with carotid endarterectomy are currently being performed.

♥ Peripheral Venous Disease

Peripheral venous disease includes chronic venous insufficiency as well as deep vein thrombosis.

CHRONIC VENOUS INSUFFICIENCY

Chronic venous insufficiency (CVI) occurs mostly after venous valvular damage secondary to remote deep thrombosis and affects up to 25% of the US population. In CVI, blood flows paradoxically from the deep to the superficial system across incompetent venous valves of the perforated veins.

CLINICAL MANIFESTATIONS AND DIAGNOSIS

Patients with CVI usually present with edema of the lower extremities. Prominent superficial veins are commonly seen as an initial sign of CVI. Some patients experience heaviness or an aching discomfort, which occurs after prolonged standing. Skin pigmentation changes, induration, and dermatitis may occur after longstanding venous insufficiency. Venous ulcers may develop in the region of the ankle. When assessing the patient with CVI, it is important to determine which venous system is involved (deep venous system, superficial venous system, or communicating veins) (Fig. 4-7), the pathologic process (valvular incompetence, obstruction or a combination or both), and the anatomic level of involvement.[29]

TREATMENT

The choice of nonsurgical versus surgical treatment depends on the severity of the disease process and the anatomic system affected. Nonsurgical management of CVI includes external compression by a variety of methods, skin care, and ulcer care. Sclerotherapy is an important adjunct to the treatment of CVI. Surgical treatment for superficial venous insufficiency includes ligation and stripping of varicose veins or subfascial ligation of incompetent perforators.

If the patient has chronic deep venous obstruction, a saphenous bypass may be performed using the greater saphenous vein. In cases of deep valvular incompetence, a vein valve transplant or valvuloplasty may be attempted.

DEEP VEIN THROMBOSIS

Virchow described deep vein thrombosis (DVT) and the predisposing risk factors of stasis, endothelial damage, and hypercoagulability more than a century ago.[30] However, DVT remains a significant clinical problem.

CLINICAL MANIFESTATIONS AND DIAGNOSIS

Patients with DVT may present with painful, swollen leg or arm. In up to 80%, patients have symptoms. Although most thrombi remain confined to the deep calf veins, approximately 20% of cases involved have extension of thrombi into the proximal deep veins and can lead to fatal pulmonary embolism.[30]

The two most important complications of DVT are pulmonary embolism and postphlebitic syndrome. Important risk factors for the development of DVT are venous stasis, injury to the vessel wall, and hypercoagulability. Other risk factors include age over 60 years, malignancy, heart failure, obesity, history of previous thrombosis, pregnancy, use of oral contraceptives, chemotherapy, varicose veins, inflammatory bowel disease, thrombocytosis, polycythemia vera, and systemic lupus erythematosus.

The clinical diagnosis of DVT is sometimes difficult, with physical examination often being unreliable. Homans' sign (pain in the upper calf during forced dorsiflexion of the foot) is insensitive and nonspecific. On rare occasions, DVT patients present with phlegmasia cerulea dolens or venous gangrene with a striking clinical picture of blue discoloration, marked swelling, and signs of arterial insufficiency.

The differential diagnosis for DVT includes superficial phlebitis, varicose veins, cellulitis, muscle tear, arterial insufficiency, ruptured Baker's cyst, vasculitis, myositis, lymphangitis, fibrositis, and panniculitis.

NONINVASIVE AND INVASIVE EVALUATION

Objective testing is important to establish the diagnosis of DVT. A variety of tests have been used for this purpose.

Impedance Plethysmography

Impedance plethysmography is a noninvasive technique that measures changes in electrical resistance of the lower leg, which in turn reflects changes in blood volume. This technique can be used to evaluate a patient with possible DVT as well as follow treatment of DVT. Disadvantages include its inability to detect isolated calf vein thrombosis, inability to visualize clot and localize the exact level of obstruction, and lack of specificity in the presence of congestive heart failure or arterial insufficiency.

Duplex Ultrasonography

Duplex Ultrasonography is now considered the most accurate noninvasive technique for the detection of DVT. It has a sensitivity and specificity as high as 95% for proximal vein thrombosis. Its sensitivity is lower for the calf vein thrombosis. Duplex scanning is considered by many the preferred diagnostic method for DVT.

Venography

Venography remains the gold standard for the diagnosis of DVT. This invasive technique outlines the entire deep venous system of the lower extremity. For lower extremity venography, a small intravenous line is placed in a pedal vein. Contrast material is injected, and images of the tibial veins, popliteal vein, femoral veins, and iliac veins are obtained. Thrombus is detected by the presence of a filling defect within the contrast medium or vessel cut-off with abnormal venous collateral filling.

TREATMENT

Heparin should be administered early to prevent extension of thrombus formation and pulmonary embolism. An intravenous bolus between 5000 and 10,000 U is given, followed by continuous-infusion heparin to maintain the activated partial thromboplastin time at two to three times that of the laboratory normal value. Warfarin should be started on the same day as heparin and should be continued for 3 months for the patient with an initial thrombotic event or for 6 months to 1 year for the patient with recurrent DVT. In patients with two or more events, warfarin should be given indefinitely.

For patients with a contraindication to anticoagulant therapy, a complication from anticoagulant therapy, or recurrent pulmonary embolism despite adequate anticoagulant therapy, an inferior vena caval filter may be required. These filters can be inserted percutaneously and are associated with excellent long-term patency rates.[31]

Low molecular weight heparins (LMWHs) are currently being used for DVT prophylaxis before hip, knee, and abdominal surgery. Recent studies have shown that LMWHs are at least as effective and safe as unfractionated intravenous heparin in the treatment of acute DVT.[32–34] Thrombolytic therapy results in greater lysis of deep vein thrombi than heparin therapy, but has not yet been definitely shown to prevent the postphlebitic syndrome. There are multiple contraindications to the use of thrombolytic therapy to include recent surgery or internal organ biopsy, trauma, active internal bleeding, pregnancy, and recent stroke.

❤ Conclusion

Coronary artery disease does not exist in isolation. Frequently patients with coronary artery disease have other clinical signs and symptoms of significant peripheral vascular disease. As the field of interventional cardiology continues to expand to include the aggressive treatment of many types of peripheral vascular disease, catheterization laboratory personnel will also expand their skills to adapt to this changing paradigm of the percutaneous treatment of atherosclerosis.

REFERENCES

1. King SB: Angioplasty from bench to bedside. *Circulation* 93:1621, 1996.
2. Spittell JA: Diagnosis and management of occlusive peripheral arterial disease. *Curr Probl Cardiol* 1:7, 1990.
3. Spittell JA Jr: Some uncommon types of occlusive peripheral arterial disease. *Curr Probl Cardiol* 8:6, 1983.

4. Young JR: Physical examination. In Young JR, Olin JW, Bartholomew JR (eds): *Peripheral Vascular Diseases*, 2nd ed. St. Louis, Mosby-Year Book, 1996.
5. Barnhost DA, Barner HB: Prevalence of congenitally absent pedal pulses. *N Engl J Med* 278:264, 1968.
6. Criqui MH, Fronek A, Klauber MR, et al: The sensitivity, specificity, and predictive value of traditional clinical evaluation of peripheral arterial disease: Results from noninvasive testing in a defined population. *Circulation* 71:516, 1985.
7. Jager KA, Ricketts HJ, Strandness DE Jr: Duplex scanning for the evaluation of lower limb arterial disease. In Bernstein EF (ed): *Noninvasive Diagnostic Techniques in Vascular Disease*, 3rd ed. St. Louis, CV Mosby, 1985.
8. Strandness DE Jr: Noninvasive vascular laboratory and vascular imaging. In Young JR, Olin JW, Bartholomew JR (eds): *Peripheral Vascular Diseases*, 2nd ed. St. Louis, Mosby-Year Book, 1996.
9. Cox GS, Young JR, Gray BR, et al: Ultrasound-guided compression repair of postcatheterization pseudoaneurysms: Results of treatment in one hundred cases. *J Vasc Surg* 19:683, 1994.
10. Cronenwett JL, Warner KG, Zelenock GB, et al: Intermittent claudication: Current results of nonoperative management. *Arch Surg* 119:430, 1984.
11. Juergens JL, Barker NW, Hines EA Jr: Arteriosclerosis obliterans. Review of 520 cases with special reference to pathogenic and prognostic factors. *Circulation* 21:188, 1960.
12. Jonason T, Jonzon B, Ringquist I, et al: Effect of physical training on different categories of patients with intermittent claudication. *Acta Med Scand* 206:253, 1979.
13. Spittell JA Jr: Pentoxifylline and intermittent claudication. *Ann Intern Med* 102:126, 1985.
14. Dotter CT, Judkins MP: Transluminal treatment of arteriosclerotic obstruction: Description of a new technique and a preliminary report of its application. *Circulation* 30:654, 1964.
15. Rooke TW, Stanson AW, Johnson CM, et al: Percutaneous transluminal angioplasty in the lower extremities: A 5 year experience. *Mayo Clin Proc* 62:85, 1987.
16. Wildus DM, Osterman FA: Evaluation and percutaneous management of atherosclerotic peripheral vascular disease. *JAMA* 261:3148, 1989.
17. Blackshear WM Jr: Surgical indications for lower extremity arterial occlusive disease. Part I and II. *Curr Probl Cardiol* 6(2):1; 6(3):1, 1981.
18. Easton JD, Sherman DG: Management of cerebral embolism of cardiac origin. *Stroke* 11:173, 1980.
19. Warlow C: Disorders of the cerebral circulation. In Walton J (ed): *Brain's Diseases of the Nervous System*, 10th ed. Oxford, Oxford University Press, 1993.
20. Sullivan TM, Hertzer NR: Extracranial cerebrovascular disease. In Young JR, Olin JW, Bartholomew JR (eds): *Peripheral Vascular Diseases*, 2nd ed. St. Louis, Mosby-Year Book, 1996.
21. Ziegler DK, Zileli T, Dick A, Sebaugh JL: Correlation of bruits over the carotid artery with angiographically demonstrated lesions. *Neurology* 21:860, 1971.

22. David TE, Humphries AW, Young JR, Beven EG: A correlation of neck bruits and arteriosclerotic carotid arteries. *Arch Surg* 107:729, 1973.
23. Chervu A, Moore WS: Carotid endarterectomy without arteriography. *Ann Vasc Surg* 8:296, 1994.
24. Gertler JP, Cambria RP, Kistler JP, et al: Carotid surgery without arteriography: Noninvasive selection of patients. *Ann Vasc Surg* 5:253, 1991.
25. Dolmatch B, Davros WL, Grist TM: Diagnostic angiography. In Young JR, Olin JW, Bartholomew JR (eds): *Peripheral Vascular Diseases,* 2nd ed. St. Louis, Mosby-Year Book, 1996.
26. Ad Hoc Committee on Guidelines for the Management of Transient Ischemic Attacks of the Stroke Council of the American Heart Association: Guidelines for the management of transient ischemic attacks. *Circulation* 89:2950, 1994.
27. North American Symptomatic Carotid Endarterectomy Trial Collaborators: Beneficial effect of carotid endarterectomy in symptomatic patients with high-grade carotid stenosis. *N Engl J Med* 325:445, 1991.
28. ACAS, Executive Committee for the Asymptomatic Carotid Atherosclerosis Study: Endarterectomy for asymptomatic carotid artery stenosis. *JAMA* 273:1421, 1995.
29. O'Donnell TF Jr, Welch HJ: Chronic venous insufficiency and varicose veins. In Young JR, Olin JW, Bartholomew JR (eds): *Peripheral Vascular Diseases,* 2nd ed. St. Louis, Mosby-Year Book, 1996.
30. Navarro F, Bartholomew JR: Deep vein thrombosis. In Young JR, Olin JW, Bartholomew JR (eds): *Peripheral Vascular Diseases,* 2nd ed. St. Louis, Mosby-Year Book, 1996.
31. Greenfield LJ, Michna BA: Twelve-year experience with the Greenfield vena cava filter. *Surgery* 104:706, 1988.
32. Hull RD, Raskob GE, Pineo GF, et al: Subcutaneous low-molecular-weight heparin compared with continuous intravenous heparin in the treatment of proximal-vein thrombosis. *N Engl J Med* 326:975, 1992.
33. Simonneau G, Charbonnier B, Decousus H, et al: Subcutaneous low-molecular-weight heparin compared with continuous intravenous unfractionated heparin in the treatment of proximal deep vein thrombosis. *Arch Intern Med* 153:1541, 1993.
34. Leizorovicz A, Simonneau G, Decousus H, et al: Comparison of efficacy and safety of low molecular weight heparins and unfractionated heparin in initial treatment of deep venous thrombosis: A meta analysis. *Br Med J* 309:299, 1994.

CHAPTER 5

Coagulation and Fibrinolysis

ANDREA S. ABIZAID, MD, ALEXANDRE ABIZAID, MD,
AND ANN GREENBERG, RN, MSN

First used by Gruentzig in 1977,[1] percutaneous transluminal coronary angioplasty (PTCA) has become a growing therapeutic modality for the treatment of coronary artery disease. Despite widespread use, its clinical success has been limited by acute reocclusion and late restenosis, which have persisted despite changes in both catheterization techniques and antithrombotic regimens.

Acute reocclusion (abrupt closure) after angioplasty is the temporary cessation of flow through the lesion, with associated chest pain or electrocardiographic (ECG) changes suggestive of transmural ischemia. This serious complication was encountered in up to 8% of balloon angioplasties.[2] It is a direct consequence of acute thrombus formation, initiated by platelet activation and often in association with an extensive tear in the coronary artery.

Coronary angioplasty exerts its effect by the application of mechanical stress to the vessel wall, which results in vascular injury, endothelial denudation, and exposure of the subendothelial surface to blood constituents. This exposed surface results in platelet adhesion to the subendothelial collagen through associations with von Willebrand factor (vWF) and fibronectin, the first step in thrombogenesis.

Restenosis, which can be defined as a greater than 50% narrowing of the diameter of the lumen at the site of a previously successful PTCA,[3] is a late process, occurring in 30% to 50% of patients in the first 6 months after the procedure.[4] In contrast to abrupt closure, in which acute thrombus formation plays a major role, the mechanisms of restenosis involve interactions among platelets, coagulation factors, vascular endothelium, and smooth muscle cells. These interactions result in varying degrees of thrombus formation, intimal hyperplasia, and vascular remodeling, leading to clinical evidence of luminal narrowing[5] (Fig. 5-1).

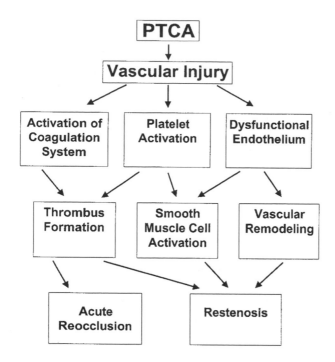

FIGURE 5–1 Mechanisms of acute and late coronary reocclusion. PTCA, percutaneous transluminal coronary angioplasty.

♥ Coagulation

The process of coagulation (appropriate clot-mediated hemostasis) and thrombosis (inappropriate clot-mediated hemostasis due to, for example, a ruptured atherosclerotic plaque) are similar in most ways, and both are intimately associated with the process of fibrinolysis (clot dissolution). Most of the key components in coagulation are the same as those in thrombosis, whereas some factors play roles in both coagula-

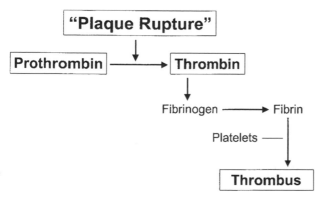

FIGURE 5–2 Steps involved in thrombus formation.

tion/thrombosis and fibrinolysis.[6] The processes of clot formation and clot dissolution may be grouped as four subprocesses: (a) procoagulation, which includes proenzymes (factor VII), enzyme cofactors (factor V), and structural proteins (fibrinogen); (b) anticoagulation with proenzymes (protein C) and enzyme inhibitor (antithrombin III); (c) profibrinolysis including plasminogen activators (t-PA) and plasmin, the main fibrinolytic enzyme; and (d) antifibrinolysis with plasminogen activator inhibitors and plasmin inhibitors. These subprocesses are organized in a way in which, under some conditions, approximates a state of pseudoequilibrium and forces the notion that coagulation and fibrinolysis are dynamically interrelated.

CLOTTING CASCADE

The coagulation system is activated by exposure of tissue factor, which occurs when atherosclerotic plaques rupture or when the endothelium is damaged by angioplasty. Regardless of the initiating factor, it concludes in the final common pathway with the activation of prothrombin to thrombin. Thrombin then catalyzes the conversion of the soluble protein fibrinogen into fibrin, an insoluble protein. A thrombus forms when fibrin traps other blood elements (red blood cells, platelets, plasminogen) into a mature clot (Fig. 5-2).

Figure 5-3 shows the physiologic pathways of blood coagulation divided into intrinsic and extrinsic pathways. In the intrinsic system, all necessary factors are present in the circulating blood, the initial reaction is triggered by contact of the blood with a negatively charged substance, such as subendothelium collagen. In most cases, blood coagulation and thrombosis are believed to be initiated by tissue factor (TF) through activation of the extrinsic pathway (after vessel injury).[7] TF acts as the receptor for factor VII and its activated form VIIa. The TF–VIIa complex is capable of activating factor IX to IXa and factor X to Xa. After activation of factor X, the two pathways merge into one. Factor Xa and factor Va participate in the generation of thrombin (T) from prothrombin (PT). Thrombin cleaves fibrinogen to fibrin, and finally the clot is formed.

♥ Fibrinolysis

The endogenous thrombolytic system is activated by the presence of an intravascular thrombus. The conversion of plasminogen to plasmin is the essential reaction in fibrinolysis. Plasmin is the final enzyme in the fibrinolytic pathway and is responsible for most actual fibrinolysis, not only

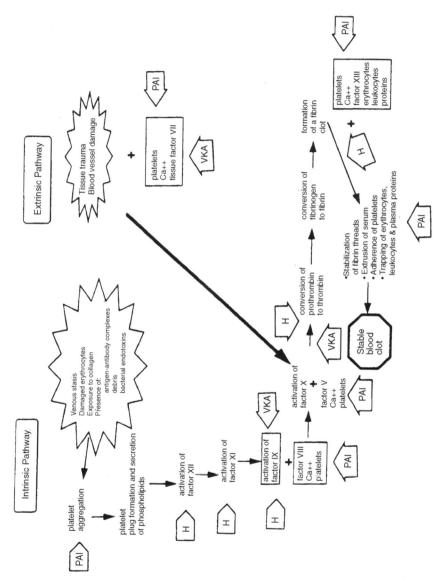

FIGURE 5–3 Intrinsic and extrinsic pathways of the coagulation cascade. H, heparin; PAI, platelet aggregation inhibitors; VKA, vitamin K antagonists. (From Workman ML: Anticoagulants and thrombolytics: What's the difference? *AACN Clin Issues Crit Care* 5:33, 1994. Used with permission.)

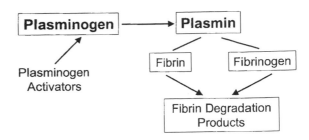

FIGURE 5-4 Steps involved in the lysis of thrombus.

by inhibiting several clotting factors (V, VII, XII) but also by lysing stable fibrin clots and degrading circulating fibrinogen (Fig. 5-4).

♥ Platelets

Over a century ago, Rudolf Virchow presented a hypothesis that three factors—vessel injury, altered blood flow, and changes in blood coagulability—were responsible for vascular thrombosis (Virchow's triad). The primary condition affecting the composition of a thrombus is the nature of blood flow.[8]

Under conditions of relatively slow flow, as in a vein or within the chambers of the heart, fibrin is the major component of such red thrombi. Thrombi that develop in areas of rapid flow, such as in coronary arteries, have a different pathogenesis and different morphologic features. Formation of such thrombi is related to the interaction of an abnormal vascular surface with elements of blood—predominantly platelets[9]—and a fibrin component with erythrocytes and leukocytes more distally.[10] The large concentration of platelets has led to the name "white thrombi." Thus, platelets play a major role in thrombus formation and can contribute both to the growth and to the progression of atherosclerotic plaques.[11]

Under normal physiologic conditions, platelets are essentially inert, their adhesion to the subendothelium is prevented by an intact vascular wall. In response to vessel trauma, platelets spontaneously adhere to exposed adhesive proteins, forming a protective monolayer of cells. Within seconds, these platelets are activated by agonists such as thrombin, collagen, and adenosine diphosphate (ADP), causing them to change shape and release materials from stored vesicles. The constituents of the vesicles are involved in the activation of platelets; ultimately these activated platelets aggregate to form a hemostatic plug. Under certain pathologic conditions, such as a rupture of an atherosclerotic plaque, these platelet aggregates can form thrombi associated with multiple cardiovascular ischemic events, including unstable angina and myocardial infarction.

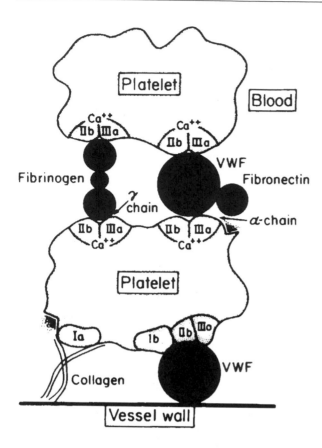

FIGURE 5–5 Platelets interact with the vessel wall directly via platelet membrane glycoprotein Ia and indirectly via glycoprotein Ib with a von Willebrand factor (vWF) protein bridge. Platelet– platelet interactions are mediated by integrin protein bridging between adjacent complexes of glycoprotein IIb/IIIa. The same sequence of events occurs on disrupted atheromatous plaques. (From Fuster V, Badimon L, Cohen M, et al: Insights into the pathogenesis of acute ischemic syndromes. *Circulation* 77(6):1213–1220, 1988. Used with permission.)

An arterial thrombi appears to develop in three phases: platelet adhesion, platelet aggregation, and activation.

PLATELET ADHESION

Platelet adhesion refers to the attachment of platelets to a surface other than another platelet. Platelets tend to adhere to damaged or disrupted endothelial surfaces. Circulating platelets do not adhere to intact endothelium. Adhesion depends on the interaction of platelet membrane glycoproteins with several components of the subendothelial matrix, such as vWF, collagen, and possibly fibronectin or vitronectin. Glycoprotein Ib appears to be important for initial contact of platelets with vWF on the subendothelium surface. This protein, exposed on the surface of nonactivated platelets, is the major receptor for platelet adhesion.[11] Glycoprotein Ia, which binds to exposed subendothelium collagen, may also be important. The glycoprotein IIb–IIIa (GP IIb–IIIa) complex binds vWF, fibronectin, and fibrinogen and is the final common pathway of the coagulation cascade (Fig. 5-5). This IIb–IIIa receptor is present in very large numbers on the platelet surface (approximately 50,000 molecules per platelet).

Platelet adhesion is determined not only by the degree of vascular injury, but also by transportation to the injured area. Transportation is determined by the wall shear rate, which is the measure of the difference in blood velocity between the center of the vessel and along the wall. At higher wall shear rates, found, for example, in medium-sized stenotic arteries, the initial platelet deposition rate and maximum extent of deposition are significantly higher.[12,13]

PLATELET AGGREGATION

In this second stage, platelets adhere to each other primarily through platelet–platelet cross-linking by fibrinogen. Platelet aggregation appears to depend primarily on an increase in cytoplasmic calcium, which is mediated by three pathways. First, concomitant with the process of platelet adhesion, there is an activation of platelets by extrinsic stimuli, specifically collagen from the vessel wall and thrombin, possibly through a platelet-activating factor that may expose the platelet membrane GP IIb–IIIa complex to fibrinogen and vWF and thus promote aggregation.[14–17] Both collagen and thrombin are strong agonists, they do not require thromboxane A_2 (TxA_2) for aggregation.

Second, during such platelet activation, the release of platelet intracytoplasmic granule constituents occurs, particularly ADP, which further activates neighboring platelets and, most important, exposes the platelet membrane GP IIb–IIIa complex, thus promoting aggregation.[14–16] ADP is a weak agonist, it causes aggregation only when TxA_2 is produced.[17] Third, also occurring during platelet activation are synthesis and release of thromboxane A_2. This pathway is mediated by arachidonic acid, which is released from the platelet membrane by the action of phospholipase A_2.[18] Cyclooxygenase converts arachidonic acid into TxA_2, the most potent platelet-aggregating agent and vasoconstrictor. It stimulates platelet aggregation by promoting the mobilization of intracellular calcium, which causes a conformational change in the GP IIb–IIIa complex. This results in exposure of sites for fibrinogen and vWF, and thus promotion of aggregation.[14–16]

In summary, collagen, thrombin, and products of platelet secretion such as ADP and TxA_2 enhance the thrombotic process by stimulating platelets and causing the exposure of platelet membrane glycoprotein receptors to fibrinogen and vWF. These reactions promote platelet aggregation and thrombus growth.

PLATELET ACTIVATION

The final common pathway of all agonist–receptor interactions is the activation of a specific receptor responsible for platelet aggregation. This receptor, GP IIb–IIIa, unlike the GP Ib receptor responsible for platelet adhesion, is active only after the platelet has been stimulated, after its intracellular calcium concentration has increased. The receptor has a high affinity for the tripeptide sequence, arginine-glycine-aspartic acid (RGD), which is found in fibrinogen, vWF, fibronectin, and vitronectin.[19] Fibrinogen, because of its high concentration in the plasma, is the substance most involved in platelet aggregation.

In summary, during platelet adhesion and aggregation, the clotting mechanism is activated and thrombin is generated. This further promotes platelet aggregation and leads to the formation of fibrin, which maintains the stability of the platelet arterial thrombus.

♥ Pharmacology

Thrombus formation on a disrupted atherosclerotic plaque is the main pathogenic mechanism for the acute coronary syndromes of myocardial infarction and unstable angina.[20] Myocardial infarction results from an acute total occlusion of the artery, whereas unstable angina is secondary in most cases to mural thrombus formation. Thrombus formation has also been implicated in chronic atherosclerotic disease progression and in restenosis after coronary angioplasty. Pharmacologic measures to treat thrombus rely on the ability of agents to prevent thrombus extension, dissolve its fibrin component, or prevent further platelet aggregation. Therefore, medications that inhibit the coagulation cascade and antagonize platelet function are fundamental to the successful treatment of acute coronary syndromes.

PLATELET INHIBITORS

The oral platelet inhibitors, such as aspirin and ticlopidine, have been shown to be helpful in improving outcomes of patients with acute coronary syndromes and in reducing ischemic complications of coronary interventions.[21] These drugs, also known as *antiplatelet agents,* inhibit platelet function and the subsequent predisposition to plaque formation.

ASPIRIN

Aspirin acts by irreversibly inactivating the enzyme cyclooxygenase, which converts arachidonic acid to thromboxane A_2, the powerful

TABLE 5–1

Effect of Antiplatelet Agents on Procedural Outcome After Coronary Angioplasty

Author	Year	Clinical Status	No. of Patients	Treatment	Procedural Outcome			
					Death (%)	MI (%)	CABG or PTCA (%)	Thrombus or Complication (%)
Schwartz[60]	1988	Elective	187	Aspirin, 330 mg TID DP, 75 mg TID	0	1.6	2.1	—
			189	Placebo	0	6.9	2.1	—
White[61]	1987	Elective	111	Aspirin, 325 mg BID DP, 75 mg TID	—	—	—	5†
			112	Ticlopidine, 250 mg TID	—	—	—	2†
			110	Placebo	—	—	—	14
Barnathan[62]	1987	All patients	32	Aspirin and DP	—	—	—	0*
			110	Aspirin alone	—	—	—	1.8†
			121	No aspirin	—	—	—	10.7
Mufson[63]	1988	Elective	253	Aspirin, 80 mg daily	0	3.6	3.6	—
			242	Aspirin, 1500 mg daily	0	3.9	3.7	—
Lembo[64]	1990	Elective	117	Aspirin, 325 mg TID DP, 75 mg TID	0.9	4.3	6.1	—
			115	Aspirin, 325 mg TID	0	1.7	2.6	—

BID, twice daily; CABG, coronary bypass surgery; DP, dipyridamole; MI, myocardial infarction; PTCA, percutaneous transluminal coronary angioplasty; TID, three times a day.
*P < 0.05 compared with placebo.
†P < 0.01 compared with placebo.
Adapted from Popma JJ, Coller BS, Ohman EM, et al: Antithrombotic therapy in patients undergoing coronary angioplasty. Chest 108(Suppl):486S, 1995.

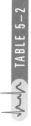 **TABLE 5–2**

Effect of Antiplatelet Agents on Restenosis After Coronary Angioplasty

| | | | | | | Late Outcome | |
| | | | | | Clinical Events | | |
Author	Year	Clinical Status	No. of Patients	Treatment	Restenosis (%)	(%)	Overall Conclusion
Schwartz[60]	1988	Elective	187	Aspirin, 330 mg TID DP, 75 mg TID	37.7	NR	Negative
			189	Placebo	38.6	NR	
Taylor[65]	1991	Elective	108	Aspirin, 100 mg/d	25*	35	Positive
			104	Placebo	38	43	
Darius[66]	1994	Elective	85	Aspirin, 500 mg/d	29*	NR	Positive
			86	Aspirin, 100 mg/d	53	NR	
			85	Aspirin, 40 mg/d	43	NR	
Mufson[63]	1988	Elective	253	Aspirin, 80 mg/d	47	NR	Negative
			242	Aspirin, 1500 mg/d	51	NR	
Bussman[67]	1987	Elective	288	Aspirin, 1500 mg/d	17	NR	Positive
			111	Aspirin, <1500 mg/d	38	NR	

DP, dipyridamole; NR, not reported; TID, three times a day.
*$P < 0.05$.
Adapted from Popma JJ, Coller BS, Ohman EM, et al: Antithrombotic therapy in patients undergoing coronary angioplasty. Chest 108(Suppl):486S, 1995.

platelet agonist and vasoconstrictor. By inactivating cyclooxygenase, aspirin also blocks the production of prostacyclin, which opposes platelet activation. Aspirin has shown beneficial results in most ischemic coronary syndromes, including primary and secondary prevention of cardiac events.[22] Its beneficial effect in reducing the frequency of ischemic complications after coronary angioplasty has been demonstrated in many controlled clinical trials (Table 5-1). However, the underlying clinical efficacy of aspirin must be considered as only partial or modest. This is because aspirin inhibits only TxA_2, and approximately 100 known agonists of platelet aggregation, including serotonin, collagen, thrombin, ADP, and shear stress, remain unaffected. Finally, aspirin does not appear to influence the restenosis rate after coronary angioplasty (Table 5-2).

THE THIENOPYRIDINES

The thienopyridines (ticlopidine and clopidogrel), orally active antiplatelet agents, inhibit platelet function by a novel mechanism. They block ADP-induced platelet activation.[23]

First to be approved for clinical use, ticlopidine has been studied and used clinically much more extensively than clopidogrel. It may be used in aspirin-sensitive patients for any indication calling for antiplatelet therapy. In interventional cardiology, its principal application is in the prevention of thrombosis in patients undergoing stent implantation. Based on two large randomized trials—one in Europe (ISAR)[24] and one in the United States (STARS)[25]—the combination of ticlopidine and aspirin has become the standard of care in patients undergoing this procedure. No benefit from this agent in the prevention of restenosis at 6 months has been demonstrated.[26]

Side effects are the principal obstacles to more general use of ticlopidine. Gastrointestinal symptoms (20%), cutaneous rash (4% to 15%), and abnormalities of liver function tests all occur.[27] There are two rare, but potentially fatal side effects. Severe leukopenia occurs in about 1% of patients.[27,28] Reversible in most instances, it has resulted in death in rare instances. An even rarer but more threatening complication is thrombotic thrombocytopenic purpura. At least 60 cases have been reported.[29] This devastating complication has been fatal in 25% to 50% of affected patients.

Clopidogrel, chemically very similar to ticlopidine, has been more recently approved for use based on the CAPRIE Trial.[30] To date, it appears to have fewer side effects than ticlopidine; for this reason, it may be preferable for patients in whom aspirin is not ideal. This drug has not had formal equivalency testing against ticlopidine for patients undergoing

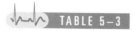

TABLE 5–3

Thirty Day and 6 Month EPIC Results in the Three Treatment Groups

Events	Placebo	c7E3 Bolus	c7E3 Bolus and Infusion
Primary end point n (%)	89 (12.8)	79 (11.4)	59 (8.3)*
Death	12 (1.7)	9 (1.3)	12 (1.7)
Q-wave MI	16 (2.3)	7 (1.0)	6 (0.8)
Emergency PTCA	31 (4.5)	25 (3.6)	6 (0.8)
Emergency CABG	35 (3.6)	16 (2.8)	17 (2.4)
Repeat revascularization (%) (6 months' follow-up)	22.3	21	16.5*

EPIC, Evaluation of c7E3 for the Prevention of Ischemic Complications[33]; Primary endpoints are death, myocardial infarction (MI), emergency coronary artery bypass surgery (CABG), emergency percutaneous transluminal coronary angioplasty (PTCA), stent placement, or intra-aortic balloon pump.
*$P < 0.01$.

stenting, but based on available experience some interventional cardiologists are using it because of its more favorable side effect profile.

GLYCOPROTEIN IIB/IIIA ANTAGONISTS

GP IIb/IIIa receptors expressed on the surface of activated platelets are involved in the final common pathway of platelet aggregation. Coller and colleagues[31] demonstrated the effectiveness of a murine monoclonal antibody to GP IIb/IIIa in preventing the binding of fibrinogen to platelets and inhibiting platelet aggregation. A modification of this agent, initially called c7E3, is now clinically available as abciximab.

The review of Madan and colleagues[32] provides a detailed description of the pharmakinetics and clinical use of abciximab and the more recently

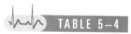

TABLE 5–4

EPILOG Trial: Results at 30 Days

Events (%)	Placebo + Standard Heparin	Abciximab + Low-dose Heparin
Death	0.8	0.4*
Death + myocardial infarction	5.7	1.6*
Major bleeding	3.1	1.8
Hemorrhagic stroke	0	0.2

EPILOG, Evaluation of PTCA to Improve Long-Term Outcome by c7E3 GP IIb/IIIa Receptor Blockade.[35]
Standard heparin = 100 U/kg; low-dose heparin = 70 U/kg.
*$P < 0.001$ compared with placebo.

released IIb/IIIa antagonists, eptifibatide and tirofiban. Unlike abciximab, the latter are synthetic agents. All three are intravenous preparations. Oral IIb/IIIa antagonists are now in clinical trials. Although similar in their ability to interfere with platelet aggregation, these agents vary in other important ways, particularly in onset and duration of action. For example, the half-life of abciximab is 6 to 12 hours, whereas those of the two synthetic agents are more nearly 2 to 3 hours.

Abciximab has had the most extensive clinical evaluation and now is widely used. The enthusiasm of interventional cardiologists for this new modality is based on a series of randomized clinical trials. The EPIC trial (Evaluation of c7E3 for the Prevention of Ischemic Complications) addressed the efficiency of abciximab in high-risk coronary angioplasty.[33] Participants were randomized in double-blind fashion to receive one of the following: (a) a bolus of 0.25 mg/kg of abciximab followed by an infusion of 10 μg/min, (b) the abciximab bolus followed by a placebo infusion, or (c) a placebo bolus followed by a placebo infusion. The 30-day and 6-month results are described in Table 5-3. Compared with placebo, the active agent administered as a bolus followed by the infusion reduced the incidence of acute adverse events by 35% and the need for subsequent revascularization by 26%. The incidence of hemorrhagic complications was, however, doubled in the treatment group. The investigators attributed this to the fact that heparin in fixed doses was administered concomitantly.

In a subsequent investigation (PROLOG), the use of weight-adjusted heparin and early sheath removal reduced the incidence of hemorrhagic complications without reducing the efficacy of abciximab treatment.[34] With these encouraging results, the EPILOG (Evaluation of PTCA to Improve Long-Term Outcome by c7E3 GP IIb/IIIa Receptor Blockade) was undertaken.[35] Patients undergoing *elective* (as opposed to high risk in the EPIC Trial) PTCA randomized to abciximab and low-dose (70 U/kg/hr) or standard-dose (100 U/kg/hr) heparin had a lower incidence of death and myocardial infarction at 30 days compared with placebo (plus standard-dose heparin) (Table 5-4). This benefit was observed without an increase in major bleeding events (1.8% compared with 3.1% for the placebo-plus-heparin group: P = ns). Data from the most recent trial of this agent in coronary angioplasty (EPISTENT) indicate that the incidence of non–Q-wave myocardial infarction after stent placement is reduced in patients treated with abciximab compared with those not so treated.[36]

The other two IIb/IIIa antagonists (eptifibatide and tirofiban) are now available for clinical use based primarily on randomized trials demonstrating their efficacy in patients with unstable angina and non–Q-wave myocardial infarction. In addition to the studies demonstrating a beneficial effect in such patients, both have been tested in randomized trials in patients undergoing angioplasty.[37,38] In these trials, both agents were superior to placebo in preventing procedural complications, but initial review of the data suggests that they may not be as effective as abciximab. Any superiority of the latter may be due to inadequate dosing with the newer agents. Credible equivalency trials await a means of evaluating the completeness of IIa/IIIb receptor blockade.

Both eptifibatide and tirofiban have shorter half-lives than abciximab. This shorter duration of action is a potential advantage if there are hemorrhagic complications or a need for the patient to go to surgery.

THROMBIN INHIBITORS

Thrombin inhibitors antagonize the actions of thrombin. Heparin, although the most commonly used antithrombotic therapy for the treatment of acute myocardial infarction or unstable angina, does have some limitations. Some of the newer thrombin inhibitors may overcome these limitations.

HEPARIN

Heparin has been traditionally used in most patients undergoing angioplasty to reduce the risk of abrupt closure. Its anticoagulant effects result from reversible binding and activation of antithrombin III, which inhibits the actions of thrombin and activated factors Xa, XIa, and XIIa.[39] In addition, heparin has been shown to inhibit migration and proliferation of smooth muscle cells within the arterial wall. Despite its clinical efficacy, heparin's antithrombotic activity is limited by (a) inability to inactivate clot-bound thrombin; (b) neutralization by platelet factor IV from platelet-rich thrombi; and (c) inactivation by fibrin II monomers, which are formed by the action of thrombin on fibrinogen.

Randomized studies comparing heparin with placebo after coronary angioplasty found no significant difference in the restenosis rates in patients 6 months after angioplasty, although the incidence of acute closure was decreased in the heparin group.[40,41] Thus, as with aspirin, the benefit of heparin appears to be achieved early after the procedure with no significant effect on late events. Inadequate dosage, failure to start treatment before the procedure and too short a period of treatment all may be relevant factors that explain why the limited clinical trials have shown no benefit.

A prospective multicenter trial, Heparin after Percutaneous Intervention (HAPI trial), recently released its preliminary results.[42] All patients undergoing interventional procedures were randomized into three groups: (a) to receive intravenous heparin overnight and removal of sheaths the next day (group I); (b) no heparin postprocedure and sheath removal and reinstitution of heparin 4 hours later for 12 hours (group II); and (c) no heparin postprocedure with early sheath removal (group III). In-hospital ischemic events, defined as death, myocardial infarction, coronary artery bypass graft, stroke, abrupt closure, and repeat PTCA were similar among groups (3.0% group I, 1.0% group II and 2.0% group III; $P = .825$). Bleeding and vascular complications were significantly higher in group I (45% compared with 10% in group II and 3% in group III; $P < .0001$), with a trend toward increased cost and length of stay. The investigators concluded that routine postprocedure heparin is not recommended.

LOW MOLECULAR WEIGHT HEPARIN

In contrast to unfractionated heparin, low molecular weight (LMW) heparin has less antithrombin activity and does not prolong the activated partial thromboplastin time; its anticoagulant effect is mediated predominantly by inhibition of factor Xa. LMW heparin has been used to prevent deep venous thrombosis and pulmonary embolism. Preliminary studies during coronary intervention suggest no benefit over unfractionated heparin. Enoxaparin, a LMW heparin, failed to reduce angiographic or clinical restenosis in a randomized trial.[43]

HIRUDIN/HIRULOG

Hirudin is a polypeptide anticoagulant originally isolated from the leech, *Hirudo medicinalis*. Hirulog is a synthetic peptide, with similar antithrombotic actions. Although it does not have direct antiplatelet effects, hirudin is a selective and potent inhibitor of thrombin. Hirudin has functional properties that confer potential advantages over heparin.[44,45] Unlike heparin, hirudin (a) can inhibit clot-bound thrombin, which is inaccessible to the heparin-antithrombin III complex; (b) is not inhibited by activated platelets; (c) does not require a cofactor for its action; and (d) provides a more stable anticoagulant response. In animal models, hirudin was more effective than heparin in preventing thrombus formation[46] and in preventing reocclusion after thrombolysis.[47]

Hirudin/Hirulog have been studied in clinical trials with effects similar to heparin.[48,49] HELVETICA (Hirudin in a European Trial versus Heparin in the Prevention of Restenosis after PTCA) showed no difference between the two drugs at 7 months in terms of restenosis and event-free survival rates, although in the hirudin group the in-hospital cardiac events were lower, with similar rates of bleeding complications.[50]

In summary, heparin is not an ideal drug, but is the anticoagulant with which the interventionalists have the greatest experience. Direct thrombin inhibitors offer a stable anticoagulant activity and a lack of direct effect on platelet function.

FIBRINOLYTICS

Despite well-documented efficiency in acute myocardial infarction, thrombolytic therapy does not have a beneficial impact on unstable angina (TIMI 3A and 2B trials).[51,52] The TAUSA (Thrombolysis and Angioplasty in Unstable Angina) trial suggested a possible detrimental effect when intracoronary urokinase was given prophylactically to patients undergoing PTCA for rest angina.[53] It appeared that thrombolytic drugs may improve resolution of intracoronary thrombus, but some lesions may become more severely stenosed or totally occluded. The mechanism by which thrombolytics may induce abrupt closure is not well understood. In vitro studies have demonstrated enhanced platelet aggregation during thrombolytic infusion.[54–56] Intimal splitting occurs in most vessels after successful PTCA. It may be associated with excessive bleeding in the plaque and media of the vessel.

In contrast, observational studies suggest that intracoronary lytics may help dissolve thrombus that forms during or after coronary intervention. Urokinase is commonly used for this purpose in doses ranging from 75,000 to 500,000 units over 15 to 45 minutes through the guiding catheter or the central lumen of a balloon.[57–59]

♥ Summary

Platelets play essential roles in normal coagulation and in coronary atherosclerotic disease and its complications. Various antiplatelet therapies, including aspirin, ticlopidine, and antithrombin therapies such as heparin have been used in patients with coronary artery disease to prevent ischemic complications.[60–67] New approaches with more potent antiaggregation effects have been accomplished by the use of GP IIb–IIIa receptor antagonists and new antithrombins. The GP IIb–IIIa antagonists seem to be the most promising of the new agents in reducing overall clinical ischemic complications rates.

REFERENCES

1. Gruentzig A: Transluminal dilation of coronary artery stenosis (Letter). *Lancet* 263:1, 1978.
2. Lincoff AM, Popma JJ, Ellis SG, et al: Abrupt closure complicating coronary angioplasty: Clinical, angiographic and therapeutic profile. *J Am Coll Cardiol* 119:926, 1992.
3. Holmes DR, Vlietstra RE, Smith HC, et al: Restenosis after percutaneous coronary angioplasty: A report from the PTCA Registry of the National Heart, Lung and Blood Institute. *Am J Cardiol* 53(Suppl):77C, 1984.
4. Melchior JP, Meier B, Urban P, et al: Percutaneous coronary angioplasty for chronic total coronary artery occlusion. *Am J Cardiol* 59:535, 1987.
5. Nobuyoshi M, Kimura T, Ohishi H, et al: Restenosis after percutaneous coronary angioplasty: Pathologic observations in 20 patients. *J Am Coll Cardiol* 17:433, 1991.
6. Mann K: Normal hemostasis. In Kelly W (ed): *Textbook of Internal Medicine,* p. 1240. Philadelphia, JB Lippincott, 1992.
7. Furie B, Furie B: Molecular and cellular biology of blood coagulation. *N Engl J Med* 326:800, 1992.
8. Baumgartner HR: The role of blood flow in platelet adhesion, fibrin deposition and formation of mural thrombi. *Microvasc Res* 5:167, 1973.
9. Davies MJ, Thomas T: The pathological basis and microanatomy of occlusive thrombus formation in human coronary arteries. *Philos Trans R Soc Lond (Biol)* 294:225, 1981.
10. Bennett JS: Mechanisms of platelet adhesion and aggregation: An update. *Hosp Pract* 27:124, 1992.
11. Wu K: Platelet activation mechanism and markers in arterial thrombosis. *J Int Med* 239:17, 1996.
12. Badimon L, Badimon JJ, Galvez A, et al: Influence of arterial damage and wall shear rate on platelet deposition: Ex-vivo study in a swine model. *Arteriosclerosis* 6:312, 1986.
13. Badimon L, Badimon JJ: Mechanisms of arterial thrombosis in non parallel streamlines: Platelet thrombi grow on the apex of stenotic severely injured vessel wall. Experimental study in the pig model. *J Clinic Invest* 84:1134, 1989.
14. Hawiger J: Formation and regulation of platelet and fibrin hemostatic plug. *Hum Pathol* 18:111, 1987.
15. Stein B, Fuster V, Israel DH, et al: Platelet inhibitor agents in cardiovascular disease: An update. *J Am Coll Cardiol* 14:813, 1989.
16. Cooler BS: Activation affects access to platelet receptor for adhesive glycoproteins. *J Cell Biol* 103:451, 1986.
17. Mruk JS, Chesebro JH, Webster MW: Platelet aggregation and interaction with the coagulation system: Implications for antithrombotic therapy in arterial thrombosis. *Coronary Artery Dis* 1:149, 1990.
18. Moncada S, Vane JR: Arachidonic acid metabolites and the interactions between platelets and blood vessel wall. *N Engl J Med* 300:1142, 1979.
19. Hirsh J, Salzman EW, Marder VJ, Colman RW: *Hemostasis and Thrombosis: Basic Principles and Clinical Practice,* pp. 1151–1163. Philadelphia, JB Lippincott, 1994.
20. Kamat SG, Kleiman NS: Platelets and platelet inhibitors in acute myocardial infarction. *Cardiol Clin* 13:435, 1995.

21. Harrington R: Trials of novel antiplatelet agents. *J Myocard Ischem* 6:20, 1994.
22. Frishman WH, Miller KP: Platelets and antiplatelet therapy in ischemic heart disease. *Curr Probl Cardiol* 11:73, 1986.
23. Flores-Runk P, Raasch RH. Ticlopidine and antiplatelet therapy. *Ann Pharmacother* 27:1090, 1993.
24. Schomig A, Neumann F-J, Kastrati A, et al: A randomized comparison of antiplatelet and anticoagulation therapy after the placement of coronary-artery stents. *N Engl J Med* 334:1084, 1996.
25. Leon MB, Baim DS, Popma JJ, et al: A clinical trial comparing three antithrombotic-drug regimens after coronary-artery stenting. *N Engl J Med* 339:1665, 1998.
26. Bertrand ME, Allain H, LaBlanche JM, et al: Results of a randomized trial of ticlopidine versus placebo for prevention of acute closure and restenosis after coronary angioplasty (PTCA). The TACT study (abstr). *Circulation* 82(Suppl 3): III-190, 1990.
27. Fernandez-Aviles F, Alonso J, Duran JM, et al: Absence of bleeding and subacute occlusion after Palmaz-Schatz coronary stenting using a new antithrombotic regimen (abstr). *J Am Coll Cardiol* 25(Suppl):197A, 1995.
28. Rodriquez JN, Fernandz-Jurado A, Dieguez JC, et al: Ticlopidine and severe aplastic anemia. *Am J Hematol* 47:332, 1994.
29. Bennett CL, Weinberg PD, Rozenberg-Ben-Dror K, et al: Thrombotic thrombocytopenic purpura associated with ticlopidine: A review of 60 cases. *Ann Int Med* 128:541, 1998.
30. CAPRIE Steering Committee: A randomized blinded, trial of clopidogrel versus aspirin in patients at risk of ischemic events (CAPRIE). *Lancet* 348:1329, 1996.
31. Coller BS, Peerschke EI, Scudderz LE, et al: A murine monoclonal antibody that completely blocks the binding of fibrinogen to platelets produces a thrombasthenic-like state in normal platelets and binds to glycoproteins IIb an/or IIIa. *J Clin Invest* 72:325, 1983.
32. Madan M, Berkowitz SD, Tcheng JE: Glycoprotein IIb/IIIa integrelin blockade. *Circulation* 98:2629, 1998.
33. EPIC investigators: Use of monoclonal antibody directed against the platelet glycoprotein IIb-IIIa receptor in high-risk coronary angioplasty. *N Engl J Med* 330:956, 1994.
34. PROLOG investigators: A multicenter, randomized, double-blind pilot trial of standard versus low dose weight adjusted heparin in patients treated with the platelet GP IIb-IIIa receptor antibody c7E3 during percutaneous coronary revascularization (abstr). *J Am Coll Cardiol* 25(Suppl):80, 1995.
35. Tcheng JE, Lincoff AM, Miller DP, et al: Benefits of Abciximab accrue in the full spectrum of coronary interventional patients: Insights from the EPILOG trial. *J Am Coll Cardiol* 29(Suppl):276A, 1996.
36. The EPISTENT investigators: Randomized placebo-controlled and balloon angioplasty controlled trial to assess safety of coronary stenting with use of platelet glycoprotein IIb/IIIa blockade. *Lancet* 352:87, 1998.
37. The IMPACT II Investigators: Randomized placebo-controlled trial of effect of eptifibatide of complications of percutaneous coronary intervention: IMPACT II. *Lancet* 349:1422, 1997.

38. The RESTORE investigators: Effects of platelet glycoprotein IIb/IIIa blockade with tirofiban on adverse cardiac events in patients with unstable angina or acute myocardial infarction undergoing coronary angioplasty. *Circulation* 96:1445, 1997.
39. Hirsh J, Fuster V: Guide to anticoagulant therapy. Part I: Heparin. *Circulation* 89:1449, 1994.
40. Ellis SG, Roubin GS, Wilentz J, et al: Effect of 18–24 hour heparin administration for prevention of restenosis after uncomplicated coronary angioplasty. *Am Heart J* 117:777, 1989.
41. Walford GD, Midei MM, Aversano TR, et al: Heparin after PTCA: Increased early complications and no clinical benefit (abstr). *Circulation* 84(Suppl 2):II-592, 1991.
42. Rabah MM, Cannon LA, Weiner BH, et al: Heparin after percutaneous intervention (HAPI): Preliminary results of a prospective multicenter randomized trial. *Circulation* 94(Suppl):I-198, 1996.
43. Faxon DP, Spiro TE, Minor S, et al: Low molecular weight heparin in prevention of restenosis after angioplasty. *Circulation* 90:908, 1994.
44. Cannon CP, Braunwald E: Hirudin: Initial results in acute myocardial infarction, unstable angina and angioplasty. *J Am Coll Cardiol* 25(Suppl):30S, 1995.
45. Lefkovits J, Topol EJ: Direct thrombin inhibitors in cardiovascular medicine. *Circulation* 90:1522, 1994.
46. Heras M, Chesebro JH, Webster MW, et al: Hirudin, heparin and placebo during arterial injury in the pig. The in vivo role of thrombin in platelet-mediated thrombosis. *Circulation* 82:1476, 1990.
47. Haskel EJ, Prager NA, Sobel BE, et al: Relative efficacy of antithrombin compared with antiplatelet agents in accelerating coronary thrombolysis and preventing reocclusion. *Circulation* 83:1048, 1991.
48. Cannon CP, McCabe CH, Henry TD, et al: A pilot trial of recombinant desulfatohirudin compared with heparin in conjunction with tissue-type plasminogen activator and aspirin for acute myocardial infarction (TIMI 5). *J Am Coll Cardiol* 23:993, 1994.
49. Bittl JA, Strony J, Brinker JA, et al: Treatment with bivalirudin (Hirulog) as compared with heparin during coronary angioplasty for unstable angina or post-infarction angina. *N Engl J Med* 333:764, 1995.
50. The HELVETICA investigators: A comparison of hirudin with heparin in the prevention of restenosis after coronary angioplasty. *N Engl J Med* 333:757, 1995.
51. The TIMI IIIA Investigators: Early effects of tissue-type plasminogen activator added to conventional therapy on the culprit coronary lesion in patients presenting with ischemic cardiac pains at rest, results of the Thrombolysis in Myocardial Ischemia (TIMI IIIA) Trial. *Circulation* 87:38, 1993.
52. The TIMI IIIB Investigators: Effects of tissue plasminogen activator and a comparison of early invasive and conservative strategies in unstable angina and non-Q wave myocardial infarction. Results of the TIMI IIIB trial. *Circulation* 89:1545, 1994.
53. Ambrose JA, Almeida OD, Sharma SK, et al: Adjunctive thrombolytic therapy during angioplasty for ischemic rest angina, results of the TAUSA trial. *Circulation* 90:69, 1994.

54. Kerins DM, Roy L, Fitzgerald GA, Fitzgerald DJ: Platelet and vascular function during coronary thrombolysis with tissue-type plasminogen activator. *Circulation* 80:1718, 1989.
55. Bennet WR, Yawn DH, Migliori PJ, et al: Activation of the complement system by recombinant tissue plasminogen activator. *J Am Coll Cardiol* 76(Suppl):IV-153, 1987.
56. Fitzgerald DJ, Roy L, Wright F, Fitzgerald GA: Functional significance of platelet activation following coronary thrombolysis. *Circulation* 76(Suppl): IV-153, 1987.
57. Goudreal E, DiSciascio G, Vetrovec GW, et al: The role of intracoronary urokinase in combination with coronary angioplasty in patients with complex lesion morphology. *J Am Coll Cardiol* 15(Suppl):154A, 1990.
58. Cohen BM, Buchbinder M, Koziina J, et al: Rethrombosis during angioplasty in myocardial infarction and unstable syndromes: Efficacy of intracoronary urokinase and redilatation. *Circulation* 78(Suppl II):II-8, 1988.
59. Schieman G, Cohen BM, Kozina J, et al: Intracoronary urokinase for intracoronary thrombus accumulation complicating percutaneous transluminal coronary angioplasty in acute ischemic syndromes. *Circulation* 82:2052, 1990.
60. Schwartz L, Bourassa MG, Lesperance J, et al: Aspirin and dipyridamole in the prevention of restenosis after percutaneous transluminal coronary angioplasty. *N Engl J Med* 318:1714, 1988.
61. White CW, Chaitman B, Lassar TA, et al: Antiplatelet agents are effective in reducing the immediate complications of PTCA. Results of the ticlopidine multicenter trial (abstr). *Circulation* 76(Suppl):IV-400, 1987.
62. Barnathan ES, Schwartz JS, Taylor L, et al: Aspirin and dipyridamole in the prevention of acute coronary thrombosis complicating coronary angioplasty. *Circulation* 76:125, 1987.
63. Mufson L, Black A, Roubin G, et al: A randomized trial of aspirin in PTCA: Effect of high versus low dose aspirin on major complications and restenosis (abstr). *J Am Coll Cardiol* 11(Suppl):236A, 1988.
64. Lembo NJ, Black AJR, Roubin GS, et al: Effect of pretreatment with aspirin versus aspirin plus dipyridamole on frequency and type of acute complications of percutaneous transluminal coronary angioplasty. *Am J Cardiol* 65:422, 1990.
65. Taylor RR, Gibbons FA, Cope GD, et al: Effects of low-dose aspirin on restenosis after coronary angioplasty. *Am J Cardiol* 68:874, 1991.
66. Darius H, Sellig S, Belz GG, Darius BN: Aspirin 500 mg/dl is superior to 100 mg and 40 mg for prevention on restenosis following PTCA (abstr). *Circulation* 90(Suppl):I-651, 1994.
67. Bussman W-D, Kaltenbach M, Kober G, Vallbracht C: The Frankfurt experience in restenosis after coronary angioplasty. *Am J Cardiol* 60(Suppl):48B, 1987.

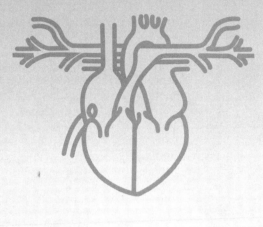

SECTION II

The
Devices

Percutaneous Transluminal Coronary Angioplasty

RAN KORNOWSKI, MD, KATIE KEHOE, RN, BSN, MS, AND MUN K. HONG, MD

❤ Historical Development

The concept of percutaneous transluminal angioplasty or mechanical alteration of the atherosclerotic plaque to increase the lumen diameter by a nonsurgical approach was first introduced by Drs. Dotter and Judkins in 1964.[1] They passed a series of stiff catheters through the atherosclerotic plaque in the iliofemoral artery from percutaneous arterial access and showed improvement in the lumen caliber. Although this initial "Dottering" technique was successful in increasing the blood flow, it was not adopted by others owing to the bleeding complications at the entry site.

A decade later, Dr. Andreas Gruentzig in Zurich, Switzerland, improved the technique by attaching a small balloon at the end of a catheter. The balloon remained deflated until positioned at the site of atherosclerotic narrowing, where it was then inflated to increase the lumen. This system reduced the overall bulkiness of the angioplasty equipment and bleeding complications at the arterial access site. This miniaturization also enabled the catheter to be inserted into the smaller coronary arteries.

Dr. Gruentzig initially tested the system in canine coronary arteries[2] and subsequently in human cadaveric vessels.[3] In 1977, he performed the first clinical case of percutaneous transluminal coronary angioplasty (PTCA) with balloons to reduce atherosclerotic narrowing without the need for bypass surgery.[4]

Since then, there has been an exponential increase in the number of PTCAs performed (estimated to be more than 500,000 annually in the Unites States), resulting from improved operator skills and the PTCA equipment. Although PTCA has performed well in most lesions, it was found to be associated with reduced procedural success and increased procedural complications in certain lesion subsets,[5] such as highly calcified, tortuous, completely occluded, or thrombus-containing lesions and degenerated saphenous vein grafts.

To overcome these limitations, new angioplasty devices have been developed to improve the procedural success and reduce the complications. These have included atherectomy catheters that actually remove the atherosclerotic plaque material, such as the directional coronary atherectomy; rotational atherectomy and transluminal extraction catheter; laser catheter to ablate the plaque material; and metallic stents to scaffold the vessel.[6]

♥ Procedure

The PTCA procedure requires high-resolution fluoroscopic equipment for angiographic visualization of the coronary arteries. The three main equipment components are a large (2 to 3 mm) lumen-guiding catheter, a flexible guidewire, and the balloon catheter itself (Fig. 6-1).[7] Vascular access is obtained using the femoral approach in most cases, although other access sites such as the brachial or radial arteries can be used. The

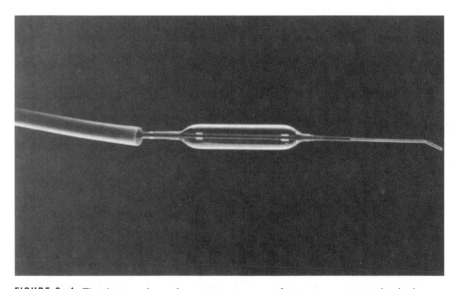

FIGURE 6–1 The three main equipment components of percutaneous transluminal coronary angioplasty: the guiding catheter (left), a flexible guidewire (right), and the balloon catheter (middle). (Figure courtesy of Cordis Corporation.)

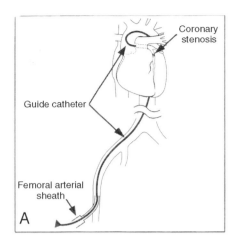
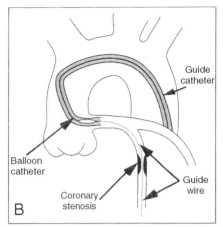
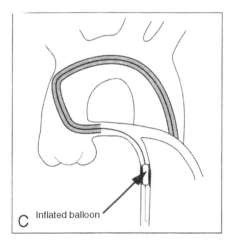
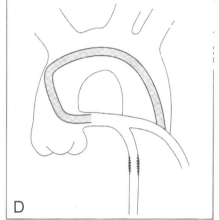

FIGURE 6–2 Procedure used in percutaneous transluminal coronary angioplasty. **(A)** The guide catheter is introduced through a femoral arterial sheath and advanced to the ostium of the diseased coronary artery. **(B)** The guidewire is advanced through the central lumen of the balloon catheter into the diseased artery and across the stenosis. **(C)** The balloon is slid forward over the guidewire, positioned adjacent to the stenosis, and inflated. **(D)** After one or more inflations, the guidewire and balloon catheter are removed, and a final angiogram is obtained. (From Landau C, Lange RA, Hillis LD: Medical progress: Percutaneous transluminal coronary angioplasty. *N Engl J Med* 330:981, 1994. Copyright 1994 Massachusetts Medical Society. All rights reserved.)

guiding catheter is advanced over a guidewire through the sheath into the ostium of the coronary artery to be treated (Fig. 6-2). Angiography of the diseased artery is performed to identify the lesion site. Then, the flexible guidewire is carefully maneuvered across the stenotic site and positioned distally. The deflated balloon catheter is then advanced over the guidewire. Once the positions of the guiding catheter (engaged in the ostium), the guidewire (far distal to the lesion), and the balloon (at the stenosis site) have been confirmed fluoroscopically, the balloon is inflated for 1 to 2 minutes at 4 to 8 atmospheres. The balloon is filled with a mixture of saline and radiocontrast so as to be visible fluoroscopically.

After the balloon is deflated and removed from the treatment site, the result is confirmed by injecting contrast material through the guiding catheter. If the angiographic result is suboptimal (the presence of more than 30% residual lumen stenosis or medial dissections), additional inflation is performed with the same or a bigger balloon. Inflation pressures may vary according to on-line fluoroscopic assessment of the lesion response (higher pressures are usually needed for calcified lesions).

During balloon inflation, which results in transient occlusion of coronary blood flow, continuous monitoring of the electrocardiographic and hemodynamic status of the patients is essential. Anginal symptoms are often provoked during the balloon inflation; however, they usually resolve spontaneously after balloon deflation.

When adequate angiographic results are achieved, the balloon and guidewire are withdrawn from the artery, and a final angiogram is obtained. Angiographic results are considered to be excellent if residual stenosis is less than 30% at the PTCA site (compared with the adjacent normal reference segment), if the radiocontrast contour is relatively smooth and without haziness, filling defects, or dissection planes, and if the distal flow is brisk (Fig. 6-3).

If angiographic results are not optimal, or if abrupt or threatened closure or extensive dissection complicates the procedure, the angioplasty procedure should be complemented by intracoronary stent implantation to improve the PTCA results and to prevent acute procedural-related ischemic complications.[8,9]

Periprocedural antithrombotic medications include aspirin (325 mg/day) and heparin (100 to 150 units/kg initial bolus with additional boluses adjusted to maintain the activated clotting time (ACT) at around 300 sec) to prevent platelet deposition and thrombin-mediated fibrin formation at the PTCA site.[10] In addition, the use of a platelet glycoprotein IIb/IIIa receptor blocker, has been shown to prevent periprocedural ischemic complications.[11,12]

Heparin administration is often terminated after the procedure, but may be continued for up to an additional 12 to 24 hours if the procedure has been complicated by dissection or thrombosis, or if the patient has been clinically unstable.

The arterial sheath is removed when the anticoagulant effect of heparin is resolving, as manifested by an ACT level of less than 150 sec-

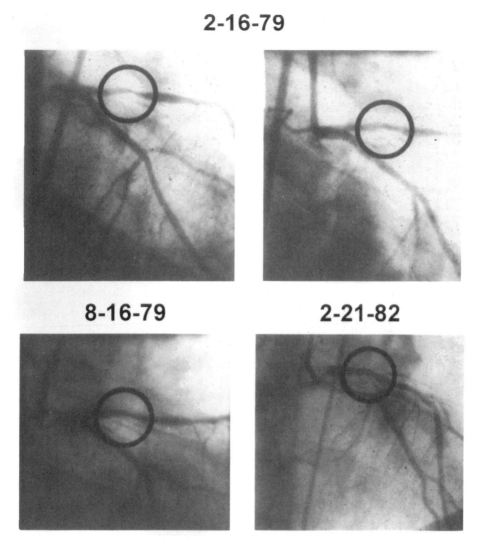

FIGURE 6–3 Angiogram before **(top left)** and immediately after **(top right)** percutaneous transluminal coronary angioplasty of the proximal left anterior descending artery. This was the first coronary angioplasty performed by Dr. Kenneth Kent. The artery remained patent at 6 months **(lower left)** and 3 years **(lower right)**. (Figures courtesy of Dr. Kent.)

onds. Manual pressure or device-based compression or both of the puncture site is essential to achieve adequate hemostasis. Discharge after a successful procedure varies according to the clinical scenario before, during, and after the PTCA, ranging from discharge the next day to a few days of hospitalization in unstable patients.

DISPLAY 6-1 Indications and Contraindications for PTCA

Indications

- Angina refractory to medical therapy
- Recurrent ischemic episodes after myocardial infarction or major ventricular arrhythmia
- Clear evidence of myocardial ischemia on resting ambulatory or exercise electrocardiography
- Objective evidence of myocardial ischemia, which increases the overall risk for noncardiac surgery
- Acute myocardial infarction, with obstructed or severely stenosed infarct-related coronary artery

Absolute or Relative Contraindications

- High-risk anatomy, including significant "unprotected" left main disease and sole remaining circulation to the myocardium, which would most likely cause hemodynamic compromise with vessel closure.
- Severe, diffuse, extensive coronary artery disease better treated surgically
- Target lesion morphology with very low anticipated success rate, unless PTCA is the only reasonable treatment option
- No coronary stenosis greater than 50% diameter reduction
- No objective clinical evidence of myocardial ischemia
- Absence of on-site surgical backup, qualified PTCA operators, or adequate radiographic imaging equipment

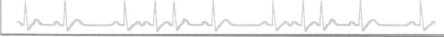

♥ Indications and Contraindications

The indications for PTCA have evolved over the years. Initially, mostly because of the limitations of the angioplasty equipment, PTCA was limited to proximal lesions in rather straight segments and usually in single-vessel coronary artery disease. Unlike coronary artery bypass surgery (CABG), which has been compared with medical therapy to identify a patient population who would benefit more from CABG,[13] PTCA has been applied empirically to treat any flow-limiting coronary artery lesions. There has been only one randomized study comparing PTCA to medical therapy in stable patients with single-vessel coronary artery disease, documenting the beneficial effect of PTCA in symptom improvement and increased exercise capacity compared with medical therapy.[14]

Because of continuing increase in operator experience and improved angioplasty equipment, the indications for angioplasty have recently broadened dramatically. Currently accepted indications for PTCA are based on angiographic findings of significant stenosis in one or more major epicardial arteries, which perfuse at least a moderate-sized area of viable myocardium, in select patients (Display 6-1).[15,16]

♥ Mechanism of Arterial Dilatation by PTCA

PTCA increases the size of the arterial lumen by barotrauma, with endothelial denudation, cracking, splitting, and disruption of the atherosclerotic plaque.[17] Dehiscence of the intima and plaque from the underlying media and stretching or tearing of the media and adventitia were noted in animal, human, and necropsy studies.[18,19] The presence of intimal flap dissections has been observed in 50% to 80% of successfully treated patients using intracoronary ultrasound imaging.[20,21] These morphologic alterations open up the coronary artery for blood flow, leading to increased lumen size and improvement in coronary flow reserve.

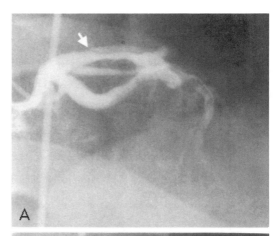

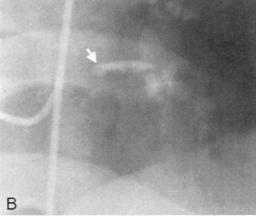

FIGURE 6–4 **(A)** Splitting and disruption of the atherosclerotic plaque occurring several hours after percutaneous transluminal coronary angioplasty with extensive dissection (*arrow*), resulting in abrupt closure of the left anterior descending artery. **(B)** Retention and extravasation of contrast occurred at the site of dissection.

(continued)

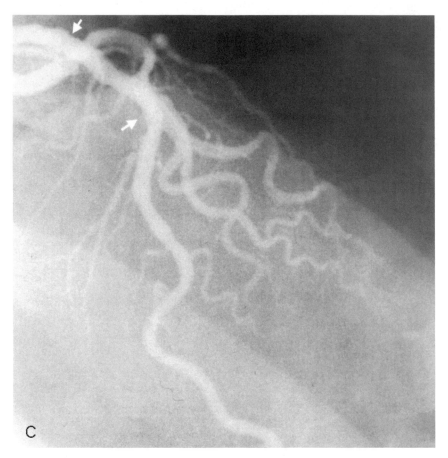

FIGURE 6-4 CONTINUED (C) Emergency (bailout) stenting was performed, resulting in a widely patent artery with restoration of flow.

Oversized or uncontrolled balloon dilatation may be deleterious, causing extensive dissection, plaque hemorrhage, and thrombus formation, with ensuing abrupt closure of the artery at the treatment site. The periprocedural use of heparin and aspirin may reduce these complications.

The acute traumatic effect of PTCA is eventually replaced by arterial healing response with reendothelization, resulting in chronic arterial dilatation (arterial remodeling) with sustained lumen patency. Nevertheless, in about 30% to 50% of treated patients, renarrowing of the PTCA site occurs, usually in the first 6 months after the procedure owing to the combined effects of arterial shrinkage ("negative" remodeling) and proliferation of neointimal tissue at the original treatment site.[22]

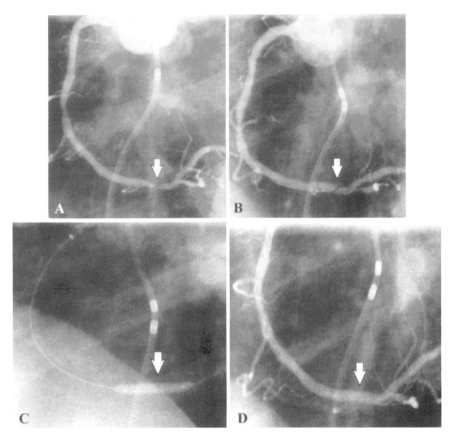

FIGURE 6–5 Distal right coronary lesion **(A)** treated with percutaneous transluminal coronary angioplasty, resulting in extensive dissection of the artery **(B)**. The dissection was treated by stenting **(C)**, resulting in an excellent angiographic result **(D)**.

♥ Limitations

Angioplasty has had three major limitations. The first consists of procedural complications, especially vessel dissections and abrupt closure. The second is restenosis, occurring usually within the first 6 months after a successful angioplasty procedure. The third is failed PTCA procedure in certain complex lesion subsets, such as very long, diffuse lesions and chronic total occlusions.

ACUTE PROCEDURAL COMPLICATIONS

Acute procedural complications, such as abrupt closure of the coronary artery after PTCA, are associated with increased morbidity and mortality (Fig. 6-4). Overall, the risk of periprocedural myocardial infarction (MI)

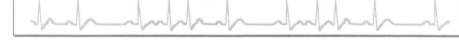

DISPLAY 6–2   Risk Factors for Abrupt Vessel Closure After PTCA

- Female gender
- Unstable angina
- Multivessel coronary artery disease
- Angiographic morphology of intracoronary thrombosis prior to intervention
- Diffuse (>10 mm), eccentric, calcified, bend or branched lesion morphology
- Procedural extensive dissection
- Use of oversized balloons for inflation

during PTCA is 3% to 5%; the risk of death is about 1%.[23,24] Extensive coronary dissection or coronary thrombosis or both have been often associated with such deleterious events.[25,26]

Other acute complications of PTCA include coronary perforation, vessel rupture, and distal embolization with slow or no flow phenomenon (usually found in saphenous vein graft interventions). Abrupt vessel closure occurs in 2% to 8% of patients undergoing PTCA, usually within minutes after the coronary intervention while the patient is still in the catheterization laboratory. In about 25% of patients, however, abrupt vessel closure is delayed up to 24 hours after the procedure.

The mechanisms of abrupt PTCA-induced vessel closure include extensive dissection, coronary thrombosis, and coronary vasospasm. The recognition of extensive dissection is crucial, because it is associated with major ischemic complications if untreated (Fig. 6-5). Thrombus formation is most likely to occur in patients with extensive dissection, owing to exposure of thrombogenic arterial wall elements to obstructed blood at the dissection site.

Several risk factors for abrupt vessel closure have been identified (Display 6-2).[27,28] The best treatment for abrupt arterial closure is immediate coronary stenting, which was shown to be effective in restoring antegrade coronary flow and reducing the need for emergent bypass surgery.[8,29]

A new pharmacologic strategy for preventing abrupt closure after PTCA has been the use of the potent platelet glycoprotein IIb/IIIa receptor antagonist, abciximab (ReoPro), which blocks the aggregation of platelets. In two large randomized trials (Evaluation of 7E3 for the Prevention of Ischemic Complications [EPIC] trial, and Evaluation in PTCA to Improve Long-Term Outcome with Abciximab GPIIb/IIIa Blockade

[EPILOG] trials), the use of abciximab caused a significant (35% to 56%) reduction in ischemic complications at 1 month after PTCA.[11,12] However, increased bleeding complications were observed in the EPIC trial, but not in EPILOG (14% compared with 2% to 3.5%) owing to reduced concomitant heparin administration in the EPILOG trial.

CORONARY RESTENOSIS

Restenosis after successful coronary angioplasty, usually within the first 6 months, continues to be the major limitation of this procedure and a therapeutic challenge. Recent randomized studies still show 32% to 57% angiographic restenosis rates after PTCA.[30]

There have been numerous randomized studies with various classes of pharmacologic agents in an effort to reduce the rate of restenosis.[31] Most of these studies intended to reduce neointimal hyperplasia, but failed to reduce restenosis. Likewise, randomized studies with new angioplasty devices, such as directional coronary atherectomy (DCA), showed no reduction in restenosis.[32,33] However, the Stent Restenosis Study (STRESS)[34] and the Belgium-Netherlands Stent Study (BENESTENT)[35] documented the efficacy of the Palmaz-Schatz tubular slotted stents in reducing restenosis compared with that which occurred with PTCA in focal lesions located in native coronary arteries.

Recent clinical studies, and especially serial intravascular ultrasound (IVUS) observations suggest possible explanations for the efficacy of stents and lack of effect with other angioplasty devices and pharmacologic agents aimed primarily to blunt cellular proliferation.[22] These studies suggest that the predominant mechanism of restenosis after non–stent PTCA procedures is chronic negative geometric remodeling of the treatment site. This results in constriction of the vessel wall rather than excessive neointimal hyperplasia causing lumen compromise.

DISPLAY 6-3   Predictors of Procedural Failure in Chronic Total Occlusions

- Older occlusions (75% <3 months old versus 35% ≥2 months old)
- Absence of any antegrade flow through the occlusion (76% with versus 58% without)
- Angiographically abrupt-appearing occlusion (50% versus 77% with tapered occlusion)
- Presence of bridging collateral vessels (23% with versus 71% without)
- Lesion > 15 mm in length

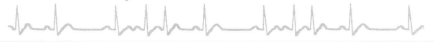

Multiple nonrandomized series of repeat PTCA for treating restenotic lesions after the original PTCA have found the second PTCA to be safer with higher procedural success.[36–38] The successful second PTCA seems to produce similar restenosis rate as the first PTCA. Several different groups have evaluated the safety and efficacy of a third PTCA for treatment of a second restenosis. Although the procedure can be performed safely with a high probability of acute success, the restenosis rate appears to be markedly higher (40% to 50%), especially if the interval between the second and third PTCAs is less than 3 months.[39–41] For these patients, more definitive therapy, such as implantation of coronary stents, is warranted.[42] A randomized study (REST) compared the Palmaz-Schatz stent with PTCA in native restenotic lesions and found a markedly reduced second restenosis rate (11.7% compared with 37%) in the stent group.[43]

A pharmacologic approach to prevent restenosis might be the use of abciximab. Although results of the EPIC trial have shown a reduced need for repeat target lesion revascularization in patients with unstable angina treated by PTCA, more recent data from the EPILOG trial failed to duplicate such findings despite a significant reduction in procedure-related ischemic complications in both trials.[12,44]

A recently published randomized controlled trial of intracoronary radiation combined with stent implantation in 55 high-risk patients with restenosis, using a hand delivery ^{192}Ir gamma source ribbon, showed a dramatic reduction in restenosis among patients treated with radiation compared with that of controls (54% versus 17%; $P = .01$).[45] The continued long-term benefit versus the potential risk of the intracoronary radiation strategy requires further clinical studies with longer follow-up.

COMPLEX CORONARY INTERVENTIONS

The treatment of diffuse coronary lesions has been identified as a factor adversely influencing both acute and long-term success rates in most reported PTCA and new angioplasty devices studies. Experiences with the treatment of diffuse lesions were associated with increased risk for acute complications (~5% to 10%) and late restenosis (~50%) in most of these studies.[46–48] Likewise, the treatment of chronic total occlusion (CTO) remains a major challenge for PTCA, with relatively low procedural success rate and high incidence of restenosis and late reocclusion.[49–51] Successful recanalization is achieved in approximately 65% of attempted procedures. Inability to cross the stenosis with a guidewire is the most common cause of procedural failure but there are several other recognized predictors of procedural failure (Display 6-3).[49] Long-term success is also limited, and restenosis is expected in more than 50% of the patients.[50,51] A recent randomized trial has shown that stent implantation for CTO can significantly reduce the occurrence of clinical and angiographic restenosis and reocclusion after successful recanalization.[52] Thus, stent implantation has become a common clinical practice in most catheterization laboratories after CTO recanalization.

❤ PTCA for Unstable Angina

Unstable angina is one of the most common indications for PTCA. Among patients with unstable angina who are treated medically, the mortality rate is between 1% and 5%; 2% to 10% sustain MI during the hospitalization course.[53-55] Aggressive anticoagulation and antithrombotic medical therapy has been used successfully in patients with unstable angina.[53-55] Nevertheless, many patients remain refractory to medical therapy and need revascularization.

The TIMI IIIB study evaluated the benefit of PTCA for patients with unstable angina or non–Q-wave MI. An "up-front" interventional strategy with early cardiac catheterization and PTCA was compared with a conservative strategy of medical therapy and cardiac catheterization for patients with rest angina or objective evidences of ischemia.[56] The invasive approach has been associated with a similar rate of mortality (4.1% versus 4.4%) and MI (9.3% versus 8.3%) during hospitalization. Postdischarge procedures and hospitalizations were required more frequently in the group assigned to the conservative strategy.[56] Overall major complications did not differ between patients assigned to the two groups. According to this study, it appears that PTCA in appropriately selected patients with unstable angina provides more rapid and sustained relief of symptoms without increasing the risk of major complications compared with medical therapy.

❤ PTCA Compared With Medical Therapy

Although PTCA has been widely used for the treatment of coronary artery disease, relatively few studies have prospectively evaluated its efficacy compared with anti-ischemic drugs. A 6-month comparison between the effect of PTCA and that of medical therapy on angina and exercise tolerance in patients with stable single-vessel coronary artery disease showed that PTCA offered an earlier and more complete relief of angina than medical therapy (64% versus 46%) and was more often associated with

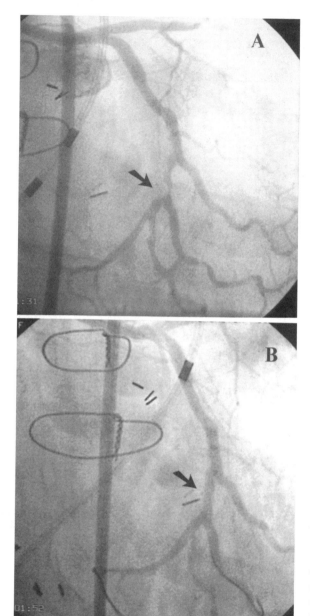

FIGURE 6–6 A representative angiogram before (**A**) and immediately after (**B**) rotational atherectomy followed by percutaneous transluminal coronary angioplasty in a 76-year-old woman with unstable angina and previous coronary artery bypass angioplasty and a critical complex stenosis of the distal left circumflex coronary artery between two marginal branches (*arrows*). The lesion was pretreated with rotational atherectomy because of calcified morphology and successfully further dilated by balloon (**B**; *straight arrow*), yielding an excellent angiographic result.

increased exercise performance.[14] In patients with ischemia during stress testing and ambulatory electrocardiographic monitoring, a therapeutic strategy of initial revascularization (PTCA or bypass surgery) was found to improve the prognosis (death, MI, or recurrent cardiac hospitalization) compared with angina-guided drug therapy (42% versus 23% event rate at 2 years).[57] According to these studies, it appears that PTCA is more effective than medical therapy alone for symptomatic improvement in appropriately selected patients with coronary artery disease.

♥ PTCA Compared With Coronary Artery Bypass Surgery

Patients with severe coronary artery disease are often eligible for either PTCA or CABG. Results from eight published randomized trials have shown no difference in prognosis comparing PTCA with CABG.[58] The combined end point of cardiac death and nonfatal MI was similar for PTCA and CABG at 1 year of follow-up. However, the treatments differ markedly in the subsequent requirement for additional revascularization procedures and in the relief of angina in favor of CABG. This is due to restenosis, with 34% need for additional reinterventions in the PTCA group compared with 2% in the surgical arm at 1-year follow-up. These results were obtained before stents were in use. Thus, both PTCA and CABG are very effective therapies for relieving angina. Patients with left main coronary artery stenosis or multiple severe stenoses, especially if associated with impaired left ventricular function or the need for valve repair or aneurysm resection, would benefit most from surgery.[59] Also, according to the Bypass Angioplasty Revascularization Investigation (BARI) trial, diabetic patients with multivessel coronary disease had better survival with CABG at 5-years compared with PTCA (81% versus

---

DISPLAY 6–4 Potential Advantages of Immediate PTCA in the Treatment of Acute Myocardial Infarction

- Immediate assessment of perfusion status before and immediately after coronary intervention
- Rapid and predictable restoration of coronary flow
- Applicability to most infarction patients, including those ineligible for thrombolytic therapy
- Prevention of intracerebral hemorrhage from thrombolytic therapy
- Ability to assess the full extent of coronary artery disease in the infarct-related artery and other coronary vessels

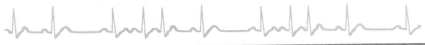

65%). Thus, diabetic patients might be better candidates for surgical revascularization strategy.[60] For other patients, PTCA is a viable strategy with favorable acute and long-term procedural success.

♥ New Device Angioplasty

Percutaneous atheroablative devices were designed to overcome some of the limitations of PTCA and to improve the acute and long-term results obtained by conventional PTCA alone. During DCA, plaque material is removed from the coronary artery with a cutting blade spinning at the tip of the atherectomy device.[61] Although using DCA has been associated with the achievement of greater initial lumen gain, in-hospital creatine kinase-MB release was found to be significantly higher after DCA (38% versus 19%), as well as one-year mortality (2.2% versus 0.8%) compared to PTCA.[62,63] The restenosis rate was similar for both DCA and PTCA groups.

Rotational atherectomy (RA) is another approach for removing atheromatous plaque from the coronary arteries. This technique uses a diamond-studded burr spinning at about 180,000 rpm to pulverize calcified or fibrotic plaque and allow microscopic debris to embolize to the coronary capillary bed and be cleared from the microcirculation.[64] RA appears to be safe and efficacious in several lesion subsets in which PTCA has proved suboptimal, such as moderately or severely calcified lesions, ostial lesions, undilatable lesions, restenotic lesions, and possibly chronic total occlusions that can be crossed with a guidewire (Fig. 6-6).[65,66]

The excimer-laser coronary angioplasty (ELCA) uses a light emitted from optical fibers through a catheter tip to vaporize atheromatous tissue.[67] In a randomized trial, comparing ELCA followed by PTCA to PTCA alone, no acute or long-term benefit was found to adjunctive ELCA therapy in the treatment of coronary artery disease.[68] The angiographic restenosis rate was high and similar in both groups (51% for ELCA and PTCA compared with 41% for PTCA alone).

A randomized comparison of PTCA and ELCA with PTCA or RA and PTCA in the treatment of complex coronary lesions has found a higher procedural success with RA compared with that in PTCA and ELCA (89% versus 80% and 77%, respectively) with similar major in-hospital complications. Clinical restenosis was high for all groups and did not differ significantly between the PTCA (32%), ELCA (46%), and RA (42%) groups.[66] According to the results of this study and others, the beneficial role of plaque debulking before balloon dilatation in PTCA or stent implantation remains to be established.

♥ PTCA in Acute Myocardial Infarction

In recent years, there has been a great interest in performing immediate cardiac catheterization and PTCA in patients with acute MI. Immediate PTCA offers several potential advantages over traditional treatment (Display 6-4).

Early nonrandomized studies of direct infarct PTCA reported high recanalization rate (>90%), low in-hospital mortality (~8%), and high 1-year survival rate (>90%).[69] These data created the background for randomized studies, comparing the strategy of direct (or "primary") infarct PTCA with the administration of thrombolytic therapy.[70–73] A trend for reduced in-hospital mortality was found in two of these studies (~2% versus ~6%), but not in others.[70–73] One study found global ejection fraction to be significantly higher in patients treated by PTCA compared with thrombolytic therapy (51% versus 45%).[70] The ability to restore brisk flow could be achieved in over 90% of patients, which has been translated into fewer recurrent ischemic episodes after the coronary event. Based on these studies, it is concluded that direct infarct PTCA is a safe and effective alternative to thrombolytic therapy for the treatment of acute MI.

It has yet to be established whether the excellent results obtained by the small trials of direct PTCA for acute MI could be reproduced in the community hospitals.[74] Also, rapid availability of the catheterization laboratory and an experienced interventional team are crucial to the success of such invasive strategy for acute MI patients.

In patients sustaining acute MI and cardiogenic shock (systolic blood pressure <90 mm Hg due to overt left ventricular failure), who received thrombolytic therapy, an aggressive strategy of early (within 24 hours from shock onset) angiography and revascularization (either PTCA or emergent CABG) might have a major beneficial impact on mortality reduction (38% compared with 62%).[75]

♥ PTCA in Saphenous Vein Grafts

Several studies have shown that approximately 50% of saphenous vein grafts (SVGs) will be occluded between 5 and 10 years after CABG.[76,77] Because repeat CABG is associated with higher rates of morbidity and mortality as well as lesser symptom improvement compared with the original surgery, PTCA has been used as an alternative to repeat CABG in selected patients with recurrent ischemia resulting from SVG disease.[78,79]

A recent review of 16 contemporary PTCA series in SVGs reported an overall procedural success rate in 88% of patients.[78] Ischemic complications were infrequent and included death (<1%), MI (4%), CABG (2%), and distal embolization (<3%). Overall procedure success was slightly lower in lesions involving the proximal (86%) compared with mid (93%) and distal (90%) segments. Proximal lesions also tended to have higher rates of angiographic restenosis (58% versus 52% and 28% for mid and distal segments, respectively).

Several variables have been associated with an increased risk of complications after PTCA of SVG lesions, principally because of increased lesion friability and propensity to distal embolization. These variables include older SVGs (>36 months), diffusely diseased SVGs, totally occluded grafts, and grafts containing intraluminal thrombus.[79-81] Therefore, PTCA has a limited role for these complex SVG lesions, although it remains the treatment of choice for distal anastomotic lesions.

As a result of these limitations, new angioplasty devices have been used in patients with symptomatic SVG disease for three general indications: (a) to improve the initial angiographic result compared with PTCA alone (e.g., DCA and stenting for aorto-ostial lesions); (b) to reduce procedural complications associated with PTCA of friable and diffusely diseased SVG lesions (e.g., transluminal extraction atherectomy for degenerated grafts); and (c) to reduce restenosis after a successful procedure (e.g., intragraft stents for ostial and body lesions).[82] Lately, intragraft stenting has replaced all other modalities in SVGs larger than 3.0 mm, using 3.0- to 4.0-mm native coronary and 4.0- to 6.0-mm biliary tubular slotted stents. These larger stents have been used without significant inflow or outflow obstruction or intragraft thrombus.[83,84]

❤ Optimal PTCA in the Stent Era

The use of coronary stents has revolutionized the field of percutaneous coronary interventions. Previously acceptable PTCA results are no longer considered optimal, and, as a result, stent implantation to improve angiographic results and to prevent restenosis has increased enormously in the last years. With increased use of stents as the primary angioplasty strategy, there are a substantial number of patients with stent-related complications, such as stent thrombosis and in-stent restenosis. Although the rate of restenosis within stents is lower compared with PTCA, the in-stent restenosis rate is still high in certain lesion subsets, such as diffuse lesions or small vessels. Thus, to avoid stent implantation, a new PTCA strategy has evolved, indicating that optimal PTCA may yield stent-like clinical outcomes.[85] Such strategy incorporating intravascular ultrasound (IVUS) guidance for balloon sizing combined with high-pressure balloon inflation to achieve greater acute lumen gain might be found effective in reducing restenosis compared with more conservative PTCA technique. Such IVUS-guided PTCA strategy has been recently shown to allow the safe use of balloons traditionally considered oversized, resulting in significantly improved luminal dimensions without increased rates of dissections or ischemic complications.[86]

♥ Conclusions

PTCA has evolved dramatically since its introduction 20 years ago and has firmly established itself as a viable, nonsurgical revascularization procedure in patients refractory to medical therapy. Its indications have been expanded to include patients with previously unapproachable lesions, acute MI, and multivessel coronary artery disease. With the complementary armamentarium of new angioplasty devices and potent pharmacologic adjunct therapy, PTCA will continue to provide benefit to patients with coronary artery disease.

REFERENCES

1. Dotter CT, Judkins MP: Transluminal treatment of arteriosclerotic obstruction: Description of a new technique and preliminary report of its application. *Circulation* 30:654–670, 1964.
2. Gruentzig AR: Perkutane dilatation von coronarstenosen-beschreibung eines neuen kathetersystems. *Klin Wochenschr* 54:543–546, 1976.
3. Gruentzig AR, Turina MI, Schneider JA: Experimental percutaneous dilatation of coronary artery stenosis. *Circulation* 54:81–86, 1976.
4. Gruentzig AR: Transluminal dilatation of coronary artery stenosis (Letter). *Lancet* 1:263, 1978.
5. Ryan TJ, Members of the Subcommittee on Percutaneous Transluminal Coronary Angioplasty: Guidelines for percutaneous transluminal coronary angioplasty: A report of the American College of Cardiology/American Heart Association task force on assessment of diagnostic and therapeutic cardiovascular procedures. *J Am Coll Cardiol* 12:529–545, 1988.
6. Bittl JA: Advances in coronary angioplasty. *N Engl J Med* 335:1290–1302, 1996.
7. Landau C, Lange RA, Hillis LD: Percutaneous transluminal coronary angioplasty. *N Engl J Med* 330:981–993. 1994.
8. Dean LS, George CJ, Roubin GS, et al: Bailout and corrective use of Gianturco-Roubin Flex Stent after percutaneous transluminal coronary angioplasty. *J Am Coll Cardiol* 29:934–940, 1997.
9. ACC expert consensus document. Coronary artery stents. *J Am Coll Cardiol* 28:782–794, 1996.
10. Popma JJ, Coller BS, Ohman EM, et al: Antithrombotic therapy in patients undergoing coronary angioplasty. *Chest* 108:486S–501S, 1995.

11. The EPIC Investigators: Use of monoclonal antibody directed against the platelet glycoprotein IIb/IIIa receptor in high-risk coronary angioplasty. The EPIC investigation. *N Engl J Med* 330:956–961, 1994.

12. The EPILOG Investigators: Platelet glycoprotein IIb/IIIa receptor blockade and low-dose heparin during percutaneous coronary revascularization. *N Engl J Med* 336:1689–1696, 1997.

13. CASS Principal Investigators: Coronary artery surgery study (CASS): A randomized trial of coronary artery bypass surgery. Survival data. *Circulation* 68:939–950, 1983.

14. Farisi AF, Folland ED, Hartigan P: A comparison of angioplasty with medical therapy in the treatment of single-vessel coronary artery disease. *N Engl J Med* 326:10–16, 1992.

15. Ryan TJ, Committee on Percutaneous Transluminal Coronary Angioplasty: Guidelines for percutaneous transluminal coronary angioplasty: A report of the ACC/AHA task force. *J Am Coll Cardiol* 22:2033–2054, 1993.

16. Baim DS: Coronary angioplasty. In Baim DS, Grossman W (eds): *Cardiac Catheterization: Angiography, and Intervention,* 5th ed, pp. 537–579. Baltimore, Williams & Wilkins, 1996.

17. Faxon DP, Weber VJ, Haudenschild C, et al: Acute effects of transluminal angioplasty in three experimental models of atherosclerosis. *Arteriosclerosis* 2:125–133, 1982.

18. Steele PM, Chesebro JH, Stanson AW, et al: Balloon angioplasty: Natural history of the pathophysiological response to injury in pig model. *Circ Res* 57:105–112, 1985.

19. Farb A, Virmani R, Atkinson JB, et al: Plaque morphology and pathologic changes in arteries from patients dying after coronary balloon angioplasty. *J Am Coll Cardiol* 16:1421–1429, 1990.

20. Potkin BN, Keren G, Mintz GS, et al: Arterial responses to balloon coronary angioplasty: An intravascular ultrasound study. *J Am Coll Cardiol* 20:942–951, 1992.

21. Tanaglia AN, Buller CE, Kisslo KB, et al: Mechanisms of balloon angioplasty and directional coronary atherectomy as assessed by intravascular ultrasound. *J Am Coll Cardiol* 20;685–691, 1992.

22. Mintz GS, Popma JJ, Pichard AD, et al: Arterial remodeling after coronary angioplasty. A serial intravascular ultrasound study. *Circulation* 94:35–43, 1996.

23. Holmes DR, Holubkov R, Vlietstra RE, et al. Comparison of complications during percutaneous transluminal coronary angioplasty from 1977 to 1981 and from 1985 to 1986: The National Heart, Lung, and Blood Institute Percutaneous Transluminal Coronary Angioplasty Registry. *J Am Coll Cardiol* 12:1149–1155, 1988.

24. Lincoff AM, Popma JJ, Ellis SG, et al: Abrupt arterial closure complicating coronary angioplasty: Clinical, angiographic and therapeutic profile. *J Am Coll Cardiol* 19:926–935, 1992.

25. Tenaglia AN, Fortin DF, Califf RM, et al: Predicting the risk of abrupt arterial closure after angioplasty in an individual patient. *J Am Coll Cardiol* 24:1004–1011, 1994.

26. Sugrue DD, Holmes DR Jr, Smith HC, et al: Coronary artery thrombus as a risk factor for acute vessel occlusion during percutaneous transluminal coronary angioplasty: Improving results. *Br Heart J* 56:62–66, 1986.

27. Laskey MAL, Deutsch E, Barnathan E, et al: Influence of heparin therapy on percutaneous transluminal coronary angioplasty in unstable angina pectoris. *Am J Cardiol* 65:1425–1429, 1990.
28. Lukas MAL, Deutsch E, Hirschfeld JW, et al: Influence of heparin on percutaneous transluminal coronary angioplasty outcome in patients with coronary arterial thrombus. *Am J Cardiol* 65:179–182, 1990.
29. Lincoff AM, Topol EJ, Chapekis AT, et al: Intracoronary stenting compared with conventional therapy for abrupt arterial closure complicating coronary angioplasty: A matched case-control study. *J Am Coll Cardiol* 21:866–875, 1993.
30. Hong MK, Mehran R, Mintz GS, et al: Restenosis after coronary angioplasty. *Curr Probl Cardiol* 22:1–36, 1997.
31. Franklin SM, Faxon DP: Pharmacologic prevention of restenosis after coronary angioplasty: Review of the randomized clinical trials. *Coron Artery Dis* 4:232–242, 1993.
32. Topol EJ, Leya F, Pinkerton CA, et al: A comparison of directional atherectomy with coronary angioplasty in patients with coronary artery disease. *N Engl J Med* 329:221–227, 1993.
33. Adelman AG, Cohen BA, Kimball BP, et al: A comparison of directional atherectomy with balloon angioplasty for lesions of the left anterior descending coronary artery. *N Engl J Med* 329:228–233, 1993.
34. Fischman DL, Leon MB, Baim DS, et al: A randomized comparison of coronary-stent placement and balloon angioplasty in the treatment of coronary artery disease. *N Engl J Med* 331:496–501, 1994.
35. Serruys PW, de Jaegere P, Kiemeneij F, et al: A comparison of balloon-expandable-stent implantation with balloon angioplasty in patients with coronary artery disease. *N Engl J Med* 331:489–495, 1994.
36. Meier B, King SB, Gruentzig AR, et al: Repeat coronary angioplasty. *J Am Coll Cardiol* 4:463–466, 1984.
37. Williams DO, Gruentzig AR, Kent KM, et al: Efficacy of repeat percutaneous transluminal coronary angioplasty for coronary restenosis. *Am J Cardiol* 53:32C–35C, 1984.
38. Dimas AP, Grigera F, Arora RR, et al: Repeat coronary angioplasty as treatment for restenosis. *J Am Coll Cardiol* 19:1310–1314, 1992.
39. Teirstein PS, Hoover CA, Ligon RW, et al: Repeat coronary angioplasty: Efficacy of a third angioplasty for a second restenosis. *J Am Coll Cardiol* 13:291–296, 1989.
40. Bauters C, McFadden EP, Lablanche JM, et al: Restenosis rate after multiple percutaneous transluminal coronary angioplasty procedures at the same site. A quantitative angiographic study in consecutive patients undergoing a third angioplasty procedure for a second restenosis. *Circulation* 88:969–974, 1993.
41. Tan KH, Sulke N, Taub N, et al: Efficacy of a third coronary angioplasty for a second restenosis: short-term results, long-term follow-up, and correlates of a third restenosis. *Br Heart J* 73:327–333, 1995.
42. Colombo A, Ferraro M, Itoh A, et al: Results of coronary stenting for restenosis. *J Am Coll Cardiol* 28:830–836, 1996.
43. Erbel R, Haude M, Hopp HW, et al: Coronary-artery stenting compared with balloon angioplasty for restenosis after initial balloon angioplasty. Restenosis Stent Study Group. *N Engl J Med* 339:1672–1678, 1998.

44. Topol EJ, Califf RM, Weisman HF, et al: Randomised trial of coronary intervention with antibody against platelet IIb/IIIa integrin for reduction of clinical restenosis: Results at six months. The EPIC Investigators. *Lancet* 343:881–886, 1994.
45. Teirstein PS, Massullo V, Jani S, et al: Catheter-based radiotherapy to inhibit restenosis after coronary stenting. *N Engl J Med* 336:1697–1703, 1997.
46. Ellis S, Vandormael M, Cowley M, et al: Coronary morphologic and clinical determinants of procedural outcome with angioplasty for multivessel coronary disease. *Circulation* 82:1193–1202, 1990.
47. Sharma SK, Israel DH, Kamean JL, et al: Clinical, angiographic, and procedural determinants of major and minor coronary dissections during angioplasty. *Am Heart J* 126:39–47, 1993.
48. Bourassa MG, Lesperance J, Eastwood C, et al: Clinical, physiologic, anatomic and procedural factors predictive of restenosis after percutaneous transluminal coronary angioplasty. *J Am Coll Cardiol* 18:368–376, 1991.
49. Puma JA, Sketch MH, Tcheng JE, et al: Percutaneous revascularization of chronic coronary occlusions: An overview. *J Am Coll Cardiol* 26:1–11, 1995.
50. Violaris AG, Melkert R, Serruys PW: Long-term luminal renarrowing after successful elective coronary angioplasty of total occlusions. *Circulation* 91:2140–2150, 1995.
51. Bell MR, Berger PB, Bresnaham JF, et al: Initial and long-term outcome of 354 patients after coronary balloon angioplasty of total coronary occlusions. *Circulation* 85:1003–1011, 1992.
52. Sirnes PA, Golf S, Myreng Y, et al: Stenting in chronic coronary occlusion (SICCO): A randomized, controlled trial of adding stent implantation after successful angioplasty. *J Am Coll Cardiol* 28:1444–1451, 1996.
53. The RISC Group. Risk of myocardial infarction and death during treatment with low dose aspirin and intravenous heparin in men with unstable coronary artery disease. *Lancet* 336:827–830, 1990.
54. Theroux P, Ouimet H, McCans J, et al: Aspirin, heparin, or both to treat acute unstable angina. *N Engl J Med* 319:1105–1111, 1988.
55. Serneri GGN, Modesti PA, Gensini GF, et al: Randomized comparison of subcutaneous heparin, intravenous heparin, and aspirin in unstable angina. *Lancet* 345:1201–1204, 1995.
56. The TIMI IIIB Investigators. Effects of tissue plasminogen activator and comparison of early invasive and conservative strategies in unstable angina and non–Q-wave myocardial infarction: Results of the TIMI IIIB trial. *Circulation* 89:1545–1556, 1994.
57. Davies RF, Goldberg D, Forman S, et al: Asymptomatic cardiac ischemia pilot (ACIP) study two-year follow-up. Outcome of patients randomized to initial strategies of medical therapy versus revascularization. *Circulation* 95:2037–2043, 1997.
58. Pocock SJ, Henderson RA, Rickards A, et al: Meta-analysis of randomized trials comparing coronary angioplasty with bypass surgery. *Lancet* 346:1184–1189, 1995.
59. White HD: Angioplasty versus bypass surgery. *Lancet* 346:1174–1175, 1995.

60. The Bypass Angioplasty Revascularization Investigation (BARI) Investigators: Comparison of coronary bypass surgery with angioplasty in patients with multivessel disease. *N Engl J Med* 335:217–225, 1996.
61. Safian RD, Baim DS, Kuntz RE: Coronary atherectomy. In Baim DS, Grossman W (eds): *Cardiac Catheterization, Angiography, and Intervention*, 5th ed, pp. 581–616. Baltimore, Williams & Wilkins, 1996.
62. Topol EJ, Leya F, Pinkerton CA, et al: A comparison of directional atherectomy with coronary angioplasty in patients with coronary artery disease. *N Engl J Med* 329:221–227, 1993.
63. Adelman AG, Cohen BA, Kimball BP, et al: A comparison of directional atherectomy with balloon angioplasty for lesions of the left anterior descending coronary artery. *N Engl J Med* 329:228–233, 1993.
64. Villa AE, Whitlow PL: Rotational coronary atherectomy. In Topol EJ (ed): *Textbook of Interventional Cardiology (Update 9)*, pp. 1–12. Philadelphia, WB Saunders, 1995.
65. MacIsaac AI, Bass TA, Buchbinder M, et al: High speed rotational atherectomy: Outcome in calcified and noncalcified coronary artery lesions. *J Am Coll Cardiol* 26:731–736, 1995.
66. Reifart N, Vandormael M, Krajcar M, et al: Randomized comparison of angioplasty of complex coronary lesions at a single center. *Circulation* 96:91–98, 1997.
67. Bittl JA: Ablative laser techniques. In Baim DS, Grossman W (eds): *Cardiac Catheterization, Angiography, and Intervention*, 5th ed, pp. 641–658. Baltimore, Williams & Wilkins, 1996.
68. Appelbaum YE, Piek JJ, Strikwerda S, et al: Randomized trial of excimer laser angioplasty versus balloon angioplasty for treatment of obstructive coronary artery disease. *Lancet* 347:79–84, 1996.
69. O'Keefe JH, Bailey L, Rutherford BD, et al: Primary angioplasty for acute myocardial infarction in 1,000 consecutive patients: Results in an unselected population and high-risk group. *Am J Cardiol* 72:107G–115G, 1993.
70. Zijlstra F, Jan de Boer M, Hoorntje JC, et al: A comparison of immediate coronary angioplasty with intravenous streptokinase in acute myocardial infarction. *N Engl J Med* 328:680–684, 1993.
71. Gibbons RJ, Holmes DR, Reeder GS, et al: Randomized trial comparing immediate angioplasty to thrombolysis followed by conservative treatment for myocardial infarction. *N Engl J Med* 328:685–691, 1993.
72. Grines CL, Browne KF, Marco J, et al: A comparison of primary angioplasty with thrombolytic therapy for acute myocardial infarction. *N Engl J Med* 328:673–679, 1993.
73. Ribiero EE, Silva LA, Carneiro R, et al: Randomized trial of direct coronary angioplasty versus intravenous streptokinase in acute myocardial infarction. *J Am Coll Cardiol* 22:376–380, 1993.
74. Every NR, Parsons LS, Hlatky M, et al: A comparison of thrombolytic therapy with primary coronary angioplasty for acute myocardial infarction. *N Engl J Med* 335:1253–1260, 1996.
75. Berger PB, Holmes DR, Stebbins AL, et al: Impact of an aggressive invasive catheterization and revascularization strategy on mortality in patients with cardiogenic shock in the global utilization of streptokinase and tissue plas-

minogen activator for occluded coronary arteries (GUSTO-1) trial. *Circulation* 96:122–127, 1997.

76. Hamby RI, Aintablian A, Handler M, et al: Aortocoronary saphenous vein bypass grafts: Long-term patency, morphology and blood flow in patients with patent grafts early after surgery. *Circulation* 60:901–909, 1979.

77. Seides SF, Borer JS, Kent KM, et al: Long-term anatomic fate of coronary artery bypass grafts and functional status of patients five years after operation. *N Engl J Med* 298:1213–1217, 1978.

78. de Feyter P, VanSuylen R, de Jaegere P, et al: Balloon angioplasty for the treatment of lesions in saphenous vein bypass grafts. *J Am Coll Cardiol* 21:1539–1549, 1993.

79. Ernst S, van der Feltz T, Ascoop C, et al: Percutaneous transluminal coronary angioplasty in patients with prior coronary artery bypass grafting. *J Thorac Cardiovasc Surg* 93:268–275, 1987.

80. Reed D, Beller G, Nygaard T, et al: The clinical efficacy and scintigraphic evaluation of post-coronary bypass patients undergoing percutaneous transluminal coronary angioplasty for recurrent angina pectoris. *Am Heart J* 117:60–71, 1989.

81. Plokker H, Meester B, Serruys P: The Dutch experience in percutaneous transluminal angioplasty of narrowed saphenous vein grafts used for aortocoronary bypass. *Am J Cardiol* 67:361–366, 1991.

82. Hong MK, Leon MB, Kent KM: Treatment for saphenous vein grafts. In Beyar R, Keren G, Leon M, et al (eds): *Frontiers in Interventional Cardiology*, pp. 29–40. London, Martin Dunitz, 1997.

83. Wong SC, Popma JJ, Pichard AD, et al: A comparison of clinical and angiographic outcomes after saphenous vein graft angioplasty using coronary versus biliary tubular slotted stents. *Circulation* 91:339–350, 1995.

84. Wong SC, Baim DS, Schatz RA, et al: Immediate results and late outcomes after stent implantation in saphenous vein graft lesions: The multicenter US Palmaz-Schatz stent experience. *J Am Coll Cardiol* 26:704–712, 1995.

85. Abizaid A, Mehran R, Pichard AD, et al: Results of high pressure ultrasound-guided "over-sized" balloon PTCA to achieve "stent-like" results. *J Am Coll Cardiol* 29:280A, 1997.

86. Stone GW, Hodgson JM, St Goar FG, et al: Improved procedural results of coronary angioplasty with intravascular ultrasound-guided balloon sizing. The CLOUT pilot trial. *Circulation* 95:2044–2052, 1997.

CHAPTER 7

Coronary Stents

ALEXANDRA J. LANSKY, MD, AND MARTIN B. LEON, MD

A dramatic increase in the worldwide use of intracoronary stents for the treatment of coronary artery disease has occurred over the past several years. It is estimated that intracoronary stents may be used in up to 25% to 60% of interventional procedures at some high-volume institutions. Along with the expanded number of patients treated with stents, the number of stent designs available for clinical use has also increased dramatically. The precise comparative advantage of any one stent design over another, however, has yet to be identified in either case-matched registry or randomized clinical trials. Furthermore, despite the immediate mechanical benefit of stent use, many questions still remain about the precise indications for stent implantation, such as in complex lesion subsets or in patients with acute coronary syndromes. The optimal postprocedure management of patients undergoing stent implantation, particularly with respect to the method and duration of anticoagulant therapy that should be given, remains at times controversial. Traditional regimens, which include use of aspirin, dipyridamole, dextran, prolonged intravenous heparin, and warfarin, have been largely replaced with "reduced" anticoagulation regimens. Standardized anticoagulation recommendations are soon needed because stent use has now expanded to patients with acute myocardial infarction and other acute ischemic syndromes.[1,2]

The major complications associated with coronary stenting, which include subacute thrombosis and vascular complications, have largely been reduced with intravascular ultrasound (IVUS)-guided implantation, high-pressure postdeployment dilation techniques, and reduced anticoagulation strategies.

The purposes of this chapter are (a) to summarize the clinical studies that have formed the basis of current stent use and indications; (b) to discuss the various stent designs currently available for worldwide clinical use; (c) to summarize complications associated with the use of stents; and (d) to review the antithrombotic regimens associated with stent use.

♥ Indications for Coronary Stenting

The understanding of the mechanisms of percutaneous transluminal coronary angioplasty (PTCA) has evolved dramatically since its first clinical report in 1979.[3] Early pathologic and ultrasound series showed that balloon arterial dilatation occurred by arterial lumen expansion, resulting from intimal and medial disruption and dissection[4,5] and, to a lesser extent, axial plaque redistribution.[6] New coronary debulking devices were developed to excise, ablate, or extract atherosclerotic plaque (e.g., directional, rotational, and extraction atherectomy, and excimer laser angioplasty, among others), particularly when the arterial or graft segment was calcified, was diffusely diseased, or contained thrombus.[7] These debulking techniques provided an advantage over balloon angioplasty in yielding a large post-treatment lumen diameter, but they did little to prevent acute vascular recoil, accounting for up to 15% to 30% of acute loss, or late arterial remodeling, now thought to account for up to 50% to 80% of late arterial lumen loss after coronary intervention.[8] Stents mechanically scaffold the arterial lumen, effectively eliminating early and late vascular recoil or remodeling,[9] although at the expense of more intimal hyperplasia than occurs after nonstent revascularization.

ELECTIVE STENT USE

The Palmaz-Schatz coronary stent was until recently the only Food and Drug Administration (FDA)–approved stent on the market for elective use in focal de novo coronary lesions to prevent restenosis. Approval was based on three well-designed randomized clinical trials demonstrating that intracoronary stent placement is associated with an improved early and late clinical outcome compared with standard balloon angioplasty in selected patients with symptomatic coronary stenosis.[10–12]

In the STent REStenosis Study (STRESS-I), 410 patients with focal (less than 15 mm), de novo stenoses in vessels between 3 and 5 mm in diameter were randomly assigned to treatment with a Palmaz-Schatz stent or balloon angioplasty.[10] Procedural success was higher in stent-treated patients (96.1% versus 89.6% in balloon-treated patients;

P = .011). The final residual percent diameter stenosis was also lower in stent-treated patients (19% versus 35% in balloon-treated patients; P < .001), resulting in a reduction in angiographic restenosis in stent-treated patients (32% versus 42% in balloon-treated patients; P = .046).

With the addition of 189 patients (STRESS-II) randomized after STRESS-I enrollment had been completed, the STRESS-I plus -II study patients further reaffirmed that stent-treated patients had improved procedural success (89.4% compared with 82.6% in balloon-treated patients; P = .02), reduced 6-month angiographic restenosis (30.4% compared with 45.4%; P = .0001), lowered rates of symptom-driven target lesion revascularization (9.8% compared with 18.2%; P = .003), and resulted in better 12-month event-free survival (80.3% compared with 71.5%; P = .008).[13]

In the Belgium Netherlands Stent (BENESTENT) Study, patients with stable angina and focal (< 15 mm) de novo lesions in native coronary arteries were randomly assigned to Palmaz-Schatz stent placement or balloon angioplasty. Angiographic restenosis (≥ 50% diameter stenosis) occurred less often in stent-treated patients (22% compared with 32% in balloon-treated patients; P = .02). Target lesion revascularization (coronary bypass operation or repeat angioplasty) also occurred less frequently in stent-treated patients (20% compared with 30% in balloon-treated patients; P = 0.02).[11]

In the Trial of Angioplasty and Stents in Canada (TASC-I), elective patients with de novo (n = 148) or restenotic (n = 122) lesions were randomly assigned to Palmaz-Schatz stent placement or balloon angioplasty. In patients with de novo lesions, there was a significant reduction in angiographic restenosis in stent-treated patients (29% compared with 49% in balloon-treated patients; P = .02).[12]

The experience from these three randomized studies, comprising nearly 1400 patients, demonstrates the clinical advantage of elective stent use over balloon angioplasty in selected patients with focal, de novo lesions located in native coronary arteries.

STENTS FOR ABRUPT/THREATENED CLOSURE

The Gianturco-Roubin™ stent (Cook, Bloomington, IN) received final approval in the United States for treatment of patients with acute and threatened closure after coronary intervention in June 1993. An extensive clinical experience has been attained demonstrating the immediate benefit of the Gianturco-Roubin (GR) stent for the management of acute and threatened vessel closure after balloon and new device angioplasty.[14–17]

The GR1 registry, which began in 1988, enrolled 518 patients with abrupt and threatened closure for which GR1 was used as a "bail-out" device. Compared with historical standards from balloon angioplasty, the GR1 stent was associated with reduced procedural mortality (2.2% compared with 2% to 8% with balloons); reduced myocardial infarctions (5.5% compared with 20% to 35% with balloons); and reduced urgent bypass surgery (4.3% compared with 20% to 35% with balloons). These results formed the basis of approval of the GR1 for the treatment of abrupt or threatened closure.

Despite clear advantages of the GR stent over conventional balloon angioplasty for the treatment of acute and threatened closures, it is uncertain whether the GR stent design confers the same long-term benefit and reduction in restenosis after bailout use as the tubular-slotted design. In a matched study of bailout GR and Palmaz-Schatz stent use, binary restenosis rates (diameter stenosis > 50% at follow-up) were higher in patients treated with the GR stent (44% compared with 15% for Palmaz-Schatz–treated patients; $P < .05$), despite similar reference sizes and residual minimal lumen diameters, and shorter dissection lengths.[18]

The second-generation Gianturco-Roubin II (GRII) stent has an improved flat-wire clam-shell design held by a single metal spine and two gold markers at each end. The GRII was evaluated in the Abrupt/Threatened Closure Registry, which demonstrated further reduction in mortality (1.5%), myocardial infarction (1.1%), emergency coronary artery bypass graft surgery (CABG; 3.6%), and subacute thrombosis (4.4%). The GRII received FDA approval in 1997. The Wiktor stent (Medtronic Inc, Minneapolis, MN), another coiled stent, has also been evaluated in a registry of abrupt/threatened closure, which demonstrated comparable results to the GRI stent. The Wiktor stent is now also approved by the FDA for treatment of acute and threatened closure. Other randomized studies are underway to assess the benefit of stent use over balloon angioplasty for failed or suboptimal results after balloon angioplasty.

STENTING IN SAPHENOUS VEIN GRAFTS

The US Palmaz-Schatz saphenous vein graft (SVG) stent registry began in 1990, enrolling patients with focal nonostial lesions in 4-mm SVGs, which were treated with one or two coronary stents. Major complications occurred in 2.9%, subacute thrombosis in 1.4%, and bleeding complications in 14%. The 6-month angiographic restenosis was 29.7%; the 12-month event-free survival was 76.3%. Compared with historical controls with balloon angioplasty, the outcome with stenting of SVG lesions appeared superior.

To further establish the benefit of the Palmaz-Schatz stent in SVG in a prospective randomized manner, the SAVED Trial (stents for SAphenous VEin graft De novo lesions), a randomized comparison of balloon angioplasty and stenting in SVGs was undertaken. The stented group had higher angiographic success (97% compared with 86%; $P < .01$), and procedural success (96% compared with 69%; $P < .001$). The 1-year event-free survival was significantly higher in the stent group. On the basis of the SAVED trial, FDA has recently granted extended approval of the Palmaz-Schatz stent for the treatment of SVGs.

The angiographic and clinical results after SVG angioplasty using coronary and biliary tubular slotted stents were compared in 231 patients.[13] Procedural success rates were high (95%), in-hospital major complications were uncommon (3%), and follow-up clinical outcomes were favorable (6-month event-free survival approximately 80%) in both groups. These data have provided support for the "off label" (not FDA-approved) use of "biliary" stent designs for larger (> 4.0 mm) SVG lesions.

STENTING IN RESTENOTIC LESIONS AND OTHER LESION SUBSETS

Stenting of restenotic lesions has been evaluated in the REST trial, which included patients randomized to Palmaz-Schatz stenting or balloon angioplasty. Although the final procedural minimal luminal diameter (MLD) and the follow-up MLD in this trial were better in the stented group, there was no difference in the follow-up target lesion revascularization (12% compared with 11%).[19]

In the Trial of Angioplasty and Stents in Canada (TASC-I), elective patients with restenotic lesions were randomly assigned to Palmaz-Schatz stent placement or balloon angioplasty. In this restenotic lesion subset, the difference in stent-treated patients was not significant either, although the study was not powered to detect differences in this subgroup.[12] Further randomized evaluation is needed to convincingly demonstrate the benefit of stenting over balloon angioplasty for the treatment of restenotic lesions.

STENTING IN ACUTE MYOCARDIAL INFARCTION

The use of intracoronary stents has also been expanded to patients with acute ischemic syndromes, including those with acute myocardial infarction.[20] Although patients undergoing stent placement for acute myocardial infarction have been deemed high-risk, acceptable rates (< 2%) of subacute thrombosis have been reported with reduced anticoagulation

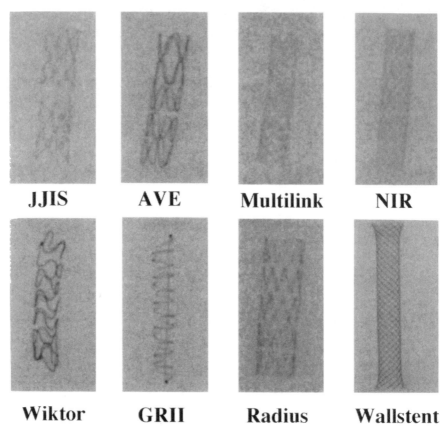

JJIS   AVE   Multilink   NIR

Wiktor   GRII   Radius   Wallstent

FIGURE 7-1 Different stent designs demonstrating relative radiopacity. (JJIS, Johnson and Johnson Stent; AVE, Arterial Vascular Engineering Micro-II Stent; Multilink, ACS Multi-Link Stent, Guidant, Inc; NIR, Medinol Ltd.; Wiktor, Wiktor Stent, Medtronic, Inc; GRII, Gianturco Roubin II Stent, Cook, Inc; Radius, Radius Stent, SciMed; Wallstent, Schneider Corporation.)

(aspirin plus ticlopidine only) regimens in a number of retrospective trials.[1,20–24]

In a series of 231 patients with stent placement for acute myocardial infarction treated with aspirin, 100 mg twice daily, and ticlopidine, 250 mg twice daily, the subacute thrombosis rate was 1.3%; the 1-month composite event rate (death, myocardial infarction, subacute thrombosis, CABG, repeat PTCA) was 3.5%.[25] Compared with balloon angioplasty, stenting appears to offer higher clinical success and lower cardiac event rates.[26] In the Primary Angioplasty in Myocardial Infarction (PAMI) stent pilot trial, patients with acute myocardial infarction underwent primary stenting; 96% were treated with aspirin and ticlopidine alone, 2% had subcutaneous heparin, and in 2% warfarin was added. In-hospital death occurred in 0.4%, reinfarction in 1.3%, repeat PTCA in 2.1%, and CABG in 1.7%, suggesting at least equal and possibly superior results with primary stenting compared with primary balloon angioplasty.[27] Clinical and angiographic follow-ups are underway. The PAMI Stent randomized trial will evaluate the early and late clinical and angiographic outcome of the heparin-coated Palmaz-Schatz stent compared with balloon angioplasty in patients with acute myocardial infarction. The CADILLAC trial will evaluate the use of the ACS Multi-Link stent compared to balloon angioplasty with or without the potent IIb/IIIa inhibitor Reopro™ in patients with acute myocardial infarction.

Although the use of stents has become virtually ubiquitous to most patient and lesion subsets, FDA approval for stent use remains limited.

♥ Contemporary Stent Designs

A number of balloon-expandable and self-expanding stents have become available for clinical use. Each of these stents varies with respect to metallic composition, design, length, delivery and deployment systems, and arterial surface coverage, among other factors (Fig. 7-1).

BALLOON-EXPANDABLE STENTS

More than seven balloon expandable stents exist, including both FDA-approved and investigation designs, in use in Canada, Europe, and the United States.

PALMAZ-SCHATZ STENT

The Johnson and Johnson Interventional Systems, Inc, Palmaz-Schatz stent is a 15-mm tubular-slotted stent composed of stainless steel, available with a 5-French (F) delivery sheath in the United States, or as a free-standing stent that is "crimped" on a standard balloon in Canada and Europe. Its major advantage is its high radial compressive strength and expansion symmetry. The Palmaz-Schatz stent is the most frequently used stent in the United States. The major disadvantages include the relative inflexibility of the sheath delivery system (in the United States), its availability in a single length, and its articulation defect. The articulation defect, which is required to improve flexibility, may result in residual stenosis from plaque protrusion through the articulation site. To improve on these limitations, a spiral articulation stent design is currently undergoing clinical evaluation in Europe.

Alternative "off-label" use of other tubular slotted stents has also been reported for the treatment of large (< 4.0- to 5.0-mm) native coronaries and SVGs,[13] in which the current Palmaz-Schatz coronary stent may be limited by significant stent shortening and deformation. The Palmaz nonarticulated stents and Palmaz-Schatz articulated "biliary" stents may provide greater radial compressive strength, enhanced visibility, and more variable length and diameter sizing than the approved coronary Palmaz-Schatz stent. Available data support the off label use of biliary stent designs for larger (> 4.0 mm) coronary and SVG lesions.

THE GIANTURCO-ROUBIN STENT

The GR stent is a balloon-expandable stent composed of a single stainless-steel wire coiled into a series of interdigitating loops in a "clam shell" design. The GR stent is available in sizes ranging from 2.0 mm to 4.0 mm. Its 25-mm length provides adequate coverage for lesions up to 20 mm long; multiple stents may be used for the treatment of longer lesions and dissections. The GR stent has two radiopaque marker bands located on either side of the stent. The compliant polyethylene balloon is slightly larger than the stent to allow full apposition of the stent coils into the vessel wall on deployment.

The major limitations of the first-generation GR stent have been its relative inflexibility, requirement for larger guiding catheters for 3.5 mm and 4.0-mm stents, and the inability to precisely locate the position of the stent after deployment. For these reasons and others, a second-generation GR stent, the GRII, has been designed and has recently completed clinical evaluation in the United States and Europe. Unique features of the GRII stent include (a) gold radiopaque markers at both ends of the stent to allow easy visualization of the proximal and distal stent margins; (b) a flat-wire design to permit more symmetric vessel expansion; (c) a central articulation spine to prevent stent axial shortening or expansion; (d) a low-profile, minimally compliant balloon, which can be deployed through most 7F guiding catheters; and (e) availability in both 20-mm and 40-mm lengths.

An initial series using 20-mm and 40-mm GRII stents reported successful deployment of the stent in all cases,[28] with minimal residual diameter stenosis despite complex lesion morphology.

THE WIKTOR CORONARY STENT

The Medtronic Wiktor stent is a balloon-expandable stent composed of a tantalum wire arranged in a sinusoidal helical wave. Its high degree of radiopacity allows precise placement. Coronary artery side branches are not significantly compromised after stent delivery because of the relatively wide sinusoidal wave. The Wiktor stent has been clinically evaluated for two primary indications: the correction of acute and threatened closure after coronary intervention and the prevention of restenosis in high-risk patients after coronary intervention.[29-31]

At least three studies have addressed the ability of the Wiktor stent to reverse ischemic events after failed coronary angioplasty. In a series of patients who developed threatened or complete occlusion after balloon angioplasty, the Wiktor stent was successfully deployed in 69 of 72 (95%) lesions. Emergency surgery was performed in three patients.

In a contemporary series of patients undergoing Wiktor stent implantation for acute or threatened closure, who were at high risk for restenosis or had a primary angioplasty result that was inadequate, Wiktor stent implantation was successful in 65 of the 67 lesions. There were no stent occlusions or myocardial infarctions during the 1- to 20-month follow-up.[32]

The comparative efficacy of the Wiktor and Palmaz-Schatz stents for the reversal of acute or threatened closure was evaluated in 65 patients randomly assigned to treatment with either the Wiktor (n = 33) or Palmaz-Schatz (n = 32) stents, with immediate success in reversing ongoing ischemia and vessel closure achieved in 60 patients (92%). At hospital discharge, rates of complications were comparable, including early vessel closure and composite clinical events (i.e., death, myocardial infarction, and surgical revascularization). Late (6-month) restenosis rates were also similar in the two groups (38% in Wiktor-treated patients compared with 27% in Palmaz-Schatz–treated patients; $P = .42$).

Both stent designs are associated with comparable early and late clinical and angiographic outcomes for treatment of acute or threatened closure.[33] The Wiktor stent recently received FDA approval for the treatment of acute and threatened closure.

THE GUIDANCE/ADVANCED CARDIOVASCULAR SYSTEMS MULTI-LINK™ STENT

The Guidance/Advanced Cardiovascular Systems (ACS) Multi-Link stent is a 15-mm balloon-expandable, stainless-steel stent designed with multiple rings connected by multiple links. This unique stent design affords unique longitudinal flexibility, high radial compressive strength, and minimal longitudinal shortening after deployment. An elastomeric balloon sheath permits concentric stent expansion.

The ACS Multi-Link recently received FDA approval for clinical use based on a randomized clinical trial with the Palmaz-Schatz stent for the prevention of restenosis in native coronary arteries. The angiographic restenosis with the ACS stent was equivalent to the Palmaz-Schatz stent and was associated with a similar late clinical outcome.

AVE MICROSTENT

The Arterial Vascular Engineering (AVE) microstent II is a second-generation AVE stent that has recently completed its clinical investigation in a large multicenter randomized trial comparing it with the Palmaz-Schatz stent. The AVE micro II stent is expected to gain FDA approval in the near future. A new-generation AVE stent, the AVE-GFX stent will be evaluated in a German multicenter clinical trial.

THE NIR® STENT

The NIR stent is a balloon-expandable cellular mesh stent composed of stainless steel. It has high longitudinal flexibility and minimal shortening on expansion. Its unique flexibility, availability in longer stent lengths, and radial compressive strength make it a very attractive alternative in patients with diffuse coronary lesions. The NIR stent is nearing completion of clinical investigation in a randomized trial comparing it with the Palmaz-Schatz stent.

THE ADVANCED CORONARY TECHNOLOGY-ONE™ STENT

The Advanced Coronary Technology (ACT)-One stent is a nitinol, balloon-expandable, tubular-slotted stent designed for use in native coronar-

---

DISPLAY 7–1   Potential Complications From Placement of Coronary Stents

- Subacute thrombosis
- Bleeding complications
- Margin dissections
- Perforation
- Side branch occlusion
- Stent embolization
- Late aneurysm formation
- Infection (rare)

ies and SVGs. Its moderate radiopacity allows precise stent positioning and adjunct balloon dilatation.

The ACT-One stent is approved for use in Europe and in phase I clinical study in the United States. To date, over 200 patients have been treated worldwide with the ACT-One stent.

In a series of 19 patients treated with the ACT-One stent reported by Nakamura and associates,[34] procedure success was achieved in 90% of lesions treated. No episodes of subacute stent thromboses were reported in this series.

SELF-EXPANDING STENTS

Self-expanding stents, as their name suggests, expand automatically as the guide or cover over the stent is removed.

THE SCHNEIDER WALLSTENT

The Schneider Wallstent is a self-expanding, wire mesh stent composed of cobalt based alloy with a platinum core. The Wallstent has excellent longitudinal flexibility, but precise localization is somewhat difficult, owing to its somewhat unpredictable shortening (up to 25%) after deployment. Its major clinical uses appear to be in tortuous and diffusely diseased native coronary and coronary bypass grafts. It is approved for use in SVGs in Europe and is being evaluated in a randomized trial with balloon angioplasty for restenotic native coronary lesions and a randomized trial with the Palmaz-Schatz stent in SVGs in the United States.

THE RADIUS STENT

The Radius stent is a self-expanding nitinol stent with multiple segments, flexible slotted tube structure, delivered by a sheath pullback mechanism. The Radius stent has excellent longitudinal flexibility, minimal shortening, and moderate radiopacity for precise placement. The SCORES Trial is an ongoing multicenter randomized clinical trial of the Radius stent to the Palmaz-Schatz stent.

❤ Complications of Coronary Stent Placement

Enthusiasm for coronary stent placement has been tempered by several major and minor complications associated with coronary stent placement (Display 7-1). Refinements in coronary stent designs and placement techniques have reduced the incidence of some of these complications, and increased awareness has reduced the clinical sequelae of others.

SUBACUTE STENT THROMBOSIS

Despite the benefits associated with stent placement in early clinical studies,[35,36] enthusiasm for stent use was tempered by two major problems: subacute thrombosis and vascular complications. Subacute stent thrombosis occurred in 3.5% to 8.6% of patients.[10,11,35-37] Furthermore, thrombosis was often delayed 2 to 14 days (average, 6 days) after stent placement[10,38] and was associated with major clinical events such as death, transmural myocardial infarction, or emergency revascularization in virtually all cases.

To define the clinical impact of subacute thrombosis, 46 of 2849 patients undergoing stent implantation were identified with this complication between 1990 and 1996. Among these patients, the mortality rate was 15%. Thirty percent had a Q-wave myocardial infarction (QMI), and the composite end point of in-hospital death, QMI, and revascularization was 54%.[38]

A very aggressive anticoagulation regimen was initially used to reduce subacute thrombosis in these early studies, which included aspirin (325 mg daily), dipyridamole (75 mg three times daily), intravenous low molecular weight dextran-40, and heparin until therapeutic systemic anticoagulation had been achieved with warfarin (Internationalized Normalized Ratio [INR] between 2.0 and 3.5). It is not surprising that this potent anticoagulation regimen resulted in more frequent major bleeding complications and vascular events (>13%) in stent-treated patients. Owing to the prolonged anticoagulation regimen, the length of hospitalization was also longer in stent-treated patients.[10,11]

INTRAVASCULAR ULTRASOUND-DETECTED INCOMPLETE STENT EXPANSION

It is now clear that anatomic factors (e.g., underdilatation of the stent, proximal and distal dissections, poor inflow or outflow obstruction, < 3 mm vessel diameter) rather than suboptimal anticoagulation regimens contributed to the development of subacute thrombosis in the early stent experience.[39,40] Sequential intravascular ultrasound (IVUS) studies have since shown that the previous stent deployment methods often resulted in incomplete apposition of the stent struts against the vessel wall, in asymmetric expansion, and in incomplete stent dilatation compared with the proximal and distal reference segments.[41-44] Complete and symmetric stent expansion occurred in less than 30% of cases after initial deployment in one study, but was noted in nearly 70% of cases after high-pressure (>12 atmospheres) balloon dilatation.[44] The relatively high (3.5% to 5.0%) rates of subacute thrombosis were possibly triggered by platelet and fibrin deposition in the region of incompletely expanded stent struts. At the very least, IVUS-guided stent deployment studies have shown that high-pressure (12 to 20 atmospheres) balloon dilatations and minimally oversized balloons are required for consistent stent apposition and expansion.[43] By optimizing these technical factors, lower (<2%) incidences of subacute stent thrombosis have been achieved, allowing a progressive reduction in the intensity of anticoagulation after stent deployment.[41–43]

REDUCED ANTICOAGULATION SERIES

At least 20 single and multicenter series have since reported the use of less aggressive anticoagulation regimens after stent placement.[20,26,43,45–69] All the regimens included aspirin and postdeployment stent dilatation using high-pressure balloons, but they have varied with respect to the type of stent used for deployment, the procedure priority (elective versus failed angioplasty), concomitant use of intravascular ultrasound, ticlopidine, postprocedural heparin, low molecular weight heparin, and warfarin. Subacute thrombosis has ranged from 0% to 3.6%; vascular complications have ranged from 0% to 4.4%.

Many reduced anticoagulation regimens have added ticlopidine (250 to 750 mg daily for 1 to 3 months) in addition to aspirin after stent deployment. The major limitations of ticlopidine are its side effects and toxicities. Although gastrointestinal symptoms, cutaneous rashes, and

---

DISPLAY 7–2 Patients at High Risk for Subacute Thrombosis After Stent Placement

- Residual proximal or distal dissection[52,76]
- Angiographic thrombus[33,77]
- Abrupt closure
- Multiple (≥3) stents[52]
- Small (<3.0-mm) vessels[68,76]
- Total occlusions
- Recent (<1 week) myocardial infarction[79]

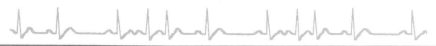

biochemical abnormalities in liver function tests may occur with ticlopidine,[65] the major side effect associated with ticlopidine use is the unpredictable occurrence of severe leukopenia (granulocyte count < 450/μL) in approximately 1% of patients.[65,70] The leukopenia is reversible after discontinuation of ticlopidine in most cases,[71] but episodes of sepsis and death have occurred. Thrombotic thrombocytopenic purpura has also been reported.[72] As a result of these issues, the risk-benefit ratio associated with ticlopidine use after stent placement is not known.

With the exception of high-risk patients undergoing stent implantation, the conventional use of warfarin, an inhibitor of vitamin K–dependent coagulation factors, has largely been abandoned, owing to increased bleeding complications, extended hospitalizations required to reach therapeutic dosing, and general inconvenience and cost associated with maintaining therapy. One recent single-center series has even suggested that use of prolonged intravenous heparin and warfarin may be associated with an increased risk of subacute thrombosis and other untoward events after stent deployment.[73]

In a series of 517 patients randomly assigned to an intensive (intravenous heparin for 5 to 10 days, warfarin for 30 days, and aspirin, 200 mg daily) or reduced (intravenous heparin for 12 hours, ticlopidine, 500 mg daily for 30 days, and aspirin, 200 mg daily) anticoagulation, a substantial reduction in 30-day cardiac events (i.e., death, myocardial infarction, and reintervention) was noted in the reduced anticoagulation group. Subacute thrombosis occurred in none of the reduced anticoagulation group compared with 5% in those in the intensive anticoagulation group. Bleeding and vascular complications were also significantly less common in the reduced anticoagulation group.[73]

RANDOMIZED ANTICOAGULATION STUDIES IN PATIENTS UNDERGOING STENT PLACEMENT

Recent randomized comparisons of antiplatelet regimens to full anticoagulation regimens have confirmed the benefits of antiplatelet therapy with aspirin and ticlopidine alone without warfarin.[74] A comparison of antiplatelet and anticoagulant therapy after successful placement of Palmaz-Schatz coronary stents was performed in which patients were randomized to aspirin and ticlopidine therapy or to heparin, warfarin, and aspirin therapy. The warfarin-treated patients had a significantly higher primary composite cardiac event rate (death, myocardial infarction, repeat PTCA, and CABG) as well as a higher subacute thrombosis rate. The aspirin and ticlopidine–treated patients had a significantly lower risk of myocardial infarction and a much lower need for repeat interventions, associated with a significant reduction in vascular complications.[74]

The Stent Antithrombotic Regimen Study (STARS) included 1650 patients undergoing successful intracoronary stent placement in low-risk lesion subsets and randomly assigned patients to treatment with aspirin alone, aspirin plus ticlopidine, or aspirin plus warfarin.[75] Patients were excluded from STARS if they had a myocardial infarction within the past 7 days, a suboptimal (> 10% residual stenosis) angiographic result, more than two stents per lesion or more than four stents per patient, a proximal or distal dissection, angiographic thrombus, or persistently reduced anterograde perfusion. The 30-day ischemic event rate (death, myocardial infarction, urgent revascularization) and the subacute thrombosis rate were significantly lower in the aspirin and ticlopidine–treated group compared with the aspirin alone or aspirin and warfarin groups.

DEFINING PATIENTS AT HIGH RISK FOR SUBACUTE THROMBOSIS AND RESTENOSIS AFTER STENT PLACEMENT

It is important to emphasize that reduced anticoagulation regimens (aspirin with or without ticlopidine) have primarily been recommended in patients at low risk for subacute thrombosis after stent placement (i.e., residual stenosis < 20%, no thrombus, recent myocardial infarction, or significant periprocedural dissection or outflow limitation). Several subgroups of patients may be at higher risk for subacute thrombosis after stent placement (Display 7-2).[76–79]

In a series of high-risk patients undergoing bail-out stenting and stenting for suboptimal results treated with aspirin and ticlopidine alone, the events related to stent implantation occurred in 5.7% after bail-out stenting, 2.1% after stenting for suboptimal results, and 0.9% after elective stenting.[52] However, because data in high-risk patient subgroups remain limited, conventional antithrombotic agents, such as warfarin for 1 month or low molecular weight heparin for 2 to 4 weeks, may be used empirically in these patients.

The use of intracoronary stents has also been expanded to patients with acute ischemic syndromes, including those with acute myocardial infarction.[26,80] Although patients undergoing stent placement for acute myocardial infarction have been deemed high-risk, acceptable rates (< 2%) of subacute thrombosis have also been reported with reduced aspirin plus ticlopidine regimens.[1,20–24,80]

In a series of patients with stent placement for acute myocardial infarction treated with aspirin 100 mg twice daily and ticlopidine 250 mg twice daily, the subacute thrombosis rate was 1.3%, the 1 month composite event rate (death, MI, subacute thrombosis, CABG, repeat PTCA) was 3.5%.[25] Compared with balloon angioplasty, stenting appears to offer higher clinical success and lower cardiac event rates.[26] In the PAMI stent pilot trial 230 of 300 (77%) patients with acute myocardial infarction underwent primary stenting; 96% were treated with aspirin and ticlopidine alone, 2% had subcutaneous heparin, and warfarin was added in 2%. In-hospital death occurred in 0.4%, reinfarction in 1.3%, repeat PTCA in 2.1%, and CABG in 1.7%, suggesting at least equal and possibly superior results with primary stenting compared with primary balloon angioplasty.[27]

BLEEDING COMPLICATIONS

As a result of the significant rates of subacute thrombosis in the early stent experience, a very aggressive anticoagulation regimen was used to lessen this often fatal complication. This regimen included aspirin, dipyridamole, intravenous low molecular weight dextran-40, and heparin until therapeutic systemic anticoagulation had been achieved with warfarin (INR between 2.0 and 3.5). This potent anticoagulation regimen resulted in more frequent major bleeding complications and vascular events (> 13%) in stent-treated patients.[10,11]

The clinical course of 1413 patients was reviewed after balloon or new device angioplasty in this early era of intracoronary stenting. Vascular complications developed after 84 (5.9%) procedures; they occurred more frequently after intracoronary stenting (14.0%) and extraction atherectomy (12.5%) than after balloon angioplasty (3.2%).

With the use of standard anticoagulation regimens after coronary stent placement, major vascular complications occurred more often after stenting than after directional coronary atherectomy (16.8% compared with 6.7%; $P = .001$). Surgical repair was required after 10.1% of stenting procedures compared with 5.1% of directional coronary arthrectomies ($P = .02$), and independent predictors of vascular complications included the use of intracoronary stenting ($P = .005$), among others.[81]

Initial attempts at curbing the vexing vascular complication rates associated with stenting procedures included percutaneous vascular closure devices, which offered a safe method of achieving prompt and effective femoral hemostasis with a low incidence of major vascular bleeding complications despite intense anticoagulation.[82] Because lower anticoagulation strategies are now advocated in conjunction with coronary stenting, the vascular complication rates have simultaneously dropped to levels of those following standard balloon angioplasty.

CORONARY MARGIN DISSECTIONS

One potential complication of an aggressive approach to stent deployment is the induction of arterial injury. It is less clear how best to ensure full stent expansion without causing significant arterial injury at the stent margin. In a series of 67 successfully stented lesions, lumen diameter at five sites within the stent was significantly reduced 6 months after stent implantation. Restenosis involving the articulation was found in 75% of the lesions, attributable to a smaller articulation site diameter both immediately and 6 months after stenting compared with that found for other stent segments. The loss index was significantly greater at the proximal and distal edges than at the bodies of the stent, suggesting that the edges of the Palmaz-Schatz stent may incur more trauma, resulting in potentially more late fibroproliferation.[83] The availability of shorter, noncompliant balloons has allowed more precise stent dilatation using high pressure.

Focal stenoses (< 5 mm) and some margin dissections have also been successfully treated with half (disarticulated) stents in some series.[84–88] Stenting with the half Palmaz-Schatz coronary stent is an effective technique, particularly when a full stent is not ideally suited.[84]

CORONARY PERFORATION

Coronary perforation is uncommon after standard balloon angioplasty, most often related to relative oversizing of the balloon to the reference artery. Coronary perforation is also uncommon after stent deployment performed without high-pressure balloon dilatation, but has been noted during poststent deployment using high-pressure or oversized balloons (Fig. 7-2).

SIDE BRANCH OCCLUSION

The occlusion of a side branch is a well-defined risk after balloon angioplasty. However, the impact of stenting on the coronary flow in side branches arising within the stented segment is unknown. To further define this complication, 45 stented coronary artery segments with 79 side branches emerging from the stented segment were analyzed. Flow worsened in six side branches (8%) after balloon dilation and in four side branches (5%) after stenting. Of the 34 side branches larger than 1 mm in diameter, two (6%) had flow impairment after stenting. Side branch occlusion was associated with transient angina in three patients, but no acute myocardial infarction.

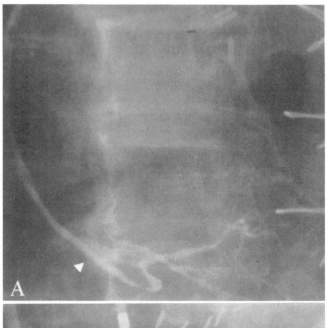

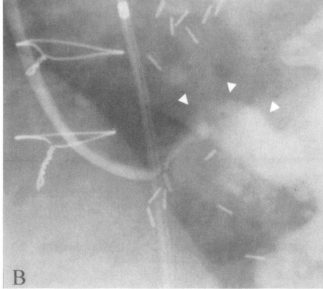

FIGURE 7–2 Stent placed in a saphenous vein graft to the right coronary artery. **(A)** During subsequent balloon inflation of the stent, dye extravasation was noted, indicating perforation of the graft (*arrow*). **(B)** A subsequent dye injection revealed an increasing area of dye extravasation (*arrows*). The patient underwent urgent surgical repair and experienced an uneventful recovery.

Coronary artery stenting does not appear to modify anterograde flow in 90% of side branches, and, although coronary flow may be reduced after stenting in a few branches, this does not appear to have major clinical relevance.[89] Late side branch occlusion after Palmaz-Schatz stent deployment occurs infrequently and is poorly predicted by angiographic or clinical factors.[90]

The coiled design of the GRII may offer an advantage in maintaining side branch patency. In a serial study of 100 consecutive patients in whom 103 GR stents were implanted for acute or threatened closure after PTCA, side branch patency was documented early (immediate) and late (6 months) after stent implantations. Seven major (>50% of stented vessel diameter) branches (6%), all of which were diseased before PTCA, and 23 minor (< 50% of stenting diameter) branches (18%) were lost after PTCA. Immediately after stent insertion, only one additional major and one minor branch were lost, whereas 2 of 7 major (29%) and 9 of 23 minor (39%) branches reappeared. Only 2 major (2%) and 5 minor (4%) branches remained occluded at follow-up.[91]

Serial coronary angiography was performed in 153 patients (167 lesions) at baseline, after conventional balloon angioplasty, immediately after Palmaz-Schatz stent placement and at 6 months. Six side branches became occluded after standard balloon angioplasty and remained occluded after stenting. Of the 60 side branches patent after conventional angioplasty, 57 (95%) remained patent immediately after stenting.[92] All three side branches that became occluded after stenting had more than 50% ostial stenosis at baseline. All 60 side branches, including the 3 initially occluded after stenting, were patent at 6-month follow-up.

Overall, these findings demonstrate that acute side branch occlusion due to coronary stenting occurs infrequently (< 10%), and when side branch occlusion occurs, it is associated with intrinsic ostial disease. In general, the patency of side branch ostia is well maintained at long-term follow-up.[92]

STENT DISLODGEMENT, EMBOLIZATION, AND INCOMPLETE STENT EXPANSION

Stent dislodgement from the delivery catheter is a major complication of both sheathed and nonsheathed delivery systems. After stent dislodgement has occurred, stent embolization may occur within the native coronary artery[93] or SVG[94] undergoing stent implantation or may embolize to the peripheral vessels including the aorta,[95] iliac,[96] or femoral arteries.[97] Removal of the stent is obviously more difficult for radiolucent stents than for radiopaque ones. Successful removal has been reported using alligator forceps and retrieval devices,[95,98,99] additional balloon catheters,[94] and coaxial wires.[93,96]

Another potential complication during stent deployment is the incomplete expansion of the stent while still on the balloon catheter, most commonly occurring after a "pinhole" balloon rupture. A number of methods have been used to fully expand the stent, including the rapid inflation of the delivery balloon with an injector and use of a fixed wire (e.g., probing catheter).[100]

LATE CORONARY ANEURYSM FORMATION

Although coronary aneurysm formation is uncommon (<1%) after standard balloon angioplasty, its incidence may be higher after stent implantation if concomitant anti-inflammatory or antiproliferative agents are also given. In a series of 29 patients undergoing late (4-month) angiography after GR stent placement for acute closure, 19 patients had been treated with intravenous or oral glucocorticoids or colchicine and 10 had been treated with aspirin, heparin, or warfarin. Six (32%) of 19 stented arteries in patients treated with anti-inflammatory agents showed evidence of coronary artery aneurysm, whereas none of the patients not receiving steroids or colchicine developed a late aneurysm.[101] These preliminary findings, which will undoubtedly require confirmation in larger prospective studies, suggest that aggressive anti-inflammatory regimens after stent implantation may impair the normal vascular healing response and result in late aneurysm formation.

INFECTION

The development of a stent abscess is a rare, but potentially devastating, complication after coronary stent placement. Formation of a fatal perivascular myocardial abscess after Palmaz-Schatz stent implantation was reported in a 66-year-old woman who developed malaise, leukocytosis, fever, and a purulent pericardial effusion 4 weeks after stent implantation.[102] The proximity of the myocardial abscess and the Palmaz-Schatz stent in the right coronary artery was demonstrated by transesophageal echocardiography, suggesting that the stent had been seeded with a bacterial source and that a myocardial empyema had subsequently developed. Although bacterial infection after stent placement is rare, meticulous sterile technique should be practiced during all stent implantation procedures, particularly when sheaths are left in place or are reinserted without sterile precautions. Antibiotic prophylaxis after stent implantation is not indicated.

♡ Conclusion

Indications for coronary stenting will continue to expand as stent designs continue to improve and ongoing clinical trials are completed. Challenges for the future include defining the optimal anticoagulation regimen, as well as exploring new methods to reduce the incidence of in-stent restenosis.

REFERENCES

1. Ahmad T, Webb JG, Carere RR, Dodek A: Coronary stenting for acute myocardial infarction. *Am J Cardiol* 76(1):77, 1995.
2. Wong PH, Wong CM: Intracoronary stenting in acute myocardial infarction. *Cath Cardiovasc Diagn* 33:39, 1994.
3. Gruentzig A, Senning A, Giegenthaler W: Nonoperative dilation of coronary-artery stenosis: Percutaneous transluminal coronary angioplasty. *N Engl J Med* 301:61, 1979.
4. Waller B: Early and late morphologic changes in human coronary arteries after percutaneous transluminal coronary angioplasty. *Clin Cardiol* 6:363, 1983.
5. Waller B, Rothbaum D, Gorfinkel H, et al: Morphologic observations after percutaneous transluminal balloon angioplasty of early and late aortocoronary saphenous vein bypass grafts. *J Am Coll Cardiol* 4:784, 1984.
6. Mintz G, Pichard A, Kent K, et al: Axial plaque redistribution as a mechanism of percutaneous transluminal coronary angioplasty. *Am J Cardiol* 77:427, 1996.
7. Waller B: "Crackers, Breakers, Stretchers, Drillers, Scrapers, Shavers, Burners, Welders, and Melters." The future treatment of atherosclerotic coronary artery disease? A clinical-morphologic assessment. *J Am Coll Cardiol* 13:969, 1989.
8. Mintz G, Popma J, Pichard A, et al: Intravascular ultrasound assessment of the mechanisms and predictors of restenosis following coronary angioplasty. *J Invas Cardiol* 1:1, 1996.
9. Hoffmann R, Mintz GS, Mehran R, et al: Intravascular ultrasound predictors of angiographic restenosis in lesions treated with Palmaz-Schatz stents. *J Am Coll* Cardiol 31:43, 1998.
10. Fischman DL, Leon MB, Baim DS, et al: A randomized comparison of coronary-stent placement and balloon angioplasty in the treatment of coronary artery disease. Stent Restenosis Study Investigators. *N Engl J Med* 331:496, 1994.
11. Serruys PW, de Jaegere PP, Kiemeneij F, et al: A comparison of balloon-expandable-stent implantation with balloon angioplasty in patients with coronary artery disease. Benestent Study Group. *N Engl J Med* 331:489, 1994.
12. Penn I, Ricci D, Almond D, et al: Coronary artery stenting reduces restenosis: Final results from the trial of angioplasty and stents in Canada (TASC I). *Circulation* 92:I-279, 1995.
13. Wong SC, Popma JJ, Pichard AD, et al: Comparison of clinical and angiographic outcomes after saphenous vein graft angioplasty using coronary versus "biliary" tubular slotted stents. *Circulation* 91:339, 1995.
14. Sutton JM, Ellis SG, Roubin GS, et al: Major clinical events after coronary stenting. The multicenter registry of acute and elective Gianturco-Roubin stent placement. The Gianturco-Roubin Intracoronary Stent Investigator Group. *Circulation* 89:1126, 1994.

15. George BS, Voorhees W, Roubin GS, et al: Multicenter investigation of coronary stenting to treat acute or threatened closure after percutaneous transluminal coronary angioplasty: Clinical and angiographic outcomes. *J Am Coll Cardiol* 22:135, 1993.

16. Fry ET, Hermiller JB, Peters TF, et al: Indications for and applications of the Gianturco-Roubin coronary stent. *Cardiol Clin* 12:631, 1994.

17. Roubin G, King SI, Douglas J, et al: Intracoronary stenting during percutaneous transluminal coronary angioplasty. *Circulation* 81:IV-92, 1990.

18. Fernandez-Ortiz A, Goicolea J, Perez-Vizcayno M, et al: Late clinical and angiographic outcome of bailout coronary stenting. A comparison study between Gianturco-Roubin and Palmaz-Schatz stents (abstr). *J Am Coll Cardiol* 27:111A, 1996.

19. Shah DC, Subramanyan K, Ramachandran P: Perfusion stenting for coronary dissection during percutaneous transluminal coronary angioplasty. *Indian Heart J* 46:45, 1994.

20. Saito S, Kim K, Hosokawa G, et al: Primary Palmaz-Schatz stent implantation without warfarin in acute myocardial infarction. *Circulation* 92:I-796, 1995.

21. Neumann F, Walter H, Schmitt C, et al: Coronary stenting as an adjunct to direct balloon angioplasty in acute myocardial infarction. *Circulation* 92:I-609, 1995.

22. Alfonso F, Hernandez R, Goicolea J, et al: Coronary stenting for acute coronary dissection after coronary angioplasty: Implications of residual dissection. *J Am Coll Cardiol* 24:989, 1994.

23. Neumann FJ, Walter H, Richardt G, et al: Coronary Palmaz-Schatz stent implantation in acute myocardial infarction. *Heart* 75:121, 1996.

24. Monassier J, Elias J, Raynaud P, Joly P: Results of early (<24 hr) and late (>24 hr) implantation of coronary stents in acute myocardial infarction. *Circulation* 92:I-609, 1995.

25. Walter H, Neuman FJ, Hadamitzky M, et al: Clinical and angiographic outcome of intracoronary stent placement in acute myocardial infarction (abstr). *J Am Coll Cardiol* 29:14A, 1997.

26. Saito S, Hosokawa G, Suzuki S, Nakamura S. Primary stent implantation is superior to balloon angioplasty in acute myocardial infarction. The result of the Japanese PASTA (primary angioplasty versus stent implantation in acute myocardial infarction) trial (abstr). *J Am Coll Cardiol* 29:390A, 1997.

27. Stone GW, Brodie B, Griffin J, et al: Safety and feasibility of primary stenting in acute myocardial infarction. In hospital and 30 day results of the PAMI stent pilot trial. *J Am Coll Cardiol* 29:389A, 1997.

28. Marco J, Fajadet J, Brunel P, et al: First use of the second-generation Gianturco-Roubin stent without warfarin (abstr). *J Am Coll Cardiol* 27:110A, 1996.

29. White CJ: Wiktor coronary stent. *Cardiol Clin* 12:665, 1994.

30. White CJ, Ramee SR, Collins TJ: Elective placement of the Wiktor stent after coronary angioplasty. *Am J Cardiol* 74:274, 1994.

31. MacIsaac AI, Ellis SG, Muller DW, et al: Comparison of three coronary stents: Clinical and angiographic outcome after elective placement in 134 consecutive patients. *Cathet Cardiovasc Diagn* 33:199, 1994.

32. Vaishnav S, Aziz S, Layton C: Clinical experience with the Wiktor stent in native coronary arteries and coronary bypass grafts. *Br Heart J* 72:288, 1994.

33. Goy JJ, Eeckhout E, Stauffer JC, et al: Emergency endoluminal stenting for abrupt vessel closure following coronary angioplasty: A randomized comparison of the Wiktor and Palmaz-Schatz stents. *Cathet Cardiovasc Diagn* 34:128, 1995.

34. Nakamura S, Degawa T, Takahiro N, et al: Preliminary experience of Act-One™ stent implantation (abstr). *J Am Coll Cardiol* 27:53A, 1996.

35. Roubin GS, Cannon AD, Agrawal SK, et al: Intracoronary stenting for acute and threatened closure complicating percutaneous transluminal coronary angioplasty. *Circulation* 85:916, 1992.

36. Hearn JA, King Sd, Douglas JJ, et al: Clinical and angiographic outcomes after coronary artery stenting for acute or threatened closure after percutaneous transluminal coronary angioplasty. Initial results with a balloon-expandable, stainless steel design. *Circulation* 88:2086, 1993.

37. Schomig A, Kastrati A, Mudra H, et al: Four-year experience with Palmaz-Schatz stenting in coronary angioplasty complicated by dissection with threatened or present vessel closure. *Circulation* 90:2716, 1994.

38. Yokoi H, Nosaka H, Kimura T, et al: Coronary stent thrombosis: Management and long term follow-up results. *J Am Coll Cardiol* 29:171A, 1997.

39. Schatz R: New challenges in coronary stenting. *J Invas Cardiol* 7:43A, 1995.

40. Serruys PW, DiMario C: Who was thrombogenic: The stent or the doctor? (Editorial). *Circulation* 91:1891, 1995.

41. Goldberg SL, Colombo A, Nakamura S, et al: Benefit of intracoronary ultrasound in the deployment of Palmaz-Schatz stents. *J Am Coll Cardiol* 24:996, 1994.

42. Hall P, Colombo A, Almagor Y: Preliminary experience with intravascular ultrasound-guided Palmaz-Schatz coronary stenting: The acute and short-term results on a consecutive series of patients. *J Intervent Cardiol* 7:141, 1994.

43. Colombo A, Hall P, Nakamura S, et al: Intracoronary stenting without anticoagulation accomplished with intravascular ultrasound guidance. *Circulation* 91:1676, 1995.

44. Kiemeneij F, Laarman G, Slagboom T: Mode of deployment of coronary Palmaz-Schatz stents after implantation with the stent delivery system: An intravascular ultrasound study. *Am Heart J* 129:638, 1995.

45. Fernandez-Aviles F, Alonso J, Duran J, et al: Absence of bleeding and subacute occlusion after Palmaz-Schatz coronary stenting using a new antithrombotic regimen (abstr). *J Am Coll Cardiol* 25:196A, 1995.

46. Blasini R, Mudra H, Schuhlen H, et al: Intravascular ultrasound guided optimized emergency coronary Palmaz-Schatz stent placement without post-procedural systemic anticoagulation (abstr). *J Am Coll Cardiol* 25:197A, 1995.

47. Colombo A, Nakamura S, Hall P, et al: A prospective study of Gianturco-Roubin coronary stent implantation without anticoagulation (abstr). *J Am Coll Cardiol* 25:50A, 1995.

48. Colombo A, Nakamura S, Hall P, et al: A prospective study of Wiktor coronary stent implantation without anticoagulation (abstr). *J Am Coll Cardiol* 25:239A, 1995.

49. Russo R, Schatz R, Sklar M, et al: Ultrasound guided coronary stent placement without prolonged systemic anticoagulation (abstr). *J Am Coll Cardiol* 25:50A, 1995.

50. Van Belle E, McFadden E, Bauters C, et al: Combined antiplatelet therapy

without anticoagulation: An effective alternative to prevent subacute thrombosis after coronary stenting (abstr). *J Am Coll Cardiol* 25:197A, 1995.

51. Lablanche J, Grollier G, Bonnet J, et al: Ticlopidine aspirin stent evaluation (TASTE): A French multicenter study. *Circulation* 92:I-476, 1995.

52. Lablanche J, Bonnet J, Grollier G, et al: Combined antiplatelet therapy without anticoagulation after stent implantation: The ticlopidine aspirin stent evaluation (TASTE) study. *J Am Coll Cardiol* 29:95A, 1997.

53. Buszman P, Clague J, Gibbs S, et al: Improved post stent management: High gain and low risk (abstr). *J Am Coll Cardiol* 25:182A, 1995.

54. Carvalho H, Fajadet J, Jordan C, et al: A lower rate of complications after Gianturco-Roubin stenting using a new antiplatelet and anticoagulation protocol (abstr). *Circulation* 90:I-125, 1994.

55. Elias J, Monassier J, Puel J, et al. Medtronic-Wiktor implantation without warfarin: Hospital outcome (abstr). *Circulation* 90:I-124, 1994.

56. Barragan P, Sainsous J, Silvestri M, et al: Ticlopidine and subcutaneous heparin as an alternative regimen following coronary stenting. *Cathet Cardiovasc Diagn* 32:133, 1994.

57. Blengino S, Maiello L, Hall P, et al: Randomized trial of coronary stent implantation without anticoagulation: Aspirin versus ticlopidine (abstr). *Circulation* 90:I-124, 1994.

58. Jordan C, Carvalho H, Fajadet J, et al: Reduction of subacute thrombosis after stenting using a new anticoagulation protocol (abstr). *Circulation* 90:I-125, 1994.

59. Morice MC, Zemour G, Benveniste E, et al: Intracoronary stenting without warfarin: One month results of a French multicenter study. *Cathet Cardiovasc Diagn* 35:1, 1995.

60. Morice M, Amor M, Benveniste E, et al: Coronary stenting without Coumadin phase II, III, IV, V. Predictors of major complications. *Circulation* 92:I-795, 1995.

61. Morice M, Breton C, Bunouf P, et al: Coronary stenting without anticoagulant, without intravascular ultrasound. Result of the French registry. *Circulation* 92:I-796, 1995.

62. Wong S, Popma J, Mintz G, et al: Preliminary results from the Reduced Anticoagulation in Saphenous Vein Graft (RAVES) Trial (abstr). *Circulation* 90:I-125, 1994.

63. Van BE, McFadden EP, Lablanche JM, et al: Two-pronged antiplatelet therapy with aspirin and ticlopidine without systemic anticoagulation: An alternative therapeutic strategy after bailout stent implantation. *Coron Artery Dis* 6:341, 1995.

64. Belli G, Whitlow P, Franco I, et al: Intracoronary stenting without oral anticoagulation: The Cleveland Clinic Registry. *Circulation* 92:I-796, 1995.

65. Hass W, Easton J, Adams H, et al. A randomized trial comparing ticlopidine hydrochloride with aspirin for the prevention of stroke in high-risk patients. Ticlopidine Aspirin Stroke Study Group. *N Engl J Med* 321:501, 1989.

66. Hall P, Colombo A, Itoh A, et al: Gianturco-Roubin stent implantation in small vessels without anticoagulation. *Circulation* 92:I-795, 1995.

67. Wong S, Hong M, Chuang Y, et al: The antiplatelet treatment after intravascular ultrasound guided optimal stent expansion (APLAUSE) trial. *Circulation* 92:I-795, 1995.

68. Goods C, Al-Shaibi K, Lyer S, et al: Flexible coil coronary stenting without anticoagulation or intravascular ultrasound: A prospective observational study. *Circulation* 92:I-795, 1995.
69. Brunel P, Jordan C, Fajadet J, et al: Successive steps in the management of coronary stenting. *Circulation* 92:I-87, 1995.
70. Rodriquez J, Fernandez-Jurado A, Dieguez J, et al: Ticlopidine and severe aplastic anemia. *Am J Hematol* 47:332, 1994.
71. Bellavance A: Efficacy of ticlopidine and aspirin for prevention of reversible cerebrovascular events. The Ticlopidine Aspirin Stroke Study. *Stroke* 25:1452, 1994.
72. Page Y, Tardy B, Seni F, et al: Thrombotic thrombocytopenic purpura related to ticlopidine. *Lancet* 337:774, 1991.
73. Schomig A, Schuhlen H, Blasini R, et al: Anticoagulation versus antiplatelet therapy after intracoronary Palmaz-Schatz stent placement. *Circulation* 92:I-280, 1995.
74. Schomig A, Neumann FJ, Kastrati A, et al: A randomized comparison of antiplatelet and anticoagulant therapy after the placement of coronary artery stents. *N Engl J Med* 334:1084, 1996.
75. Leon MB, Baim DS, Popma JJ, et al: A clinical trial comparing three antithrombotic-drug regimens after coronary-artery stenting. *N Engl J Med* 339:1665, 1998.
76. Liu MW, Voorhees WR, Agrawal S, et al: Stratification of the risk of thrombosis after intracoronary stenting for threatened or acute closure complicating coronary balloon angioplasty: A Cook registry study. *Am Heart J* 130:8, 1995.
77. Herrmann HC, Buchbinder M, Clemen MW, et al: Emergent use of balloon-expandable coronary artery stenting for failed percutaneous transluminal coronary angioplasty. *Circulation* 86:812, 1992.
78. Benzuly K, O'Neil W, Gangadharan V, et al: Stenting in acute myocardial infarction (STAMI): Bailout, conditional and planned stents. *J Am Coll Cardiol* 29:456A, 1997.
79. Moussa I, Di Mario C, Di Francesco L, et al: Subacute stent thrombosis and the anticoagulation controversy: Changes in drug therapy, operator technique, and the impact of intravascular ultrasound. *Am J Cardiol* 78:13, 1996.
80. Saito S, Hosokawa FG, Kim K, et al: Primary stent implantation without warfarin in acute myocardial infarction. *J Am Coll Cardiol* 28:74, 1996.
81. Popma JJ, Satler LF, Pichard AD, et al: Vascular complications after balloon and new device angioplasty. *Circulation* 88:1569, 1993.
82. Bartorelli AL, Sganzerla P, Fabbiocchi F, et al: Prompt and safe femoral hemostasis with a collagen device after intracoronary implantation of Palmaz-Schatz stents. *Am Heart J* 130:26, 1995.
83. Ikari Y, Hara K, Tamura T, et al: Luminal loss and site of restenosis after Palmaz-Schatz coronary stent implantation. *Am J Cardiol* 76:117, 1995.
84. Mehan VK, Salzmann C, Kaufmann U, Meier B: Coronary stenting without anticoagulation. *Cathet Cardiovasc Diagn* 34:137, 1995.
85. Mehan VK, Kaufmann U, Urban P, et al: Stenting with the half (disarticulated) Palmaz-Schatz stent. *Cathet Cardiovasc Diagn* 34:122, 1995.
86. Hadjimiltiades S, Gourassas J, Louridas G, Tsifodimos D: Use of half of the Palmaz-Schatz stent in a stent-related dissection. *Cathet Cardiovasc Diagn* 29:35, 1993.

87. Colombo A, Hall P, Thomas J, et al: Initial experience with the disarticulated (one-half) Palmaz-Schatz stent: A technical report. *Cathet Cardiovasc Diagn* 25:304, 1992.

88. Nordrehaug JE, Priestley K, Chronos N, et al: Implantation of half Palmaz-Schatz stents in short aorto-ostial lesions of saphenous vein grafts. *Cathet Cardiovasc Diagn* 29:141, 1993.

89. Iniguez A, Macaya C, Alfonso F, et al: Early angiographic changes of side branches arising from a Palmaz-Schatz stented coronary segment: Results and clinical implications. *J Am Coll Cardiol* 23:911, 1994.

90. Pan M, Medina A, Suarez deLezo J, et al: Follow-up patency of side branches covered by intracoronary Palmaz-Schatz stent. *Am Heart J* 129:436, 1995.

91. Mazur W, Grinstead WC, Hakim AH, et al: Fate of side branches after intracoronary implantation of the Gianturco-Roubin flex-stent for acute or threatened closure after percutaneous transluminal coronary angioplasty. *Am J Cardiol* 74:1207, 1994.

92. Fischman DL, Savage MP, Leon MB, et al: Fate of lesion-related side branches after coronary artery stenting. *J Am Coll Cardiol* 22:1641, 1993.

93. Veldhuijzen FL, Bonnier HJ, Michels HR, et al: Retrieval of undeployed stents from the right coronary artery: Report of two cases. *Cathet Cardiovasc Diagn* 30:245, 1993.

94. Rozenman Y, Burstein M, Hasin Y, Gotsman MS: Retrieval of occluding unexpanded Palmaz-Schatz stent from a saphenous aorto-coronary vein graft. *Cathet Cardiovasc Diagn* 34:159, 1995.

95. Berder V, Bedossa M, Gras D, et al: Retrieval of a lost coronary stent from the descending aorta using a PTCA balloon and biopsy forceps. *Cathet Cardiovasc Diagn* 28:351, 1993.

96. Cishek MB, Laslett L, Gershony G: Balloon catheter retrieval of dislodged coronary artery stents: A novel technique. *Cathet Cardiovasc Diagn* 34:350, 1995.

97. Mohiaddin RH, Roberts RH, Underwood R, Rothman M: Localization of a misplaced coronary artery stent by magnetic resonance imaging. *Clin Cardiol* 18:175, 1995.

98. Eeckhout E, Stauffer JC, Goy JJ: Retrieval of a migrated coronary stent by means of an alligator forceps catheter. *Cathet Cardiovasc Diagn* 30:166, 1993.

99. Foster SK, Garratt KN, Higano ST, Holmes DJ: Retrieval techniques for managing flexible intracoronary stent misplacement. *Cathet Cardiovasc Diagn* 30:63, 1993.

100. Pitney MR, Cumpston N: A solution to the problem of an unexpanded Palmaz-Schatz stent following balloon rupture. *Cathet Cardiovasc Diagn* 24:246, 1991.

101. Rab ST, King Sd, Roubin GS, et al: Coronary aneurysms after stent placement: A suggestion of altered vessel wall healing in the presence of anti-inflammatory agents. *J Am Coll Cardiol* 18:1524, 1991.

102. Gunther HU, Strupp G, Volmar J, et al: [Coronary stent implantation: Infection and abscess with fatal outcome]. *Z Kardiol* 8:521, 1993.

CHAPTER 8

Coronary Atherectomy Devices

RAINER HOFFMANN, MD

Although percutaneous transluminal coronary angioplasty (PTCA), also known as *balloon angioplasty,* is a highly safe and effective procedure, significant limitations do exist.[1-3] These may result in immediate or long-term failure of PTCA. The main reasons for immediate failure are occlusive dissections and abrupt closure. Restenosis accounts for a 30% to 50% long-term failure rate.[4-8]

Balloon angioplasty enlarges the lumen by splitting and shifting the atherosclerotic plaque and stretching the coronary vessel (Fig 8-1).[9,10] However, because plaque material is not removed by this procedure, acute recoil and chronic remodeling of the artery result in renarrowing or restenosis. Furthermore, it has been proved that the greater the plaque burden at the treatment site, the higher the risk of subsequent restenosis.[11]

These findings led to the development of new devices that (a) remove atherosclerotic plaque in hopes of obtaining a larger and smoother lumen free of dissection planes and that (b) exert less trauma to the deeper components of the arterial vessel wall. Thus, less intimal hyperplasia with subsequent decreased lumen loss and a lower restenosis rate was anticipated.

This chapter reviews atherectomy devices, including directional, rotational atherectomy, transluminal extraction, and excimer laser angioplasty.

♥ Directional Atherectomy

The directional coronary atherectomy (DCA) catheter was approved by the Food and Drug Administration (FDA) for the treatment of coronary artery disease in 1991 as the first non–balloon interventional device. Its side-cutting head can be directed toward the area of the vessel wall with

135

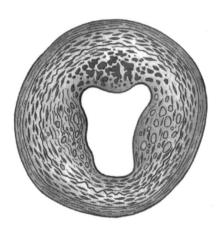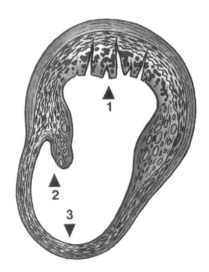

FIGURE 8–1 Cross-section of a coronary artery before **(left)** and after **(right)** successful percutaneous transluminal coronary angioplasty (PTCA). The lumen is enlarged by fissuring of the plaque (*1*), separation of the plaque from the underlying layers (*2*), and stretching of the less diseased portion of the artery (*3*). (From Landau C, Lange RA, Hillis LD: Medical progress: Percutaneous transluminal coronary angioplasty. *N Engl J Med* 330:981, 1994. Copyright 1994 Massachusetts Medical Society. All rights reserved.)

the thickest atherosclerotic plaque by rotating the shaft of the catheter. The term directional atherectomy resulted from this ability to orient the cutting device toward the thickest plaque accumulation. By debulking the obstructive tissue, a large smooth lumen is created (Fig. 8-2).

The Simpson coronary AtheroCath (SCA) is available in sizes from 5 French (F) to 7F. There are presently three generations of AtheroCath, of which the newer designs address some of the limitations of the earlier models. The nose-cone design has been improved for gentler passage through the coronary vessel; the redesigned shaft provides better support and torque control. However, the basic design has not been changed. All

FIGURE 8–2 The principle of directional atherectomy for lumen enlargement. **(A)** The Simpson coronary AtheroCath device is placed within the stenotic lesion. **(B)** The balloon is inflated pushing the housing window against the lesion. **(C)** The plaque protruding into the housing window is excised by the rotating cup-shaped cutter. The cutting head is rotated, and multiple cuts are performed. **(D)** The excised plaque material is stored in the distal collecting chamber. **(E)** After directional atherectomy. (From Baim DS: Percutaneous transluminal coronary angioplasty and newer treatments for coronary heart disease. In Willerson JT (ed): *Treatment of Heart Diseases*. London, Gower Medical Publishing. Copyright 1992, Gower Medical Publishing.)

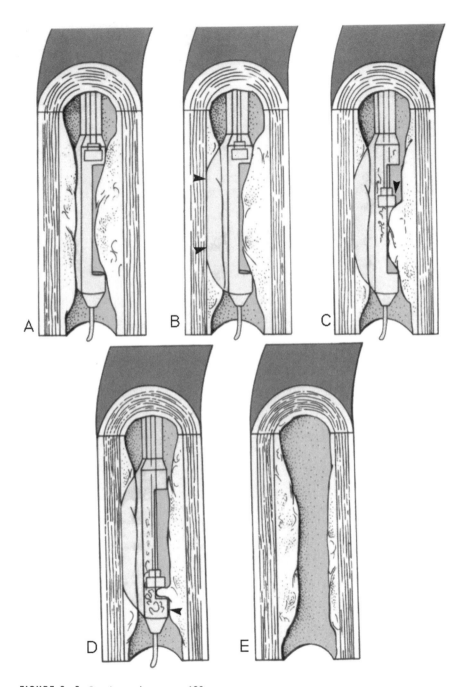

FIGURE 8—2 See legend on page 136.

three versions contain a flexible nose cone, cutter housing, cylindrical cutter, torque tube, support balloon, catheter shaft, and battery-operated motor drive unit.

TECHNIQUE

The cylindrical cutter housing has an eccentric, longitudinal window occupying a 120-degree arc on one side. The window is directed by the operator toward the atherosclerotic plaque. The support balloon is attached outside the cutter housing opposite to the cutting window. Its inflation results in plaque being pushed into the cutter housing. The cup-shaped cutter can be moved manually by a lever located along the window of the cutter housing while it is rotated at 2000 rpm by the motor drive unit by a torque cable. The excised atheroma is stored in the distal nose-cone collection chamber.

The high profile of the rigid housing demands guiding catheters with large lumens and no acute bends. Thus, special guiding catheters that are more rigid than analogous angioplasty guiding catheters have been designed for use of the DCA device. Guiding catheter manipulation has to be done with special care to avoid ostial dissections. Soft tip wires are used to cross the lesion in a standard fashion to prevent vessel trauma. However, stiffer wires with more shaft support may be useful if the passage of the atherectomy device into the coronary artery is difficult. Advancement of the SCA into the vessel should always be done with gentle pressure and with constant rotating movements. Predilatation of the coronary lesion with an undersized balloon may be helpful to allow passage through the coronary stenosis with the atherectomy device. Otherwise, a smaller or shorter cutter device might be used.

After the cutter housing is positioned across the coronary lesion, the cutter window is oriented toward the atherosclerotic plaque. Initially, the balloon is inflated to 10 to 15 pounds per square inch (psi) to press the device against the opposite wall to the balloon, thereby forcing the plaque to invaginate into the window of the cutter housing. The cutter head, which until this point has been kept in the forward position of the housing, is now pulled back into its backward position, and cutter head rotation is started by the motor drive. The cutter is then advanced from the backward to the forward position. Plaque that is cut is pushed forward into the nose-cone collection chamber. The balloon is deflated, and the cutter housing is rotated slightly before the balloon is inflated again. Only then is the cutter head retracted to prevent embolization of plaque material from the collection chamber. After approximately 10 cuts, the AtheroCath is removed and emptied. If the wire mobility is lost or the cutter head cannot be advanced to the end of the cutter housing, the collection chamber is full and should be emptied.

DCA produces a smoother endoluminal surface with distinct cuts in the plaque compared with the dissected surface after balloon angioplasty. If the angiographic result after several cuts at low balloon pressure is inadequate, additional cuts at higher balloon pressures (up to 50 psi) may be performed. If these additional cuts still do not result in an adequate final result, a larger atherectomy device, additional balloon angioplasty, or stent placement may be performed. A residual angiographic diameter stenosis of 0% to 15 % compared with the reference vessel segment is ideal. Using intravascular ultrasound–guided directional atherectomy, a residual plaque burden (plaque/vessel area) of less than 50% should be obtained.

The mechanism of lumen enlargement has been studied in detail by intravascular ultrasound studies. Matar and colleagues[12] demonstrated that 75% of the luminal improvement after DCA is due to tissue removal, whereas the remaining 25% is due to Dotter effect and vessel stretching similar to that produced by balloon angioplasty.

DCA provides a unique opportunity for obtaining atherosclerotic vascular tissue from peripheral and coronary arteries. Histologic analysis of the vascular tissue allows an assessment of the content of the atherosclerotic tissue. De novo lesions consist primarily of fibrosis, calcium, thrombus, necrotic material, cholesterol, and foam cells. There is a higher incidence of mural thrombus and plaque hemorrhage in unstable angina compared with stable angina.[13] Restenotic lesions consist of mural thrombus and plaque hyperplasia.[14]

INDICATIONS

Indications for DCA include the following:

1. Ostial lesions. DCA has been successfully used for noncalcified ostial lesions of large vessels, particularly for lesions of the left anterior descending (LAD) ostium. In these lesions, balloon angioplasty frequently results in suboptimal results, whereas DCA has a procedural success rate exceeding 85%.[15]

2. Eccentric lesions. The directional control allowing atherectomy plaque removal from one side of the vessel circumference is unique, and DCA may be ideal for eccentric lesions. A high success rate (95%) has been reported for lesions with an angiographic appearance of plaque mass on only one side.[16] However, intravascular ultrasound studies have demonstrated that the angiographic appear-

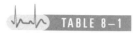

TABLE 8–1

Procedural Results After Directional Coronary Atherectomy

Study	Number of Lesions	Procedure Success	Final DS	In-Hospital Outcomes (Death MI, CABG, Abrupt Closure)
BOAT[21]	497	99%	15%	2.8%
CAVEAT-I[18]	512	89%	29%	11%
CCAT[20]	138	94%	25%	5%
OARS[22]	213	98%	7%	2.5%

DS, diameter of stenosis; MI, myocardial infarction; CABG, coronary artery bypass grafting; BOAT, Balloon Versus Optimal Atherectomy Trial; CAVEAT, Coronary Angioplasty Versus Directional Atherectomy; CCAT, Canadian Coronary Atherectomy Trial; OARS, Optimal Atherectomy Restenosis Study.

ance and the actual distribution of plaque mass may be totally different.[17] Thus, angiography may be misleading for the direction of the DCA device, whereas intravascular ultrasound imaging may be helpful in directing the window of the cutting head toward the thickest atherosclerotic plaque.

3. Bifurcation lesions. Balloon angioplasty of bifurcation lesions is frequently complicated by "shifting plaque" with subsequent occlusion or compromise of a side branch. DCA avoids the shifting of plaque. In CAVEAT-I (Coronary Angioplasty Versus Excisional Atherectomy Trial), DCA had a higher success rate (88% compared with 74%, $P < 0.001$) for bifurcation lesions than balloon angioplasty, but resulted in more ischemic complications (9.5% compared with 3.7%, $P < 0.01$).

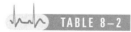

TABLE 8–2

Procedural Results After Directional Coronary Atherectomy in Vein Grafts

Study	Number of Lesions	Procedure Success	Final DS	In-Hospital Death	In-Hospital Q-Wave MI	In-Hospital CABG
CAVEAT-II[19]	149	89%	32%	2.0%	1.3%	0.7%
Cowley*	363	86%		0.9%	1.3%	0.9%

DS, diameter of stenosis; CABG, coronary artery bypass graft; MI, myocardial infarction.
*Data from Cowley MJ, et al: Directional coronary atherectomy of saphenous vein graft narrowings. *Am J Cardiol* 72:30E, 1993.

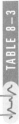

TABLE 8–3

Comparison of Acute and Follow-Up Results of Directional Coronary Atherectomy (DCA) and Percutaneous Transluminal Coronary Angioplasty (PTCA)

	BOAT[19]			CAVEAT[18]			CCAT[20]		
	DCA (%) (n = 497)	PTCA (%) (n = 492)	P	DCA (%) (n = 512)	PTCA (%) (n = 500)	P	DCA (%) (n = 138)	PTCA (%) (n = 136)	P
Success	99	97	0.02	82	76	0.016	94	88	0.061
Final DS	15	28	<0.0001	29	36	<0.001	25	33	<0.0001
Abrupt closure				7	3	0.1914	4.3	5.1	0.98
Major complication	2.8	3.3	0.72	5	4.4	0.06	2.1	4.4	
Follow-up restenosis rate*	31.4	39.8	0.016	50	57	0.41	46	43	0.71
Follow-up TLR*	15.3	18.3	0.23	36.5	37.2	0.49	28.3	26.4	
Follow-up EFS*			ns	63	60		71	71	1.0

BOAT, Balloon Versus Optimal Atherectomy Trial; CAVEAT, Coronary Angioplasty Versus Excisional Atherectomy Trial; CCAT, Canadian Coronary Atherectomy Trial; DS, diameter of stenosis; TLR, target lesion revascularization; EFS, event-free survival.
*Follow-up period was 6 months in CAVEAT and CCAT and 1 year in BOAT.

PROCEDURAL SUCCESS

The results of DCA have been studied in several single and multicenter studies (Tables 8-1 and 8-2). The success rate of DCA has been reported to be about 90%. This rate improves with increased operator experience.

Five major randomized studies compared acute and follow-up results of DCA with balloon angioplasty for treatment of native vessels and saphenous vein grafts: the Coronary Angioplasty Versus Excisional Atherectomy Trials (CAVEAT) I[18] and II,[19] the Canadian Coronary Atherectomy Trial (CCAT),[20] the Balloon Versus Optimal Atherectomy (BOAT) Trial,[21] and the "Optimal" Directional Coronary Atherectomy (OARS) Study.[22] In each study, DCA resulted in better immediate lumen enlargement and higher procedural success (Table 8-3). However, DCA was associated with a trend to a higher procedural complication rate, especially regarding the rate of non–Q-wave myocardial infarctions.

COMPLICATIONS

Abrupt vessel closure during the procedure or immediately thereafter has been reported in 0% to 7% of cases. In CAVEAT-I, abrupt closure occurred in 7% of cases, 42% at a site other than the target lesion indicating guiding catheter or atherectomy device related trauma. In the Optimal Atherectomy Restenosis Study (OARS),[23] abrupt closure rate was only 1%. In a series of 1020 DCA procedures in the US Directional Atherectomy Investigator Group Registry, abrupt vessel closure was encountered in 4.2% of patients and was attributed to thrombosis in 51.5%, dissections in 30.3%, and guide catheter dissections in 9.3%.

Abrupt vessel closure is associated with a significant increase in procedure-related myocardial infarction and mortality. Treatment of abrupt closure usually requires coronary stenting. Other treatment options involve immediate coronary artery bypass surgery (CABG) or additional medical therapy. In addition to abrupt closure, other less common complications are encountered. Thrombus formation after DCA complicates 2% of DCA procedures.

Distal embolization causing no flow in the target vessel beyond the original target lesion has been reported in up to 13.4%. Such embolization is a complication more frequently observed when the target lesion is in saphenous vein graft, owing to the frequent presence in such conduits of loose friable atherothrombotic debris. After DCA, the incidence of vessel perforation is less than 1%. Perforations resulting in hemopericardium or tamponade are very rare, occurring in less than 0.1%. Milder forms of perforation may result in focal ectasia and pseudoaneurysms.

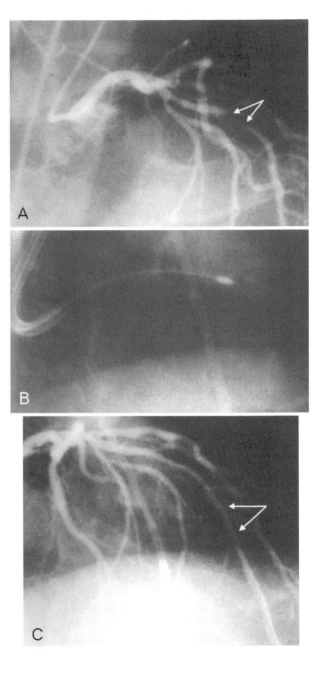

FIGURE 8-3 (A) Rotational atherectomy of a mid left anterior descending (LAD) coronary lesion (*arrows*). **(B)** Burr crossing the lesion. **(C)** Final angiographic result.

CONTRAINDICATIONS

Contraindications to DCA include small vessel size, lesion calcification, lesion angulation, proximal tortuosity of the vessel, and lesion length. Popma and colleagues[24] studied the clinical, angiographic, and procedural factors affecting angiographic results after directional angiography. Heavy calcification was found to be the most powerful predictor for a procedural failure. In an intravascular ultrasound study, lesion calcification was also found to be a major adverse predictor for luminal gain after DCA.[25]

FOLLOW-UP OUTCOME/RESTENOSIS

Restenosis rates of 25% to 58% have been reported after DCA. Comparison of restenosis rates between PTCA and DCA in CAVEAT and BOAT as well as the CCAT study demonstrated similar restenosis and event-free survival rates (see Table 8-3).[18–20]

♡ Rotational Atherectomy

PTCA has been shown to have significant shortcomings in specific lesion types. Heavily calcified lesions may not dilate at all and are associated with a high rate of dissection.[7] Lesions in the aorto-ostial location are frequently fibrotic and may immediately recoil. Thus, an interventional device such as rotational atherectomy, which ablates plaque material instead of stretching the vessel is desirable.

TECHNIQUE

Percutaneous rotational atherectomy (Rotablator™) uses a high-speed (160 to 190,000 rpm) metal burr coated with diamond chips to abrade and pulverize atheromatous plaque into fine microparticles (5-10 μm in size) (Fig. 8-3). Unlike other devices, rotational atherectomy removes harder, calcific-fibrous atherosclerotic plaque while deflecting more elastic, normal tissue. In vitro studies[26,27] showed that the damage to normal arterial wall was largely confined to the intima without evidence of medial dissection, whereas noncompliant plaque material, especially calcium, was selectively removed. The resulting vessel surface after rotational atherectomy is smooth, shiny, and polished.

The use of intravascular ultrasound after rotational atherectomy has confirmed that the plaque lumen surface is smooth, especially in calcified plaque and that a cylindrical lumen results.[28] The ratio of lumen to burr size is greater than 1 because of nonaxial rotation of the burr. The ratio is larger in calcified vessels because such arteries do not recoil. Thus, rotational atherectomy causes lumen enlargement by ablation of atherosclerotic plaque and not arterial expansion. Dissections were reported to occur in only 26% to 32% of lesions after pure rotational atherectomy by intravascular ultrasound.[28,29] This is in sharp contrast to findings after balloon angioplasty of highly calcified lesions that show dissections in up to 100% of instances.

Because most rotational atherectomy burrs are small in relation to the target vessel, adjunctive therapy is normally required to obtain an adequate procedural result. Balloon angioplasty has frequently been used to further enlarge the lumen. Kovach and associates[29] evaluated the effect of additional balloon angioplasty using intravascular ultrasound, finding that adjunct balloon angioplasty results in a further increase in lumen area by a combination of arterial dissection and arterial expansion, especially of the compliant, noncalcified plaque elements. However, even after additional balloon angioplasty, residual diameter stenosis remains significant in a number of patients.[30] Thus, other device synergies have been applied to obtain a larger final angiographic result. DCA as well as stent therapy has been used with rotational atherectomy. The combination of Rotablator followed by stent implantation has been shown to result in a larger acute angiographic result, as well as a lower follow-up event rate.[31]

The rotational atherectomy device consists of a control console that allows adjustment of the rotational speed; a turbine system that receives compressed air from the control console; a flexible drive shaft; and an olive-shaped, nickel-plated, brass burr, coated with micron-sized diamond chips at the tip of the drive shaft. The turbine system is controlled by the control console and activated by a foot pedal. The control console contains a monitor of the rotational speed by means of a fiberoptic tachometer. The drive shaft is enclosed in a flexible Teflon sheath. It protects the vessel wall from the inner rotating drive shaft and provides a conduit for a constant saline flush to cool the burr tip. Rotational atherectomy burrs are available in diameters of 1.25 to 2.5 mm. The Rotablator burrs are forwarded over a specially designed 0.009-inch stainless-steel Rotablator guidewire. Floppy and stiff distal tips are available, which are 0.017-inch thick and radiopaque. The burr cannot be advanced over this thicker diameter tip.

After placement of the guidewire tip in the distal coronary artery, the burr-drive shaft unit is advanced over the wire just proximal to the coronary stenosis. While infusing saline flush through the sheath, the rotating burr is advanced slowly through the lesion using a control knob on the top of the turbine system-advancer unit. Rotablator speed should be set, depending on the burr size, between 160,000 and 200,000 rpm with higher speeds used for smaller burrs. The Rotablator speed is adjusted proximal to the lesion in the platform segment and is called the *platform speed*. The Rotablator speed should be controlled during burr advancement to prevent a fall by more than 5000 rpm below the platform speed during forceful push of the burr, because this might create larger microparticles with potentially more harm to the left ventricular function in the dependent myocardial perfusion bed and a greater risk of vessel trauma.

Initial burr size selection depends on whether a one-burr or two-burr approach is selected. A two-burr approach normally starts with a burr size slightly larger than the minimal lumen diameter of the lesion, with the second burr aiming at a burr-to-artery ratio of 0.75 to 0.8. With a one-burr approach, a slightly larger initial burr size might be selected. The burr is advanced to a platform position, where it must have unimpeded rotation. This decreases the risk of vessel trauma from burr injury due to vessel wall contact while activating the system. Free flow of contrast around the burr confirms adequate positioning.

Vessel spasm and slow-flow or no-reflow phenomenon occur in up to 15% of cases. Adenosine, verapamil, and nitroglycerin have been administered to reduce the incidence of this problem or reverse it. Adequate hydration of the patient and preprocedure administration of calcium channel blockers have also been recommended to reduce the occurrence of vasospasm.

The application of rotational atherectomy may be accompanied by development of severe bradyarrhythmias or even heart block, especially if the target lesion is a dominant right coronary or dominant left circumflex artery. The bradycardia usually lasts 5 to 60 seconds after termination of rotational atherectomy. Insertion of a temporary pacemaker is warranted for lesions in which a high incidence of bradyarrhythmias can be anticipated.

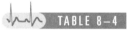 **TABLE 8-4**

Procedural Results After Rotational Atherectomy

Series	No. of Lesions	Procedure Success (%)	Final DS (%)	Death (%)	Q-Wave MI (%)	CABG (%)
Warth[33]	874	94.7		0.8	0.9	1.7
MacIsaac[38]	2161	94.5	22	0.8	0.7	2.0
Ellis*	400	89.9	27	0.3	0.9	0.9
Safian†	116	95.2	30	1.0	4.8	1.9

DS, diameter of stenosis; CABG, coronary artery bypass graft; MI, myocardial infarction.
*Ellis SG, et al: Relation of clinical presentation, stenosis morphology, and operator technique to the procedural results of rotational atherectomy and rotational artherectomy-facilitated angioplasty. *Circulation* 89:882, 1994.
†Safian RD, et al: Detailed angiographic analysis of high-speed mechanical rotational atherectomy in human coronary arteries. *Circulation* 88:961, 1993.

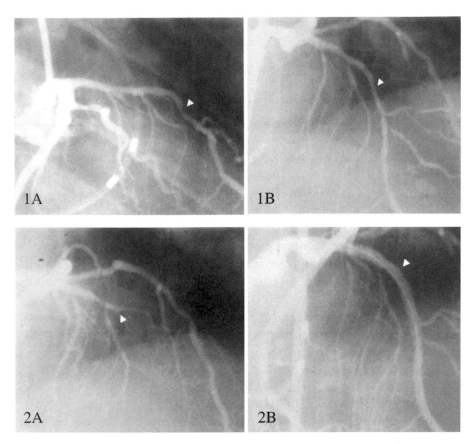

FIGURE 8–4 Mid left anterior descending lesion before **(1A)** and after **(1B)** successful rotational atherectomy. Several hours later, the patient developed chest pain with typical ischemic electrocardiographic changes in the precordial leads. A repeat catheterization revealed abrupt closure of the treated site **(2A)**, which was successfully treated with a stent **(2B)**.

INDICATIONS

1. Calcified lesions. Because it abrades the arterial plaque, rotational atherectomy is the device of choice for heavily calcified stenoses, lesions for which balloon angioplasty and directional atherectomy have been shown to have unsatisfactory results. Success rates of 82% and 94% have been reported for this type of plaque.[32,33]

2. Ostial lesions. Aorto-ostial lesions are frequently heavily calcified or of a fibrotic-elastic nature, characteristics associated with an unfavorable result after balloon angioplasty because of high rates of dissection, acute occlusion, or restenosis. Rotational atherectomy, by

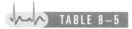

TABLE 8–5

Follow-Up Results After Rotational Atherectomy

Series	Number of Lesions	Restenosis Rate (%)
Warth[33]	874	38
Vandormael[55]	215	62

ablating plaque material, effectively treats ostial lesions with a high success rate (96%) and an acceptable restenosis rate (40%).[34]

3. Lesion length. A success rate of 92% has been reported for rotational atherectomy in the multicenter registry for lesions 15 to 25 mm in length. However, after Rotablator in long lesions, left ventricular wall motion abnormalities increase, mortality increases, and rate of restenosis increases.[35] Thus, judicious case selection is required in this setting. It is reasonable to use rotational atherectomy in patients with well-preserved left ventricular function in whom other devices are not applicable. However, rotational atherectomy should be used very carefully in patients with long lesions and a poor ventricular function.

4. In-stent restenosis. Recently, rotational atherectomy has been recommended for treatment of in-stent restenosis with a better acute procedural result than balloon angioplasty.[36] The immediate and long-term effect of the Rotablator on the metallic stent is unclear at this time.

SUCCESS

Several small studies indicated a high procedural success rate for rotational atherectomy.[37–39] Moreover, data from a multicenter registry including 3424 patients demonstrated that rotational atherectomy has a high success rate even in complex lesions.[40] Thus, a high success rate could be obtained even in lesions deemed to have suboptimal results with balloon angioplasty (Table 8-4).

COMPLICATIONS

Despite concern about the myocardial effects of microparticle embolization, major in-hospital complications such as death, myocardial infarction, abrupt closure, and the need for CABG are infrequent with rotational atherectomy (see Table 8-4) (Fig. 8-4). Teirstein and associates[35] did report on a small subgroup of patients who developed severe wall-motion abnormalities after treatment of very long lesions. However, other studies did not confirm these findings, suggesting that rotational atherectomy has little deleterious effect on myocardial function if short segments are treated.[37,38,41,42]

"Coronary no-reflow," presumed to occur as the sequela of distal microparticle embolization, is a significant complication. This phenomenon is not a mechanical problem and therefore cannot be corrected with a mechanical device, such as another Rotablator or stent. Fortunately, it is a transient phenomenon, which usually resolves over a period of 5 to 15 minutes. A less significant version of no-reflow is "slow-reflow," associated also with symptoms and electrocardiographic evidence of ischemia. Microembolization might also cause microinfarction with resulting creatine phosphokinase (CPK) elevation. Data of a multicenter registry[42] indicated that CPK elevations more than 1.5 times normal occurred in 8.5% of patients and occurred most frequently when long lesions were treated and in patients who developed abrupt closure and coronary spasm.

The risk of coronary artery injury has been addressed in several studies. Satler and Warth,[43] analyzing a multicenter registry, found that eccentric lesions, lesions in tortuous vessels, and long lesions are at increased risk of undergoing dissection. In addition, Leon and colleagues[32] found that calcified lesions had a dissection rate of 10.5% compared with 5.1% for noncalcified lesions.

In summary, lesion length increases the risk of myocardial dysfunction and coronary dissection, whereas lesion eccentricity and lesion calcification increase the risk of dissection.

CONTRAINDICATIONS

Rotational atherectomy should be undertaken with caution in patients with severe left ventricular dysfunction because further compromise of myocardial function can occur and produce left ventricular failure. Rotational atherectomy should not be used in the presence of visible thrombus in the target artery. Lesions in saphenous vein grafts are also a contraindication for the use of rotational atherectomy. In both of the latter situations, friable debris or thrombus material results in a considerable risk of distal embolization with subsequent adverse effects.

FOLLOW-UP OUTCOME/RESTENOSIS

Restenosis rates of up to 62% have been reported after rotational atherectomy. Long lesions and noncalcified lesions seem to be predictors of higher restenosis rates (Table 8-5).

❤ Transluminal Extraction Atherectomy

Balloon angioplasty increases luminal dimensions by stretching the coronary artery. It does not reduce the amount of plaque material. The transluminal extraction catheter (TEC) increases luminal dimensions by cutting plaque material and aspirating it. The system consists of a conical cutting head with two stainless-steel blades bound to the distal end of a hollow flexible torque tube. Attached to the proximal end of the hollow lumen are suction bottles that collect the excised material. Also attached to the proximal end of the catheter is a battery-powered motor drive unit, which rotates the cutting blade and activates aspiration. The cutting head can be advanced and retracted by an external lever. A stainless-steel guidewire designed for the TEC device is passed in the central lumen of the cutting device. The guidewire has a radiopaque floppy tip with a terminal ball that prevents wire tip entrapment or advancement of the cutting blades beyond the guidewire. The stiffer proximal part of the wire ensures that the cutting device keeps a central position in the artery.

Cutter heads of 5.5 to 7.5F are available. The cutting blades are rotated at 750 rpm from the external motor drive unit. Special TEC guiding catheters are available from 8 to 10F. Because of the stiffness of these guiding catheters, special care must be taken not to induce vessel injury while engaging the coronary ostium.

TECHNIQUE

The selected cutter head size is normally 1 mm smaller than the reference vessel diameter to obtain a cutter-to-artery ratio of 0.5 to 0.7. The TEC cutter is positioned just proximal to the lesion. Pressurized flush is turned on, and the TEC cutter is activated and advanced slowly through the lesion (1 mm/3 sec). During advancement of the cutter, a continuous stream of blood should enter the vacuum bottle to lower the risk of dissection and distal embolization. Depending on the length and the severity of the lesion, five to ten vacuum bottles may be necessary for adequate removal of thrombus and atheroma from the artery. Angioscopy has been used to evaluate thrombus removal after TEC, demonstrating partial or complete thrombus removal in 75% to 100%.[44] Adjunct PTCA, DCA, or stenting should be performed when residual stenosis is significant.

INDICATIONS

The TEC device is indicated for lesions in which thrombus or debris has to be removed from the artery. Thus, TEC has been used with success in

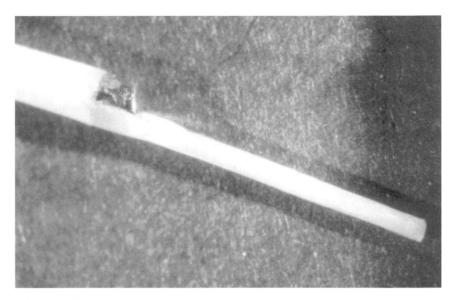

FIGURE 8-5 The directional excimer laser catheter. The eccentric arrangement of fiberoptic wires allows the laser beam to be directed, thus allowing selective ablation of the plaque.

acute ischemic syndromes including acute myocardial infarctions, after failed thrombolysis, and in unstable angina associated with thrombotic lesions. The TEC device has also been successfully used for degenerated saphenous vein grafts that are filled with thrombus and friable debris.

PROCEDURAL SUCCESS

Procedural success after the TEC device has been reported to be 82% to 94%.[45,46] However, adjunct PTCA is required in most patients to enlarge lumen dimensions or manage TEC-induced vessel occlusion.

COMPLICATIONS

Major clinical complications after use of the TEC device include death in 0% to 3.2% of patients, Q-wave myocardial infarction in 0.7% to 3.4%, and emergency coronary bypass in 0.2% to 3.4%.[46-48] Serious angiographic complications include dissections, abrupt closure, coronary artery perforation, distal embolization and no-reflow. Distal embolization and no-reflow occur more frequently after treatment of saphenous vein grafts than in native arteries. Angiographic restenosis occurs in 56% to 69% of patients, higher for vein graft lesions.

CONTRAINDICATIONS

Contraindications to the use of the TEC device include moderate to heavily calcified lesions, severely angulated lesions, highly eccentric lesions, bifurcation lesions, lesions in vessels smaller than 2.5 mm in diameter, and dissections.

FOLLOW-UP OUTCOME/RESTENOSIS

Restenosis rates after transluminal extraction atherectomy have been reported to be as high as 61% for native vessels. Safian and associates[48] reported an event rate of 29% after transluminal extraction atherectomy.

♥ Coronary Laser Angioplasty

The term *laser* is an acronym for light amplification by the stimulated emission of radiation. Specific properties characterize laser: (a) Laser radiation is monochromatic, which means that it is produced at a single specific wavelength. (b) Laser photons are characterized by spatial and temporal coherence owing to collimation and synchronization of the photons both in space and time. This results in constancy of energy density of the laser beam, regardless of distance to the laser source.

Several laser systems using different active mediums to form the radiation have been described, including solid-state crystals (ruby, Nd:YAG, erbium, holmium, and thulium), liquid (tunable dye), and gas (argon, CO_2, excimer). Laser energy has three types of tissue effect: thermal ablation, photoacoustic ablation, and photodecomposition. Photodecomposi-

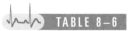 TABLE 8–6

Procedural Results After Excimer Laser Angioplasty

Series	No. of Lesions	Procedure Success (%)	Final DS (%)	Death (%)	Q-Wave MI (%)	CABG (%)
Bittl[51]	215	91.5	14 (n = 21)	0.0	3.5	3.0
Litvack[53]	3592	90.0	17 (n = 24)	0.5	2.1	3.8

DS, diameter of stenosis; CABG, coronary artery bypass graft; MI, myocardial infarction.

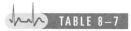

TABLE 8–7

Follow-up Results After Excimer Laser Angioplasty

Series	Number of Lesions	Restenosis Rate (%)
Bittl[50]	858	46
Bittle[51]	215	48

tion (i.e., direct breakage of molecular bond) can produce precise, scalpel-like excision and ablation of tissue.

Only the excimer laser systems have obtained approval for coronary revascularization. Its primary effect is photodecomposition. *Excimer* is an acronym for excited dimer. It is a pulsed laser, meaning that energy is emitted at brief bursts of ultraviolet light separated by relatively long periods of silence, during which laser emission is switched off.

The mechanism by which excimer laser coronary angioplasty enlarges the coronary lumen has been investigated in detail by intravascular ultrasound. Mintz and colleagues[49] found that the lumen cross-sectional area increased by both ablation of atherosclerotic plaque and vessel expansion. In most cases, adjunct therapy after laser therapy is necessary. Most frequently, adjunct balloon angioplasty is used. The mechanism of progressive lumen enlargement after adjunct angioplasty is additional vessel expansion. Intravascular ultrasound did not demonstrate calcium ablation after laser angioplasty. Vessel wall dissections were demonstrated in 39% of lesions.

TECHNIQUE

Concentric excimer laser angioplasty catheters are available in diameters of 1.4, 1.7, and 2.0 mm, and one directional excimer laser catheter, 1.7 mm in size. The catheters have small fibers concentrically arranged around the guidewire lumen. Because of this concentric fiber arrangement, there is a risk of vessel perforation in highly eccentric lesions or bend lesions as the tip of the catheter might be directed into the normal vessel wall. The directional excimer laser catheter has an eccentric fiberoptic arrangement opposite the guidewire lumen (Fig. 8-5). The catheter tip can be rotated. Thus, directional laser therapy should allow more selective ablation of eccentric plaque. Furthermore, because the laser tip can be rotated, a larger final lumen diameter can be achieved.

Laser interventions should be performed using a stiff guiding catheter, which provides coaxial alignment and support. Furthermore, the tip of the guidewire should be kept as distal as possible to have the stiff position of the wire at the lesion side. These precautions decrease the risk of vessel perforation due to guidewire deflection.

The laser beam generated is initially set to provide an energy density of 40 mJ/mm^2 at a frequency of 20 to 25 Hz. If the lesion cannot be crossed with the laser catheter, the laser energy density can be increased to 60 mJ/mm^2, and the frequency can be increased to 30 Hz. The laser catheter should always be in contact with the lesion to reduce the risk of blood vaporization and the subsequent increased risk of vessel trauma.

INDICATIONS

The results of a multicenter trial of 764 patients with 858 coronary stenosis indicate that favorable success rates with excimer laser coronary angioplasty can be achieved for saphenous vein graft lesions, long lesions, ostial lesions, and total occlusions.[50] This same trial also reported favorable outcomes when the excimer laser was used after initial unsuccessful balloon dilatation.[50] These indications are the result of a finding that excimer laser therapy has a higher success rate in saphenous vein graft lesions than in native coronary arteries. Also, lesions larger than 20 mm in length, total occlusions, ostial stenosis, and moderately calcified lesions were treated as successfully as all other lesion types. Successful treatment was also achieved in 15 of 16 patients after unsuccessful balloon angioplasty, and in certain lesions not ideal for balloon angioplasty.[51,52]

The results of the Excimer Laser Coronary Angioplasty Registry on 3000 patients[53] confirmed these findings, showing that excimer laser angioplasty can be safely and effectively applied to aorto-ostial lesions, long lesions, total occlusions crossable with a wire, diffuse disease, and vein grafts.

Excimer laser coronary angioplasty has been successfully applied to in-stent restenosis.[54] Balloon angioplasty has been disappointing for this purpose, and excimer laser tissue ablation was associated with a significantly better acute lumen diameter gain as well as better clinical follow-up outcomes.

PROCEDURAL SUCCESS

In a multicenter study reported by Bittl and associates,[50] successful passage of the laser catheter through a lesion reduced stenosis severity by

20% or more in 79% of lesions, but in only 60% was a residual stenosis of less than 50% achieved after excimer laser alone. Adjunctive balloon angioplasty, was used in 83% of lesions to achieve an optimal result. In 657 of 764 patients (86%) clinical success, defined as 50% or less residual-diameter stenosis and no major complications (death, Q-wave or non–Q-wave myocardial infarction, abrupt vessel closure, repeat PTCA, or need for bypass surgery at any time during hospitalization) was obtained (Table 8-6).

COMPLICATIONS

Initial reports from a multicenter study showed that major complications after excimer laser angioplasty (myocardial infarction, need for coronary bypass surgery, and death) occurred in 7.6%.[50] Further complications reported in this first multicenter report were dissections (18%), significant perforation of the vessel (1%), spasm (5.2%), abrupt closure (5.4%), embolization (1.4%), and aneurysm formation (0.2%). Treatment of bifurcation lesions was associated with an increased risk of acute complications. Further predictors of acute complications were multivessel disease and calcified lesions.

The results of a larger multicenter study of 3000 patients had similar complication rates with necessity for in-hospital bypass surgery in 3.8%, Q-wave myocardial infarction in 2.1%, and death in 0.5%.[53] Coronary artery perforation occurred in 1% of lesions, angiographic dissections in 13%, transient occlusions in 3.4%, and sustained occlusion in 3.1%.

The incidence of frequently occurring vessel dissections after laser angioplasty can be lowered by the use of saline injections into the coronary artery via the guiding catheter directly before laser application. A commonly recommended practice is to inject a 10-mL bolus of saline via the guide catheter and continue a slow injection at 1 to 3 mL per second during each lasing run. The laser catheter should be advanced at 1 mm per second.

CONTRAINDICATIONS

Contraindications for application of excimer laser angioplasty are bifurcation lesions, highly eccentric lesions, severe lesion angulation, vessel tortuosity, and prior dissections. Each of these lesion characteristics is associated with an increased risk for subsequent vessel perforation after application of the laser device.[55]

FOLLOW-UP OUTCOME/RESTENOSIS

The angiographic restenosis rate is 40% to 50% with a clinical event rate of 20% to 30% at 6-month follow-up. However, these data have to be seen in context of the relatively unfavorable lesion morphology for which excimer laser angioplasty has been used (Table 8-7).

♥ Conclusion

Although the devices described in this chapter do not improve the restenosis rate after transcatheter procedures, each has specific applications with regard to the characteristics of the lesions being treated. These devices make possible successful transcatheter treatment of stenoses with characteristics that make them unsuitable for balloon angioplasty. Use of these devices for plaque mass reduction (debulking) before stenting is often a particularly attractive option.[56]

REFERENCES

1. Faxon DP, Kelsey SF, Ryan TJ, et al: Determinants of successful percutaneous transluminal coronary angioplasty: Report from the National Heart, Lung, and Blood Institute Registry. *Am Heart J* 108:1019, 1984.
2. Tan K, Sulke N, Taub N, Sowton E: Clinical and lesion morphologic determinants of coronary angioplasty success and complications: Current experience. *J Am Coll Cardiol* 25:855, 1995.
3. Detre K, Holubkov R, Kelsey SF, et al: Percutaneous transluminal coronary angioplasty in 1985–86 and 1977–81: The National Heart, Lung, and Blood Institute Registry. *N Engl J Med* 318:265, 1988.
4. Gruentzig AR, King SB III, Schlumpf M, Siegenthaler W: Long-term follow-up after percutaneous transluminal coronary angioplasty: The early Zurich experience. *N Engl J Med* 316:1127, 1987.
5. Leimgruber PP, Roubin GS, Hollman J, et al: Restenosis after successful coronary angioplasty in patients with single-vessel disease. *Circulation* 73:710, 1986.
6. Hirshfeld JW Jr, Schwartz JS, Jugo R, et al: Restenosis after coronary angioplasty: A multivariate statistical model to relate lesion and procedure variables to restenosis. *J Am Coll Cardiol* 18:647, 1991.
7. Ellis S, Roubin G, King S, et al: Angiographic and clinical predictors of acute closure after native vessel coronary angioplasty. *Circulation* 77:372, 1988.
8. Lincoff AM, Popma JJ, Ellis SG, et al: Abrupt vessel closure complicating coronary angioplasty: Clinical, angiographic and therapeutic profile. *J Am Coll Cardiol* 19:926, 1992.
9. Landau C, Lange RA, Hillis LD: Percutaneous transluminal coronary angioplasty. *N Engl J Med* 330:981, 1994.
10. Gravanis MB, Roubin GS: Histopathologic phenomena at the site of percutaneous transluminal coronary angioplasty: The problem of restenosis. *Hum Pathol* 20:477, 1989.

11. Mintz GS, Popma JJ, Pichard AD, et al: Intravascular ultrasound predictors of restenosis after percutaneous transcatheter coronary revascularization. *J Am Coll Cardiol* 27:1678, 1996.
12. Matar FA, Mintz GS, Farb A, et al: The contribution of tissue removal to lumen improvement after directional coronary atherectomy. *Am J Cardiol* 74:647, 1994.
13. Rosenschild U, Ellis S, Haudenschild C, et al: Comparison of histopathologic coronary lesions obtained from directional atherectomy in stable angina versus acute coronary syndromes. *Am J Cardiol* 73:508, 1994.
14. Miller M, Kuntz R, Friedrich S, et al: Frequency and consequences of intimal hyperplasia in specimens retrieved by directional atherectomy of native primary coronary artery stenoses and subsequent restenoses. *Am J Cardiol* 71:652, 1993.
15. Stephan W, Bates E, Garratt K, et al: Directional atherectomy of coronary and saphenous vein graft ostial stenoses. *Am J Cardiol* 75:1015, 1995.
16. Hinohara T, Rowe M, Robertson, et al: Directional atherectomy for the treatment of coronary lesions with abnormal contour. *J Invas Cardiol* 2:57, 1990.
17. Mintz GS, Popma JJ, Pichard AD, et al: Limitations of angiography in the assessment of plaque distribution in coronary artery disease. *Circulation* 93:924, 1996.
18. Topol EJ, Leya F, Pinkerton CA, et al: A comparison of directional atherectomy with coronary angioplasty in patients with coronary artery disease: The CAVEAT Study Group. *N Engl J Med* 329:221, 1993.
19. Holmes DR, Topol EJ, Califf RM, et al: A multicenter, randomized trial of coronary angioplasty versus directional atherectomy for patients with saphenous vein bypass graft lesions. CAVEAT II. *Circulation* 91:1966, 1995.
20. Adelman AG, Cohen EA, Kimball BP, et al: A comparison of directional atherectomy with balloon angioplasty for lesions of the left anterior descending coronary artery. CCAT. *N Engl J Med* 329:228, 1993.
21. Baim DS, Cutlip DE, Sharma S, et al: Final results of the Balloon vs Optimal Atherectomy Trial (BOAT). *Circulation* 97:322, 1998.
22. Simonton CA, Leon MB, Baim DS, et al: 'Optimal' directional coronary atherectomy: Final results of the Optimal Atherectomy Restenosis Study (OARS). *Circulation* 97:332, 1998.
23. Lansky A, Mintz GS, Popma JJ, et al: Remodeling after directional coronary atherectomy (with and without adjunct percutaneous transluminal coronary angioplasty): A serial angiographic and intravascular ultrasound analysis from the Optimal Atherectomy Restenosis Study (OARS). *J Am Coll Cardiol* 32:329, 1998.
24. Popma JJ, Decesare NB, Ellis SG, et al: Clinical angiographic and procedural correlates of quantitative coronary dimensions following directional coronary atherectomy. *J Am Coll Cardiol* 18:1183, 1991.
25. Matar FA, Mintz GS, Pinnow E, et al: Multivariate predictors of intravascular ultrasound end points after directional coronary atherectomy. *J Am Coll Cardiol* 25:318, 1995.
26. Fourrier JL, Stankowiak C, Lablanche JM, et al: Histopathology after rotational angioplasty of peripheral arteries in human beings (abstr). *J Am Coll Cardiol* 11(Suppl):109A, 1988.

27. Ahn S, Auth DC, Marcud D: Removal of focal atheromatous lesions by angiographically guided high-speed rotary atherectomy. *J Vasc Surg* 7:292, 1988.
28. Mintz GS, Potkin BN, Keren G, et al: Intravascular ultrasound evaluation of the effect of rotational atherectomy in obstructive atherosclerotic coronary artery disease. *Circulation* 86:1383, 1992.
29. Kovach JA, Mintz GS, Pichard AD, et al: Sequential intravascular ultrasound characterization of the mechanisms of rotational atherectomy and adjunct balloon angioplasty. *J Am Coll Cardiol* 22:1024, 1993.
30. MacIsaac A, Whitlow P, Cowley M, et al: Angiographic predictors of outcome of coronary rotational atherectomy from the completed multicenter registry. *J Am Coll Cardiol* 23:353A, 1994.
31. Hoffmann R, Mintz GS, Kent KM, et al: Is there an optimal therapy for calcified lesions in large vessels? Comparative acute and follow-up results of rotational atherectomy, stents, or the combination. *J Am Coll Cardiol* 29:68A, 1997.
32. Leon M, Kent K, Pichard A, et al: Percutaneous transluminal coronary rotational angioplasty of calcified lesions. *Circulation* 84:II-521, 1991.
33. Warth DC, Leon MB, O'Neill W, et al: Rotational atherectomy multicenter registry: Acute results, complications and 6-month angiographic follow-up in 709 patients. *J Am Coll Cardiol* 24:641, 1994.
34. Koller P, Freed M, Niazi K, et al: Success, complications and restenosis following atherectomy of coronary ostial stenosis. *J Am Coll Cardiol* 19:333A, 1992.
35. Teirstein PS, Warth DC, Haq N, et al: High speed rotational coronary atherectomy for patients with diffuse coronary artery disease. *J Am Coll Cardiol* 18:1694, 1991.
36. Sharma SK, Duvvuri S, Kakarala V, et al: Rotational atherectomy (RA) for in-stent restenosis (ISR): Intravascular ultrasound (IVUS) and quantitative coronary analysis (QCA). *Circulation* 94:I454, 1996.
37. Bertrand ME, Lablanche JM, Leroy F, et al: Percutaneous transluminal coronary rotary ablation with Rotablator (European experience). *Am J Cardiol* 69:470, 1992.
38. MacIsaac AI, Bass TA, Buchbinder M, et al: High speed rotational atherectomy: Outcome in calcified and noncalcified coronary artery lesions. *J Am Coll Cardiol* 26:731, 1995.
39. Stertzer S, Rosenblum J, Shaw R, et al: Coronary rotational ablation: Initial experience in 302 procedures. *J Am Coll Cardiol* 21:287, 1992.
40. Davis KE, Foreman RD, Buchbinder M: Rotational atheroablation/atherectomy. In Ellis S, Holmes DR (eds): *Strategic Approaches in Coronary Intervention*, pp. 17–26. Baltimore, Williams & Wilkins, 1996.
41. Fourrier JL, Bertrand ME, Auth DC, et al: Percutaneous coronary rotational angioplasty in humans: Preliminary report. *J Am Coll Cardiol* 14:1278, 1989.
42. Popma J, Leon M, Buchbinder M, et al: Predictors and prognostic significance of CPK elevations after percutaneous transluminal rotational coronary atherectomy. *J Am Coll Cardiol* 19:77A, 1992.
43. Satler LF, Warth D: Dissections after high-speed rotational atherectomy: Frequency, predictive factors and clinical consequences. *Circulation* 86:I-3124, 1992.

44. Annex BH, Larkin TJ, O'Neill WW, Safian RS: Evaluation of thrombus removal by transluminal extraction coronary atherectomy by percutaneous coronary angioscopy. *Am J Cardiol* 74:606, 1994.

45. Safian RD, May MA, Lichtenberg A, et al: Detailed clinical and angiographic analysis of complex lesions in native coronary arteries. *J Am Coll Cardiol* 25:848, 1995.

46. Meany TB, Leon MB, Kramer BL, et al: Transluminal extraction catheter for the treatment of diseased saphenous vein grafts: A multicenter experience. *Cathet Cardiovasc Diagn* 34:112, 1995.

47. Popma JJ, Leon MB, Mintz GS, et al: Results of coronary angioplasty using the transluminal extraction catheter. *Am J Cardiol* 70:1526, 1992.

48. Safian RD, Grines CL, May MA, et al. Clinical and angiographic results of transluminal extraction coronary atherectomy in saphenous vein bypass grafts. *Circulation* 89:302, 1994.

49. Mintz GS, Kovach JA, Javier SP, et al: Mechanism of lumen enlargement after excimer laser coronary angioplasty. An intravascular ultrasound study. *Circulation* 92:3408, 1995.

50. Bittl JA, Sanborn TA, Tcheng JE, et al: Clinical success, complications and restenosis rates with excimer laser coronary angioplasty. *Am J Cardiol* 70:1533, 1992.

51. Bittl JA, Sanborn TA: Excimer laser-facilitated coronary angioplasty. Relative risk analysis of acute and follow-up results in 200 patients. *Circulation* 86:71, 1992.

52. Cook SL, Eigler NL, Shefer A, et al: Percutaneous excimer laser coronary angioplasty of lesions not ideal for balloon angioplasty. *Circulation* 84:632, 1991.

53. Litvack F, Eigler N, Margolis J, et al: Percutaneous excimer laser coronary angioplasty: Results in the first consecutive 3000 patients. *J Am Coll Cardiol* 23:323, 1994.

54. Mehran R, Mintz GS, Popma JJ, et al: Excimer laser angioplasty in the treatment of instent restenosis: An intravascular ultrasound study. *J Am Coll Cardiol* 27:362A, 1996.

55. Vandormael M, Reifart N, Preusler W, et al: Six months follow-up results following excimer laser angioplasty, rotational atherectomy and balloon angioplasty for complex lesions: ERBAC study. *J Am Coll Cardiol* 23:57A, 1994.

56. Lindsay J Jr, Pinnow EE, Pichard AD: New devices enhance hospital results of coronary angioplasty. *Cathet Cardiovasc Diagn* 43:1, 1998.

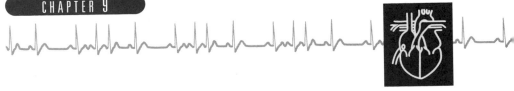

CHAPTER 9

Intravascular Ultrasound Imaging

GARY S. MINTZ, MD, FACC, AND CAROL WALSH, RCVT

Bom and associates[1] in Rotterdam designed the first true intravascular ultrasound (IVUS) system in 1971. It was conceived as an improved technique for visualizing cardiac chambers and valves. Yock and associates[2] recorded the first transluminal images of human arteries in 1988.

Two basic technical approaches to catheter-based ultrasound imaging are available: solid state and mechanical. With solid-state technology, an array of transducer elements is mounted in a cylinder at the tip of the catheter. By sequentially firing the multielement array, a beam is created and rotated in a 360-degree arc to produce the tomographic image. With mechanical technology, a single element transducer is located within the tip of a polyethylene imaging catheter or sheath. By means of a flexible drive shaft the transducer is then rotated "mechanically" to create the tomographic image. The solid-state approach is advantageous because of the lack of moving parts.

♥ Intravascular Ultrasound Basics

Transducers are devices that convert one type of energy into another. IVUS transducers convert electrical energy into ultrasound energy and ultrasound energy back into electrical energy. Assuming that ultrasound travels through all tissues at a fixed speed, the time that it takes for the transmitted ultrasound impulse to be backscattered and returned to the transducer is a measure of distance. The intensity of the signal depends on a number of factors (Display 9-1). These factors can affect not only the overall appearance of an image slice, but also the relative appearance of different sectors of the image.[3,4]

> ### DISPLAY 9-1   Factors Affecting the Intensity of the Transmitted IVUS Signal
>
> - Intensity of the transmitted signal
> - Attenuation of the signal as it passes through tissue (tissue attenuates ultrasound energy)
> - Distance from the transducer to the target (intensity is inversely related to distance)
> - Angle of the signal relative to the target (the closer the angle is to 90 degrees, the more intense is the reflected signal)[3,4]
> - Density or reflectivity of the tissue (which determines how much ultrasound energy passes through the tissue and how much is backscattered)
>
>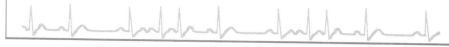

Resolution is the ability to discriminate two closely adjacent objects. Because IVUS creates images in three-dimensional space, there are three resolutions: (a) axial resolution (the ability to discriminate two closely adjacent objects located along the axis of the ultrasound beam), (b) lateral resolution (the ability to discriminate two closely adjacent objects located along the axis of the ultrasound catheter), and (c) angular or circumferential resolution (the ability to discriminate two closely adjacent objects located along the circumferential sweep of the ultrasound beam as it generates the planar image). Because ultrasound beams diverge, the optimal resolution is in the near field, the area closest to the transducer. In general, the higher the frequency, the greater the resolution; for a given frequency, the larger the size of the transducer aperture, the better the resolution.

Appropriate use of system controls can improve an image, whereas misuse of the available controls can degrade an image. Increasing overall gain increases overall image brightness. Overall gain that is set too low limits the detection of low-amplitude signals. Gain that is set too high compresses the gray scale and causes all tissue to appear echoreflective.

The approximate axial position of the images can be determined from the position of the transducer as seen fluoroscopically. However, the precise location and reproducible identification of individual image slices are optimized by the use of a motorized transducer pullback device, which withdraws the transducer at a constant speed, especially when combined with careful attention to vascular and perivascular markings. There is no absolute rotational orientation (anterior versus posterior; left versus right) of the image. Instead, side branches are useful markers during clinical IVUS imaging, and the image is described as if viewing the face of a clock.

♥ Measurements

The IVUS image is not identical with a histologic image. Cross-sectional images are created when the ultrasound beam encounters an interface between tissues or structures of different density.

Truly normal coronary arteries are rare in the practice of interventional cardiology.[5] The adventitia of coronary arteries has a high collagen content and is echoreflective. Conversely, the media of coronary arteries has a low collagen content, is mostly muscular, and is typically echolucent. Because the ultrasound beam is attenuated as it passes through the overlying plaque, the echolucent zone seen in vivo is almost always thicker than the true anatomic media. Because the adventitia and periadventitial structures have similar echoreflectivity, it is not possible to discriminate the adventitia from periadventitial structures.

The first "structure" that the IVUS beam sees is the blood-filled arterial lumen. Blood has a speckled, low-intensity, and continuously changing pattern that is distinct from tissue. The intensity of the blood

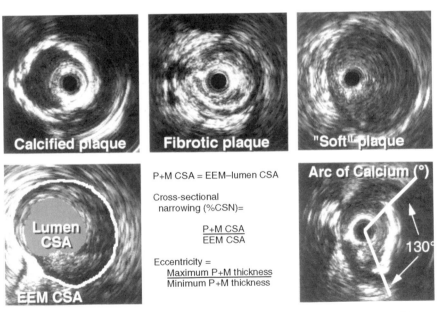

FIGURE 9–1 Intravascular ultrasound cross-sectional images of three types of intracoronary plaque **(top)** and intracoronary calcium **(lower right)**. **(Lower left)** Quantitative IVUS measurements are shown. The EEM CSA is a reproducible measure of total arterial area. Media thickness cannot be measured accurately; therefore, P+M CSA is used as a measure of plaque. Cross-sectional narrowing (% CSN) equals the percentage of area occupied by plaque. (CSA, cross-sectional area; EEM, external elastic membrane; P+M, plaque plus media.)

speckle increases exponentially with the frequency of the transducer and stasis. Saline (or contrast) injection through the guiding catheter is useful in clearing the lumen of blood (even static blood), in differentiating blood speckle from tissue, and in defining true lumen borders. Both blood speckle and saline injection are useful for identifying dissection planes.

During clinical IVUS imaging of nonstented lesions, there are only two distinct boundaries that have consistent histologic correlates: the lumen–plaque interface and the media–adventitia interface. Thus, only two cross-sectional area (CSA) measurements can be reproducibly performed: arterial CSA and lumen CSA (Fig. 9-1). Because the media cannot be quantified accurately, the cross-sectional measurement of atherosclerotic plaque is usually reported as the plaque + media (P+M) CSA. The P+M CSA is often divided by the total arterial CSA to generate a measurement called *plaque burden,* which is also sometimes referred to as the cross-sectional narrowing or percent plaque area or cross-sectional area obstruction. In addition, motorized transducer pullback through a stationary imaging sheath (as is available with mechanical IVUS systems) permits accurate length measurements.

Because endovascular stents are intensely echoreflective, the metallic prosthesis creates a third IVUS boundary between the lumen and the media–adventitia interface. In stented lesions, stent CSA can be measured, and neointimal tissue CSA can be calculated as stent CSA minus lumen CSA. Sometimes, the media–adventitia border can be seen through stents.

❤ Plaque Composition

Atherosclerotic lesions are heterogeneous and include varying amounts of calcium, dense fibrous tissue, lipid, smooth muscle cells, thrombus, and other material. In general, although IVUS cannot provide biochemically accurate information regarding plaque composition, IVUS imaging can separate lesions into subtypes according to echodensity (using the collagen-rich adventitia as a reference) and presence or absence of shadowing and reverberations (see Fig. 9-1).[6–12] The terminology used to describe specific plaque types has been the subject of much debate. Terms that have been used include calcific, echodense, fibrocalcific, fibrotic, soft, echolucent, fatty, and fibrofatty. Because atherosclerosis is a heterogeneous process, many lesions are mixed, containing more than one plaque type. Regardless of the classification used, it is clear that from the standpoint of therapeutic device response, a calcific, fibrocalcific, or echodense plaque behaves differently from a soft, echolucent, or fibrofatty plaque.

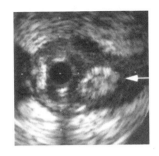

FIGURE 9–2 Intravascular ultrasound image of intracoronary thrombus (*arrow*).

Calcium (Fig. 9-1) is a powerful reflector of ultrasound; essentially none of the beam penetrates through or even into the calcium. Thus, calcium casts a shadow over deeper arterial structures, and even calcium thickness cannot be measured. In practice, the signature of calcium is echodense plaque (brighter than the reference adventitia) that shadows. However, dense fibrous tissue without calcium is also echodense and can sometimes cast a shadow. Infrequently, calcium (but not dense fibrous tissue) produces reverberations: one or more equidistantly spaced rings at intervals that are a multiple of the distance from the transducer to the leading edge of the calcium.[13,14]

Echolucent plaques are less bright compared with the reference adventitia. Although echolucent plaques are commonly referred to as "soft" (to differentiate them from echoreflective plaques that are labeled "hard"), these plaques are not soft or compliant to the touch, but are as firm as hard plaques.[15] Furthermore, the lesion compliance—that is, its response to balloon angioplasty or stent implantation—is dependent on many factors, including histologic plaque composition or ultrasound plaque classification, patient age, compliance of the adventitia and periadventitial structures, and vessel size.[16]

Varying amounts of fibrous and fatty tissue are contained in echolucent plaques. Pure fat is much more echolucent than muscle. A lipid pool, therefore, should appear as a dark or echolucent zone within a lesion. Neointimal hyperplasia within restenotic stents is usually echolucent, especially within the first 6 months after stent implantation.

Thrombus identification is one of the more difficult aspects of IVUS imaging.[17,18] The presence of thrombus can include the following: (a) a sparkling "scintillating" appearance; (b) a lobulated mass projection into the lumen (Fig. 9-2); (c) a distinct interface between the suspected thrombus and underlying plaque; (d) identification of blood speckle within the thrombus, indicating microchannels through the thrombus; and (e) mobility. Routine IVUS diagnosis of thrombus in native coronary arteries is difficult, and the diagnosis of thrombus in saphenous vein is unreliable because degenerated tissue of grafts can have many of these same features.

♥ Intravascular Ultrasound and Angiography Differences

Angiography has been the traditional gold-standard for evaluating coronary artery disease and for catheter-based interventions. However, there are limitations to the information that can be obtained from the angiogram. Angiography studies the arterial lumen; atherosclerosis is a disease of the arterial wall. Coronary arteries are complex three-dimensional structures with branch points, tortuous segments, and bends. Angiography is a shadow-graph technique that visualizes the lumen in multiple projected longitudinal planes. Atherosclerosis is a diffuse process. Angiography assesses coronary artery disease by comparing "diseased" segments with supposedly normal segments.

ATHEROSCLEROSIS IN ANGIOGRAPHIC REFERENCE SEGMENTS

IVUS routinely shows significant atherosclerosis in angiographically normal reference segments. In a study of 884 native vessel target lesions and their angiographically normal reference segments, only 6.8% of the reference segments were normal.[19] The explanation for angiographic silent atherosclerosis accumulation is as follows. Adaptive remodeling of the wall of diseased arterial segments (increase in arterial CSA) occurs to compensate for the accumulation of atherosclerotic plaque in direct relation to the CSA of the accumulated plaque.

REFERENCE SEGMENT MEASUREMENTS

IVUS routinely measures reference segment dimensions that are different from angiography. The IVUS measurements can be used to safely upsize intracoronary devices. Although IVUS measurements of reference dimensions are usually larger than angiographic measurements, this can be highly variable.

TARGET LESION CALCIUM

Using IVUS, calcium can be localized to the lesion vs the reference segment, characterized as superficial (closer to the tissue–lumen interface) versus deep (closer to the media–adventitia junction), and quantified according to its arc and length.[20,21]

IVUS routinely detects target lesion calcification that is angiographically silent. In a study of 1155 native vessel target lesions, IVUS detected calcium in 73%, twice as often as angiography. [22,23]

ECCENTRICITY

An eccentricity index can be calculated with the IVUS measurement of maximum and minimum plaque plus media thicknesses (see Fig. 9-1). Few lesions are truly concentric (eccentricity index = 1.0). Although almost all lesions show some degree of eccentric plaque distribution, there is no consensus as to the exact IVUS definition of an eccentric plaque. In a large series of native vessel lesions, the angiographic classification of lesions as eccentric or concentric was not related to plaque distribution as measured by the IVUS eccentricity index.[24] Furthermore, the concordance rate between IVUS and angiography was only 53.8%. Angiographic classification of a lesion as concentric or eccentric is primarily determined by the lesion length (as well as by the absolute measurement of maximum and minimum P+M thicknesses, but not by their ratio). Angiographic classification requires a visual interpolation of the course of the normal coronary artery and its lumen. Interpolation is more difficult in longer lesions and in those with more atherosclerotic plaque.

IVUS studies have also related plaque distribution to side branches and bifurcations. These studies have shown that regardless of the angiographic appearance, plaque is deposited preferentially opposite to the major branch.[25]

LUMEN DIMENSIONS

Several studies have compared IVUS and quantitative coronary angiography in measurement of lesion site lumen dimensions before and after intervention. Before intervention, the correlation between the IVUS and angiographic lumen diameters ranged from 0.77 to 0.98.[26–29] However, after percutaneous transluminal coronary angioplasty (PTCA) the correlation fell to 0.28 to 0.42.[30,31] Nakamura and associates[32] have indicated that the post-PTCA discrepancy is greater in the presence of deep vessel injury than with superficial lesion injury.

♥ Atherogenesis and Lesion Formation

The conventional concept of development and progression of a focal coronary artery stenosis in stable coronary artery disease is that there is a balance between plaque accumulation and adaptive remodeling until plaque accumulation outstrips the ability of the artery to compensate. Several IVUS studies suggest that there is a spectrum in the magnitude of arterial remodeling and that in some lesions inadequate remodeling or arterial shrinkage may contribute to the development of focal stenoses.[33] Pasterkamp and colleagues[34,35] showed that in most diseased femoral arteries, significant arterial remodeling could not be demonstrated. Instead, arterial shrinkage accelerated the luminal narrowing caused by plaque accumulation. Nishioka and colleagues[36] studied 35 primary lesions and showed that 54% had compensatory enlargement (lesion arterial CSA greater than proximal reference), 26% had inadequate compensatory remodeling (lesion arterial CSA less than distal reference), and 20% had intermediate compensatory enlargement (lesion arterial CSA intermediate between the proximal and distal references).

♥ Mechanisms, Results, and Complications of Catheter-Based Interventions

All catheter-based interventions increase lumen dimensions by one of the following mechanisms: vessel expansion, plaque dissection, plaque embolization, plaque redistribution, or plaque ablation/removal. In treating in-stent restenosis, two additional mechanisms can be invoked: neointimal tissue extrusion out of the stent and additional stent expansion. By comparing IVUS images before and after intervention, the mechanisms and results of catheter-based interventions can be delineated.

PERCUTANEOUS TRANSLUMINAL CORONARY ANGIOPLASTY

Plaque compression was the mechanism of balloon angioplasty originally proposed by both Dotter and Gruentzig[37,38]—an analogy was drawn to "footprints in the snow." However, IVUS studies have indicated that balloon angioplasty increases lumen dimensions primarily by vessel expansion and plaque dissection.[26–29,31,39,40] Some of these IVUS studies seemed to confirm the presence of plaque compression because quantitative cross-sectional IVUS analysis post-PTCA consistently showed a decrease in plaque CSA compared with preintervention. More recent studies suggest that apparent plaque compression was, in reality, plaque redistribution along the axis of the lesion, analogous to footprints in the sand.[41] Plaque has liquid and solid elements, which are not compressible. A special case is that of PTCA in the setting of thrombus. Thrombus embolization may contribute to the increase in acute lumen dimensions during PTCA of acute myocardial infarction[42]; thrombus embolization can also masquerade as plaque compression on IVUS analysis.

The most vulnerable sites for plaque dissection are the junctions of focal differences in lesion distensibility, the transition from plaque to normal vessel, and the junction of calcified and noncalcified plaque elements. In vitro modeling and clinical IVUS studies indicate that localized calcium deposits increase the vulnerability to dissection.[43–46] Typically, a tear is seen to start immediately adjacent to a localized calcium deposit and then extend into the lumen. However, because dissections are one of the mechanisms of successful PTCA, the presence of dissection by IVUS should not automatically be viewed as a complication. Detecting dissections can be enhanced by visualizing blood speckle or microbubbles from injected saline or contrast in the false lumen. Other unusual complications after PTCA, such as deep wall hematomas, can be detected by IVUS.

Several studies have shown that with the routine use of IVUS-guided balloon sizing, acute results during balloon angioplasty procedures can be optimized,[47] especially in an era of routine "bail-out" stent availability.[48,49]

DIRECTIONAL CORONARY ATHERECTOMY

Most IVUS studies have indicated that tissue removal accounts for over 75% of the improvement in lumen dimensions after stand-alone directional coronary atherectomy (DCA).[50,51] The addition of adjunct PTCA reduces the relative contribution of tissue removal and increases the contribution of vessel expansion to overall lumen improvement.[52,53] Dissections, especially superficial dissections, are common.[54] Regardless of the mechanism, the amount of plaque removed during DCA is low.[52]

The most important factors affecting delivery of the DCA device are vessel size, vessel tortuosity, and vessel compliance. The most consistent factor affecting vessel compliance is calcium, which magnifies the limits imposed by all other unfavorable lesion and vessel characteristics. Calcium also affects the ability of DCA to cut and remove tissue.[51,55,56]

Other lesion characteristics important for optimal performance of the DCA procedure include eccentricity, plaque thickness, and length. For example, plaque thickness defines the margin of safety for performing DCA. IVUS can also be used to exclude potentially unsafe lesions: extensive or spiral dissections outside the confines of the original lesions, dissections in areas of minimal plaque, or guidewires that are in false lumens.

To perform IVUS-guided DCA, the first step is to correlate the IVUS with the angiographic images, particularly the relation of the maximum and minimum plaque thicknesses to major side branches.[57] These side branches can then be used to orient the DCA device toward the maximum plaque thickness and away from the minimum plaque thickness (or, more important, away from normal vessel wall in a highly eccentric lesion). IVUS is also useful in determining whether the target end points (lumen dimension and plaque burden) have been achieved, identifying complications of DCA such as dissection or perforation and selecting adjunct device use.

ROTATIONAL ATHERECTOMY

There have been few systematic studies of rotational atherectomy (RA) using IVUS, and the ideal IVUS end points after RA are not known. RA effectively ablates calcified atherosclerotic plaque. Stand-alone RA increases lumen dimensions almost exclusively by atheroablation; however, the plaque burden after stand-alone RA is large. Adjunct PTCA increases the lumen almost exclusively by vessel expansion and plaque dissection. Like primary PTCA, dissections typically occur at the junction of calcified and noncalcified plaque.[58] Although initial studies suggested that atheroblation was limited in noncalcified compared with calcified plaque,[59] recent volumetric IVUS analysis indicates that this device is equally effective in the absence of calcium.[60] The final burr/artery ratio measured by IVUS is variable and depends primarily on changes in vascular tone, which is greater in noncalcified vessels.[59,60]

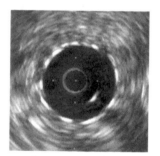
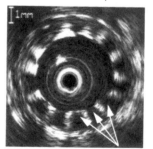

Palmaz-Schatz
stent

Stent-vessel wall
nonapposition

FIGURE 9–3 Cross-sectional intravascular ultrasound images of a Palmaz-Schatz stent fully opposed against the coronary wall **(A)** and a stent not fully apposed **(B)**. The area between the nonapposed stent and the coronary wall is a nidus for thrombus formation.

The measured arc of calcium has been shown to decrease after RA; however, this decrease is modest.[61] Full-thickness calcium removal is necessary to decrease the arc measured by IVUS. In heavily calcified plaques, full-thickness calcium removal is unusual.

EXCIMER LASER CORONARY ANGIOPLASTY

Only one report has studied the mechanism of lumen enlargement after excimer laser coronary angioplasty (ELCA).[62] After primary ELCA, lumen enlargement was found to result from a combination of tissue ablation and vessel expansion with a large residual plaque burden. The lumen CSA was often larger than the CSA of the laser catheter. However, these findings were extremely variable. In some lesions, lumen improvement was entirely due to tissue ablation, whereas in others it was entirely due to vessel expansion. There was no detectable change in calcium. Dissections into superficial calcium had an appearance that was unique to ELCA, consisting of a fragmented or shattered appearance with newly created sharp-edged gaps in a previously solid deposit of superficial calcium. The nonatheroablative IVUS findings after primary ELCA were attributed to laser-induced shock waves and forced expansion of vapor bubbles into tissue.[63–65] As with other devices, adjunct PTCA improved lumen dimensions by a combination of dissection at the junction of calcified and noncalcified plaque and by vessel expansion.

STENTS

Most IVUS reports have involved tubular slotted stents, primarily for fear of compressing the first-generation coiled stents. Even with tubular slotted stents, few IVUS studies have attempted to evaluate the mechanism of lumen improvement during stent implantation. One recent study has indicated that lumen improvement is the result of axial plaque redistribution during stenting.[66] This is similar to what has been observed during PTCA.[41]

There are two potential reasons to advocate routine use of IVUS guidance during stent implantation procedures: avoiding subacute thrombosis and reducing restenosis. Seminal observations by Colombo and colleagues[67] showed that using conventional implantation techniques, stents were typically underexpanded, asymmetric, and not fully apposed to the vessel wall (Fig. 9-3). These findings were linked to subacute thrombosis and led to the routine use of aggressive high-pressure adjunct PTCA with IVUS guidance. As a result of IVUS-guided high-pressure adjunct PTCA, lumen CSA increased by an average of 33% to 50%,[68,69] and subacute thrombosis became rare.[68,70]

Since then, the need for routine IVUS use during stent implantation procedures has become a matter of intense debate. A number of studies have shown that with routine high-pressure PTCA, subacute thrombosis is rare even without IVUS guidance, especially if ticlopidine is used after stent implantation.[71–73]

Will IVUS guidance decrease restenosis after stenting? Two concurrent observational studies, both using high-pressure adjunct PTCA—one using IVUS guidance and one not using IVUS guidance—have reported similarly low restenosis rates (~7%).[74,75] Nevertheless, numerous studies continue to show that even with routine high-pressure adjunct PTCA, minimum-lumen CSA can be further increased with IVUS guidance in tubular-slotted[76,77] and more recently in coiled stents.[78,79]

TREATMENT OF IN-STENT RESTENOSIS

IVUS studies before and after PTCA of in-stent restenosis showed that tissue extrusion out of the stent contributed 44% to lumen enlargement and additional stent expansion (even in stents initially implanted using high-pressure adjunctive PTCA) contributed 56%.[80] In that study, (a) PTCA achieved only 85% of the minimum-lumen CSA of the original stent implantation procedure, (b) after PTCA, there was significant residual neointimal tissue within the stent, and (c) residual stenosis was relatively high. These IVUS findings have been confirmed by two reports.[81,82] In-stent dissections may occur because the junction of neointimal tissue, and stent metal is an effective plane of cleavage.

More recently, atheroablative techniques have been used, typically followed by adjunct PTCA in an attempt to improve the acute and long-term results of PTCA for in-stent restenosis.[83–86] Both ELCA and RA increase lumen dimensions through ablation of neointimal tissue, although tissue ablation with RA appears to be greater, which is partly related to the larger burr sizes available. Adjunct PTCA is needed with both ELCA and RA to optimize final lumen dimensions. As with primary PTCA for in-stent restenosis, (a) the increase in lumen dimensions during adjunct PTCA is a combination of tissue extrusion out of the stent and additional stent expansion, (b) final lumen dimensions do not recover the lumen dimensions achieved during the initial stent implantation procedure, and (c) in-stent dissections can be observed.

♥ Restenosis

The major contributions of IVUS to the understanding of restenosis have been (a) identifying remodeling (the change in arterial CSA) as a mechanism of restenosis in nonstented lesions, (b) identifying the residual plaque burden as a predictor of restenosis in nonstented lesions, and (c) identifying neointimal hyperplasia (and eliminating chronic stent recoil) as the mechanism of in-stent restenosis.[20,87–90]

In the Washington Hospital Center's initial study,[89] the decrease in lumen CSA in nonstented lesions was due more to a decrease in arterial CSA than to an increase in P+M CSA. These findings have been confirmed in the Optimal Atherectomy Restenosis Study (OARS)[90] and in the SURE (Serial Ultrasound REstenosis) trial.[91] An exception is in diabetic patients: Remodeling appears to be similar to nondiabetics; but tissue growth is exaggerated.[92,93]

In the SURE Trial,[94] patients were treated with PTCA and DCA and studied before and immediately after intervention, 24 hours after intervention, after 1 month of follow-up, and after 6 months of follow-up. Little change was found in arterial CSA within the first 24 hours after intervention, but an increase was seen in arterial CSA between 24 hours and 1 month and a decrease in arterial CSA between 1 and 6 months. Thus, the decrease in arterial CSA resulting in restenosis was shown to be a late event, distinct from early passive elastic recoil. Two studies have shown that the most powerful predictor of restenosis in nonstented lesions is the residual plaque burden.[61,79] It has been suggested that the residual plaque burden acts as an amplifier of the remodeling process.[94]

Conversely, serial IVUS studies have shown that stents almost never chronically recoil (although they may acutely recoil).[88,95] In an analysis of stented lesions, the decrease in lumen correlated more strongly with the increase in neointimal tissue than with the change in stent dimensions.[88] In-stent neointimal tissue proliferation was exaggerated in diabetic patients.[92] Recent studies suggest that in stented lesions the final lumen CSA is the most important IVUS predictor of subsequent restenosis.[96,97]

❤ Clinical Practice

In general, current imaging catheters fit well into the interventional environment. Imaging should be performed only after administration of intracoronary nitroglycerin (to minimize catheter-induced spasm) and only after adequate heparinization. Anticoagulation during interventional procedures is usually dictated by the intervention. During diagnostic imaging, typically 5000 to 7500 U heparin is administered intravenously. When the activated clotting time (ACT) is checked at the end of the diagnostic study, it is usually less than 150 seconds, allowing removal of the sheaths and same-day patient discharge, if clinically advisable.

Routine clinical IVUS imaging begins with a careful understanding of the coronary angiogram so that the IVUS imaging run can be related to the angiographic anatomy. The imaging run should include careful interrogation of the vessel: distal reference, lesion site, and proximal reference back to the aorto-ostial junction. It is important to cross the lesion, ideally by at least 10 mm. One common pitfall is that there may be so much plaque in the reference segment proximal to the lesion that the operator may not be aware that he or she has not crossed the lesion. With current IVUS catheters, preintervention imaging can be performed routinely in more than 90% of studies. The major limitations to preintervention imaging are vessel tortuosity (hampering delivery of the imaging catheter) and lesion calcification (impeding crossing of the lesion). Lesion severity (even a total occlusion) does not appear to be a limitation as long as the lesion is not too rigid (usually indicating calcification).

Preintervention IVUS is useful in assessing lesion severity (lumen compromise and plaque burden), lesion length, reference vessel size, reference segment plaque burden, plaque composition (especially calcium), lesion eccentricity, and unusual morphology (e.g., aneurysms, ulcers, and dissections).[98] Of particular interest is the assessment of angiographically ambiguous, unusual, or intermediate lesions. Common sites for ambiguous or intermediate lesions include vessels with significant tortuosity, kinking, or bending; ostial (especially aorto-ostial) locations; segments of diffuse disease; or bifurcations or trifurcations. Many "intermediate" or difficult-to-assess lesions are readily shown to contain either insignificant or severe disease. Aneurysms can be differentiated from pseudoaneurysms or ulcerated plaques. Filling defects can occasionally be shown to be calcific "nodules," not thrombi.

Preintervention IVUS is also useful in assessing restenotic stents to determine whether the stent was implanted correctly. Before the atheroablative treatment of in-stent restenosis, IVUS can be used to determine the largest atheroablative device that can be used safely.

During intervention, IVUS is useful in understanding and managing complications, after crossing a total occlusion to determine whether the guidewire is in the true or false lumen, and in evaluating adequacy of stent placement.

After intervention, IVUS is useful in determining whether the targeted end points have been reached, in determining the residual plaque burden, and in determining the final stent or lumen dimensions.

🫀 Practical Considerations

The major resistance to the routine use of IVUS is the limited information that can link IVUS to improved patient outcomes, procedural cost, physician education (both how to interpret the images and how to use the information), equipment complexity, and difficulties in integrating IVUS into a busy catheterization laboratory environment. IVUS will be used routinely only if it is quick to set up and easy to perform and if it does not slow down the flow of the clinical cases. Each catheterization laboratory is organized differently, and each presents unique problems. Tasks performed by the same health care professionals vary from laboratory to laboratory. However, it is possible to integrate clinical IVUS imaging into a busy laboratory, maintain image acquisition standards, and not add significant time to the overall procedure. The integration of IVUS will be most successful if it is under the administrative structure of the cardiac catheterization laboratory.

Even in a busy laboratory with constant IVUS use, it is difficult to train all laboratory personnel. Many practical aspects of IVUS imaging (e.g., handling of videotapes) are foreign to traditional "cath lab" practices. IVUS imaging is facilitated by designating specific IVUS technologists, who become responsible for all practical aspects of IVUS imaging, such as (a) equipment and catheter setup, (b) image optimization, (c) proper recording of IVUS imaging runs, (d) accurate voice and on-screen alphanumeric documentation, (e) patient and procedure logs, (f) equipment maintenance, and so on. With time, technologists can be trained to interpret images accurately, to provide the iterative feedback necessary for IVUS-based decision making, and to answer questions posed by the primary operators. Measurements should be made off-line (from videotape after the imaging run is complete), not when the catheter is in the vessel; this saves procedure time and minimizes patient ischemia.

The angiographic (e.g., "road-map") monitors can be wired to display the IVUS images. Angiographic monitors offer superior resolution, are convenient and readily visible to the operator, and allow the IVUS machine to be placed in a position away from the patient table and out of the way of the nurses providing patient care.

In a busy laboratory with many operators, image acquisition and analysis should be standardized. The use of a motorized transducer pullback device aids (in fact, enforces) discipline and acquisition standards. There is no question whether the transducer is being advanced or withdrawn. At this laboratory, we prefer a pullback speed of 0.5 mm/sec. However, with very focal stenoses, especially ostial stenoses, a pullback speed of 0.25 mm/sec is preferable. Conversely, we never use a speed of 1 mm/sec for fear of missing important information. Motorized transducer pullback also does not preclude additional, careful manually controlled interrogation of the lesion. Standardization of image acquisition facilitates off-line image analysis and comparison of serial (pre- versus postintervention or postintervention versus follow-up) studies. It is essential for multicenter studies.

Accurate procedure information is critical. Even when recording verbal commentary, it is helpful if on-line procedural information is annotated onto the ultrasound system's video screen. The ideal on screen labeling should contain three elements: (a) the timing of IVUS imaging (e.g., preintervention), (b) the procedure being performed, and (c) the target vessel and location. All IVUS instruments have internal clocks, and the time is automatically recorded onto the videotape. It is helpful to note the time that corresponds to the center of the lesion. In the absence of systematic preintervention imaging, voice annotation or recording the time corresponding to the lesion may be the only way to identify the target lesion on subsequent review. After some procedures, it may be difficult to identify the target lesion without this information.

Good-quality videotapes are essential. It is recommended that virgin (never-used) broadcast quality VHS tapes be used. There is a quality difference, and the cost differential is minimal. Videotapes should be stored in a secure place. If there is voice annotation information, then the audio circuit must be linked as well. The first-generation copy loses some image quality, but is usually acceptable. The second-generation copy (copy of a copy) loses too much image information to be useful. Videotape storage can become unwieldy if each patient has his or her own tape. In general, 20 studies can be recorded on each 120-minute tape. Individual tapes (for each patient) should be reserved for multicenter studies in which the videotape must be sent away to a core laboratory.

Many catheterization laboratories have excessive ambient electrical or radio frequency (RF) noise, which can produce artifacts on the ultrasound image. Offenders include monitoring equipment, intra-aortic balloon pumps, and other devices. Eliminating these problems requires troubleshooting and working with both the IVUS and non-IVUS equipment vendors. The Doppler FloWire can cause two types of interference. One is electrical, but the other is cross-talk between the two signals. Ultrasonic *cross-talk* is present whenever two sources of ultrasonic signals are used simultaneously. In addition, in some hospitals the paging system generates an RF signal that momentarily "blanks out" the IVUS image. Inexpensive, custom filters solve this problem.

SAFETY

There have been three large studies of the safety of IVUS.[99-101] Other than transient spasm, complications appear to be rare. The Washington Hospital Center experience has been similar to these reports.

♥ Conclusion

The introduction of IVUS into the catheterization laboratory has greatly expanded the understanding of both coronary artery disease and the mechanisms by which interventional devices remove plaque and expand the lumen. It has become an essential clinical tool that will help guide practice into the future.

REFERENCES

1. Bom N, Lancee CT, van Egmond FC: An ultrasonic intracardiac scanner. *Ultrasonics* 10:71, 1972.
2. Yock PG, Johnson EL, Linker DT: Intravascular ultrasound: Development and clinical potential. *Am J Cardiac Imag* 2:185, 1988.
3. Picano E, Landini L, Distante A, et al: Angle dependence of ultrasonic backscatter in arterial tissues: A study in vitro. *Circulation* 72:572, 1985.
4. DiMario C, Madretsma S, Linker D, et al: The angle of incidence of the ultrasonic beam: A critical factor for the image quality in intravascular ultrasonography. *Am Heart J* 125:442, 1993.
5. Fitzgerald PJ, St. Goar FG, Connolly AJ, et al: Intravascular ultrasound imaging of coronary arteries. Is three layers the norm? *Circulation* 86:154, 1992.
6. Gussenhoven EJ, Essed CE, Lancee CT, et al: Arterial wall characteristics determined by intravascular ultrasound imaging: An in vitro study. *J Am Coll Cardiol* 14:947, 1989.
7. Potkin BN, Bartorelli AL, Gessert JM, et al: Coronary artery imaging with intravascular high-frequency ultrasound. *Circulation* 81:1575, 1990.
8. Nishimura RA, Edwards WD, Warnes CA, et al: Intravascular ultrasound imaging: In vitro validation and pathologic correlation. *J Am Coll Cardiol* 16:145, 1990.
9. Kimura BJ, Bhargava V, De Maria AN: Value and limitations of intravascular ultrasound imaging in characterizing coronary atherosclerotic plaque. *Am Heart J* 130:386, 1995.
10. Hodgson JMcB, Reddy KG, Suneja R, et al: Intracoronary ultrasound imaging: Correlation of plaque morphology with angiography, clinical syndrome and procedural results in patients undergoing coronary angioplasty. *J Am Coll Cardiol* 21:35, 1993.
11. Tobis JM, Mallery J, Mahon D, et al: Intravascular ultrasound imaging of human coronary arteries in vivo. Analysis of tissue characterizations with comparison to in vitro histological specimens. *Circulation* 83:913, 1991.

12. Gussenhoven EJ, Essed CE, Frietman P, et al: Intravascular echographic assessment of vessel wall characteristics: A correlation with histology. *Int J Card Imaging* 4:105, 1989.

13. Friedrich GJ, Moes NY, Muhlberger VA, et al: Detection of intralesional calcium by intracoronary ultrasound depends on the histologic pattern. *Am Heart J* 128:434, 1994.

14. Gutfinger DE, Leung CY, Hiro T, et al: In vitro atherosclerotic plaque and calcium quantitation by intravascular ultrasound and electron-beam computed tomography. *Am Heart J* 131:899, 1996.

15. Hiro T, Leung CY, de Guzman S, et al: Are "soft echoes" really soft? Ultrasound assessment of mechanical properties in human atherosclerotic tissue (abstr). *Circulation* 92:I-649, 1995.

16. Kok WE, Peters RJ, Prins MH, et al: Contribution of age and intimal lesion morphology to coronary artery wall mechanics in coronary artery disease. *Clin Sci* 89:239, 1995.

17. Chemarin-Alibelli MJ, Pieraggi MT, Elbaz M, et al: Identification of coronary thrombus after myocardial infarction by intracoronary ultrasound compared with histology of tissues sampled by atherectomy. *Am J Cardiol* 77:344, 1996.

18. Frimerman A, Miller HI, Hallman M, et al: Intravascular ultrasound characterization of thrombi of different composition. *Am J Cardiol* 73:1053, 1994.

19. Mintz GS, Painter JA, Pichard AD, et al: Atherosclerosis in angiographically "normal" coronary artery reference segments: An intravascular ultrasound study with clinical correlations. *J Am Coll Cardiol* 25:1479, 1995.

20. Mintz GS, Douek P, Pichard AD, et al: Target lesion calcification in coronary artery disease: An intravascular ultrasound study. *J Am Coll Cardiol* 20:1149, 1992.

21. Mintz GS, Popma JJ, Pichard AD, et al: Patterns of calcification in coronary artery disease. A statistical analysis of intravascular ultrasound and coronary angiography in 1155 lesions. *Circulation* 91:1969, 1995.

22. Ge J, Gorge G, Haude M, et al: Doesn't diseased human coronary saphenous vein bypass grafts undergo compensatory enlargement? An intravascular ultrasound study (abstr). *J Am Coll Cardiol* 29:178A, 1997.

23. Mintz GS, Pichard AD, Popma JJ, et al: Determinants and correlates of target lesion calcium in coronary artery disease: A clinical, angiographic, and intravascular ultrasound study. *J Am Coll Cardiol* 29:268, 1997.

24. Mintz GS, Popma JJ, Pichard AD, et al. Limitation of angiography in the assessment of plaque distribution in coronary artery disease. A systematic study of target lesion eccentricity in 1446 lesions. *Circulation* 93:924, 1996.

25. Kimura BJ, Russo RJ, Bhargava V, et al: Atheroma morphology and distribution in proximal left anterior descending coronary artery: In vivo observations. *J Am Coll Cardiol* 27:825, 1996.

26. Tenaglia AN, Buller CE, Kisslo KB, et al: Mechanisms of balloon angioplasty and directional coronary atherectomy as assessed by intracoronary ultrasound. *J Am Coll Cardiol* 20:685, 1992.

27. Braden GA, Herrington DM, Downes TR, et al: Qualitative and quantitative contrasts in the mechanisms of lumen enlargement by coronary balloon angioplasty and directional coronary atherectomy. *J Am Coll Cardiol* 23:40, 1994.

28. Suneja R, Nair RN, Reddy KG, et al: Mechanisms of angiographically successful directional coronary atherectomy: Evaluation by intracoronary ultrasound and comparison with transluminal coronary angioplasty. *Am Heart J* 126:507, 1993.
29. Honye J, Mahon DJ, Jain A, et al: Morphological effects of coronary balloon angioplasty in vivo assessed by intravascular ultrasound imaging. *Circulation* 85:1012, 1992.
30. Tobis JM, Mahon DJ, Honye J, McRae M: Intravascular ultrasound imaging following balloon angioplasty. *Int J Card Imaging* 6:191, 1991.
31. Davidson CJ, Sheikh KH, Kisslo KB, et al: Intracoronary ultrasound evaluation of interventional technologies. *Am J Cardiol* 68:1305, 1991.
32. Nakamura S, Mahon DJ, Maheswaran B, et al: An explanation for discrepancy between angiographic and intravascular ultrasound measurements after percutaneous transluminal coronary angioplasty. *J Am Coll Cardiol* 25:633, 1995.
33. Wong CB, Porter TR, Xie F, Deligonul U: Segmental analysis of coronary arteries with equivalent plaque burden by intravascular ultrasound in patients with and without angiographically significant coronary artery disease. *Am J Cardiol* 76:598, 1995.
34. Pasterkamp G, Borst C, Post MJ, et al: Atherosclerotic arterial remodeling in the superficial femoral artery. Individual variation in local compensatory enlargement response. *Circulation* 93:1818, 1996.
35. Pasterkamp G, Wensing PJW, Post MJ, et al: Paradoxical arterial wall shrinkage may contribute to luminal narrowing of human atherosclerotic femoral arteries. *Circulation* 91:1444, 1995.
36. Nishioka T, Luo H, Eigler NL, et al: Contribution of inadequate compensatory enlargement to development of human coronary artery stenosis: An in vivo intravascular ultrasound study. *J Am Coll Cardiol* 27:1571, 1996.
37. Dotter CT, Judkins MP: Transluminal treatment of arteriosclerotic obstruction: Description of new technique and a preliminary report of its application. *Circulation* 30:654, 1964.
38. Grüntzig A: Transluminal dilatation of coronary artery stenosis. *Lancet* 1:263, 1978.
39. Tobis JM, Mallery JA, Gessert J, et al: Intravascular ultrasound cross-sectional arterial imaging before and after balloon angioplasty in vitro. *Circulation* 80:873, 1989.
40. Potkin BN, Keren G, Mintz GS, et al: Arterial responses to balloon coronary angioplasty: An intravascular ultrasound study. *J Am Coll Cardiol* 20:942, 1992.
41. Mintz GS, Pichard AD, Kent KM, et al: Axial plaque redistribution as a mechanism of percutaneous transluminal coronary angioplasty. *Am J Cardiol* 77:427, 1996.
42. Boksch WG, Schartl M, Beckmann SH, et al: Intravascular ultrasound imaging in patients with acute myocardial infarction: Comparison with chronic angina pectoris. *Coron Artery Dis* 5:727, 1994.
43. Lee RT, Richardson G, Loree HM, et al: Prediction of mechanical properties of human atherosclerotic tissue by high-frequency ultrasound imaging. An in vitro study. *Arteriosclerosis and Thrombosis* 12:1, 1992.
44. Lee RT, Loree HM, Cheng GC, et al: Computational structural analysis

based on intravascular ultrasound imaging before in vitro angioplasty: Prediction of plaque fractures. *J Am Coll Cardiol* 21:777, 1993.

45. Fitzgerald PJ, Ports TA, Yock PG: Contribution of localized calcium deposits to dissection after angioplasty. An observational study using intravascular ultrasound. *Circulation* 86:64, 1992.

46. Tenaglia AN, Buller CE, Kisslo KB, et al: Intracoronary ultrasound predictors of adverse outcomes after coronary artery interventions. *J Am Coll Cardiol* 20:1385, 1992.

47. Stone GW, Hodgson JB, St Goar FG, et al: Improved procedural results of coronary angioplasty with intravascular ultrasound-guided balloon sizing: The CLOUT Pilot Trial. Clinical Outcomes With Ultrasound Trial (CLOUT) Investigators. *Circulation* 95:2044, 1997.

48. Abizaid A, Mehran R, Pichard AD, et al: Results of high-pressure ultrasound-guided "over-sized" balloon PTCA to achieve "stent-like" results (abstr). *J Am Coll Cardiol* 29:280A, 1997.

49. Hodgson JMcB, Muller C, Roskamm H, Frey AW: Ultrasound (IVUS)-guided PTCA and stenting improves acute angiographic results: Acute analysis of the Strategy of IVUS-guided PTCA and Stenting (SIPS) Trial (abstr). *J Am Coll Cardiol* 29:96A, 1997.

50. Matar FA, Mintz GS, Farb A, et al: The contribution of tissue removal to lumen improvement after directional coronary atherectomy. *Am J Cardiol* 74:647, 1994.

51. Umans VA, Baptista J, DiMario C, et al: Angiographic, ultrasonic, and angioscopic assessment of the coronary artery wall and lumen area configuration after directional atherectomy: The mechanism revisited. *Am Heart J* 130:217, 1996.

52. Baim DS, Simonton CA, Popma JJ, et al: Mechanism of luminal enlargement by optimal atherectomy: IVUS insights from the OARS Study (abstr). *J Am Coll Cardiol* 27:291A, 1996.

53. Hosokawa H, Kato O, Tamai H, et al: Role of adjunct balloon angioplasty following coronary atherectomy: A serial intravascular ultrasound analysis from the ABACAS Trial (abstr). *J Am Coll Cardiol* 29:281A, 1997.

54. Popma JJ, Mintz GS, Satler LF, et al: Clinical and angiographic outcome after directional coronary atherectomy: A qualitative and quantitative analysis using coronary arteriography and intravascular ultrasound. *Am J Cardiol* 72:55E, 1993.

55. Matar FA, Mintz GS, Pinnow E, et al: Multivariate predictors of intravascular ultrasound endpoints after directional coronary atherectomy. *J Am Coll Cardiol* 25:318, 1995.

56. Dussaillant GD, Mintz GS, Pichard AD, et al: Mechanisms and acute and long term results of adjunctive directional atherectomy after rotational atherectomy. *J Am Coll Cardiol* 27:1390, 1996.

57. Yock PG, Fitzgerald PJ, Linker DT, Angelsen BAJ: Intravascular ultrasound guidance for catheter-based coronary interventions. *J Am Coll Cardiol* 17:39B, 1991.

58. Kovach JA, Mintz GS, Pichard AD, et al: Sequential intravascular ultrasound characterization of the mechanisms of rotational atherectomy and adjunct balloon angioplasty. *J Am Coll Cardiol* 22:1024, 1993.

59. Fitzgerald PJ, Stertzer SH, Hidalgo BO, et al: Plaque characteristics affect lesion and vessel response to coronary rotational atherectomy: An intravascular ultrasound study. *J Am Coll Cardiol* 23:353A, 1994.

60. Dussaillant GR, Mintz GS, Pichard AD, et al: Effect of rotational atherectomy in noncalcified atherosclerotic plaque: A volumetric intravascular ultrasound study. *J Am Coll Cardiol* 28:856, 1996.

61. The GUIDE Trial Investigators: IVUS-determined predictors of restenosis in PTCA and DCA: Final report from the GUIDE Trial, Phase II (abstr). *J Am Coll Cardiol* 27:156A, 1994.

62. Mintz GS, Kovach JA, Javier SP, et al: Mechanisms of lumen enlargement after excimer laser coronary angioplasty: An intravascular ultrasound study. *Circulation* 92:3408, 1995.

63. Isner JM, Rosenfield K, Losordo DW: Excimer laser atherectomy (The Greening of Sisyphus). *Circulation* 81:2018, 1990.

64. van Leeuwen TG, van Erven L, Meertens JH, et al: Origin of arterial wall dissections induced by pulsed excimer and mid-infrared laser ablation in the pig. *J Am Coll Cardiol* 19:1610, 1992.

65. van Leeuwen TG, Meertens JH, Velema E, et al: Intraluminal vapor bubble induced by excimer laser pulse causes microsecond arterial dilation and invagination leading to extensive wall damage in the rabbit. *Circulation* 87:1258, 1993.

66. Honda Y, Yock CA, Hermiller JB, et al: Longitudinal redistribution of plaque is an important mechanism for lumen expansion in stenting (abstr). *J Am Coll Cardiol* 29:281A, 1997.

67. Nakamura S, Colombo A, Gaglione A, et al: Intracoronary ultrasound observations during stent implantation. *Circulation* 89:2026, 1994.

68. Colombo A, Hall P, Nakamura S, et al: Intracoronary stenting without anticoagulation accomplished with intravascular ultrasound guidance. *Circulation* 91:1676, 1995.

69. Garge G, Haude M, Ge J, et al: Intravascular ultrasound after low and high inflation pressure coronary artery stent implantation. *J Am Coll Cardiol* 26:725, 1995.

70. Hall P, Nakamura S, Maiello L, et al: A randomized comparison of combined ticlopidine and aspirin versus aspirin therapy alone after successful intravascular ultrasound-guided stent implantation. *Circulation* 93:215, 1996.

71. Goods CM, Al-Shaibi KF, Yadav SS, et al: Utilization of the coronary balloon expandable coil stent without anticoagulation or intravascular ultrasound. *Circulation* 93:1803, 1996.

72. Roy PR, Lowe HC, Walker BW, et al: Intracoronary stenting without intravascular ultrasound guidance followed by antiplatelet therapy with aspirin alone in selected patients. *Am J Cardiol* 77:1105, 1996.

73. Leon MB, Baim DS, Popma JJ, et al: A clinical trial comparing three antithrombotic-drug regimens after coronary-artery stenting (STARS). *N Engl J Med* 339:1665, 1998.

74. Mudra H, Sunamura M, Figulla H, et al: Six month clinical and angiographic outcome after IVUS-guided stent implantation (abstr). *J Am Coll Cardiol* 29:171A, 1997.

75. Morice MC, Duman P, Voudris V, et al: The MUST Trial. In-hospital and clinical events at six months. Final results (abstr). *J Am Coll Cardiol* 29:93A, 1997.

76. Akiyama T, DiMario C, Reimers B, et al: Do we need intracoronary ultrasound after high-pressure stent expansion? (abstr). *J Am Coll Cardiol* 29:59A, 1997.

77. Roberts DK, Arthur A, Bellinger RL, et al: The impact on coronary stent implantation of intravascular ultrasound guidance following "aggressive" angiographic stent implantation (abstr). *J Am Coll Cardiol* 29:275A, 1997.
78. Werner GS, Schunemann S, Ferrari M, et al: Comparison of slotted-tube and coil stents after high-pressure stent deployment by intravascular ultrasound (abstr). *J Am Coll Cardiol* 29:275A, 1997.
79. Itoh A, Hall P, Moussa I, et al: Comparison of quantitative angiography and intravascular ultrasound after stent implantation with 6 different stents (abstr). *Circulation* 94:I-263, 1996.
80. Mehran R, Mintz GS, Popma JJ, et al: Mechanisms and results of balloon angioplasty for the treatment of in-stent restenosis. *Am J Cardiol* 78:618, 1966.
81. Schiele F, Meneveau N, Vuillemenot A, et al: Intracoronary ultrasound assessment of balloon angioplasty in intrastent restenosis (abstr). *J Am Coll Cardiol* 29:240A, 1997.
82. Gorge G, Konorza E, Voegle E, et al: Incomplete restoration of luminal dimensions after PTCA in restenotic stented segments: An intravascular ultrasound analysis (abstr). *J Am Coll Cardiol* 29:311A, 1997.
83. Sharma SK, Duvvuri S, Kakarala V, et al: Rotational atherectomy for in-stent restenosis: Intravascular ultrasound and quantitative coronary analysis (abstr). *Circulation* 94:I-454, 1996.
84. Mehran R, Mintz GS, Popma JJ, et al: Treatment of in-stent restenosis: An intravascular ultrasound study in 159 stented lesions (abstr). *J Am Coll Cardiol* 29:77A, 1997.
85. Mehran R, Mintz GS, Popma JJ, et al: Mechanisms of lumen enlargement during atheroblation of in-stent restenosis: A volumetric intravascular ultrasound analysis (abstr). *J Am Coll Cardiol* 29:497A, 1997.
86. Schiele F, Meneveau N, Vuillemenot A, et al: Rotational atherectomy followed by balloon angioplasty for treatment of intra stent restenosis. A pilot study with quantitative angiography and intracoronary ultrasound (abstr). *J Am Coll Cardiol* 29:498A, 1997.
87. Mintz GS, Popma JJ, Pichard AD, et al: Intravascular ultrasound predictors of restenosis following percutaneous transcatheter coronary revascularization. *J Am Coll Cardiol* 27:1678, 1996.
88. Hoffmann R, Mintz GS, Dussaillant GR, et al: Patterns and mechanisms of in-stent restenosis: A serial intravascular ultrasound study. *Circulation* 94:1247, 1996.
89. Mintz GS, Popma JJ, Pichard AD, et al: Arterial remodeling after coronary angioplasty. A serial intravascular ultrasound study. *Circulation* 94:35, 1996.
90. Lansky AJ, Mintz GS, Popma JJ, et al: Remodeling after directional coronary atherectomy with and without adjunct percutaneous transluminal coronary angioplasty): A serial angiographic and intravascular ultrasound analysis from the Optimal Atherectomy Restenosis Study (OARS). *J Am Coll Cardiol* 32:329, 1998.
91. Stiel GM, Stiel LSG, Schofer J, et al: Impact of compensatory enlargement of atherosclerotic coronary arteries on angiographic assessment of coronary heart disease. *Circulation* 80:1603, 1989.

92. Kornowski R, Mintz GS, Kent KM, et al: Increased restenosis in diabetes mellitus after coronary interventions is due to exaggerated intimal hyperplasia: A serial intravascular ultrasound study. *Circulation* 95:1366, 1997.

93. de Vrey E, Mintz GS, Kimura T, et al: Arterial remodeling after directional coronary atherectomy: A *volumetric* analysis from the Serial Ultrasound REstenosis (SURE) Trial (abstr). *J Am Coll Cardiol* 29:280A, 1997.

94. Currier JW, Faxon DP: Restenosis after percutaneous transluminal coronary angioplasty: Have we been aiming at the wrong target? *J Am Coll Cardiol* 25:516, 1995.

95. Painter JA, Mintz GS, Wong SC, et al: Serial intravascular ultrasound studies fail to show evidence of chronic Palmaz-Schatz stent recoil. *Am J Cardiol* 75:398, 1995.

96. Ziada KM, Kim MH, Potts W, et al: Predictors of target vessel revascularization following coronary stent deployment (abstr). *J Am Coll Cardiol* 29:239A, 1997.

97. Moussa I, DiMario C, Moses J, et al: The predictive value of different intravascular ultrasound criteria for restenosis after coronary stenting (abstr). *J AM Coll Cardiol* 29:60A, 1997.

98. Mintz GS, Pichard AD, Kovach JA, et al: Impact of pre-intervention intravascular ultrasound imaging on transcatheter treatment strategies in coronary artery disease. *Am J Cardiol* 73:423, 1994.

99. Hausmann D, Erbel R, Alibelli-Chemarin M-J, et al: The safety of intracoronary ultrasound: A multicenter survey of 2207 examinations. *Circulation* 91:623, 1995.

100. Batkoff BW, Linker DT: The safety of intracoronary ultrasound: Data from a multicenter European registry (abstr). *J Am Coll Cardiol* 25:143A, 1995.

101. Gorge G, Peters RJG, Pinto F, et al: Intravascular ultrasound: Safety and indications for use in 7085 consecutive patients studied in 32 centers in Europe and Israel (abstr). *J Am Coll Cardiol* 27:155A, 1996.

CHAPTER 10

Percutaneous Direct Myocardial Revascularization

RAN KORNOWSKI, MD, NANCY MORRIS, RN, BSN, RCVT,
AND MARTIN B. LEON, MD

Although coronary artery bypass surgery (CABG) and percutaneous transluminal coronary angioplasty (PTCA) can successfully treat most patients with symptomatic coronary artery disease (CAD), an increasing number of patients with anginal syndromes are refractory to medical therapy and cannot be treated using these conventional revascularization techniques. This includes patients with diffuse or small-vessel CAD, chronic total occlusions, no available bypass conduits, or incomplete revascularization by the conventional revascularization techniques alone. For such patients, a novel revascularization approach is needed.

♥ Historical Overview

Direct myocardial revascularization (DMR), also known as transmyocardial revascularization (TMR), represents a nonconventional approach aimed at improving myocardial perfusion by applying a laser energy source directly into the ischemic myocardium. The goal of DMR is to treat the endocardium directly without increasing the blood flow through the epicardial coronary arteries. This is a new concept, based on the finding of "myocardial sinusoids" and "arteriosinusoidal" vessels, which seemed to connect the coronary arteries with the left ventricular chamber in human cadaveric hearts.[1]

Based on these findings, Mirhoseini and colleagues[2] proposed the use of laser energy to create the transmural channels. They demonstrated in the canine coronary occlusion model that the CO_2 laser channels can remain patent, become chronically functional, and protect against myocardial ischemia.[2] For patients who could not be completely revascularized by CABG, the researchers used surgical myocardial revascularization as an adjunct to CABG.[3-5]

Since these early reports, various investigators have used laser-assisted DMR either as a sole therapy in patients not amenable to CABG or as an adjunct to CABG.[6-9] These investigators have uniformly reported improved symptoms and have shown some evidence of increased myocardial perfusion, either by positron emission tomography (PET) imaging or nuclear studies.[6-9]

Preliminary results from randomized studies comparing medical therapy with surgical DMR in patients not amenable to conventional revascularization supports initial experiences regarding improvement in symptoms and possible improvement in myocardial perfusion in the treated areas.[10,11]

The mechanism of DMR, even if it provides improved myocardial perfusion, is not known.[12,13] Initially, it was hypothesized that the blood flow through the patent channels would provide myocardial perfusion. However, the available data regarding the long-term patency of the channels are conflicting.[14,15] There are reports of neovascularization and increased collateral flow possibly contributing to increased myocardial perfusion.[16,17]

❤ Catheter-Based Direct Myocardial Revascularization

If surgical DMR could improve myocardial perfusion, then percutaneous DMR may provide equal benefit without the need for thoracotomy or general anesthesia. The hypothesis for percutaneous DMR is that it could generate endomyocardial channels from the left ventricular cavity to the subepicardial myocardium using catheter-based laser energy. This therapy may also reach regions not approachable with surgical DMR, such as the ventricular septum and the posterior wall. It may also provide an opportunity for multiple treatment sessions using a less invasive approach.

Various investigators have used Holmium (Ho):YAG laser energy to perform catheter-based DMR.[18,19] System requirements for catheter-based DMR include the integration of catheter guidance with an ablative laser system using the optimal laser parameters. By modifying the lasing parameters (e.g., number of pulses, energy per pulse, and laser fiber configuration), resultant tissue responses can vary dramatically and predictably.[20] Thus, specific laser-tissue interactions must be carefully evaluated to design the optimal parameters for DMR. Most important, the percutaneous approach must ensure penetrating energy

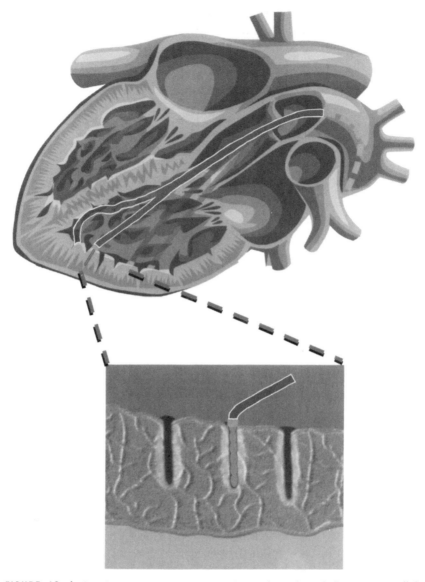

FIGURE 10-1 A schematic representation of a catheter-based direct myocardial revascularization procedure. The energy source is Ho:YAG laser. The catheter tip is equipped with a laser fiber. The catheter tip is in contact with the endocardial surface. After activation of the laser system, the endomyocardial channel is being created.

delivery to prespecified viable treatment zones without perforation or application of laser energy multiple times into the same location.

The catheter design for percutaneous DMR is in a rapid stage of evolution. The catheter should include a laser fiber and should permit access to all endocardial zones. This requires adequate torque response, tip deflection, and endocardial contact stability as well as a tip configuration that minimizes surface trauma (Fig. 10-1).

Three commercially available catheter-based laser DMR systems (CardioGenesis, Sunnyvale, CA; Eclipse, Sunnyvale, CA; and Biosense Johnson & Johnson, Tirat-Hacarmel, Israel) are undergoing evaluation in investigational clinical trials.[21] The energy source for all three systems is a Ho:YAG laser with differing energy parameters, fiber diameters, and catheter design. These clinical studies were designed to prove the safety and feasibility of percutaneous DMR and will be followed by randomized, controlled clinical trials. Initially, patient cohorts will include patients with chronic refractory ischemia, who are poor candidates for angioplasty or CABG revascularization procedures. The clinical end points in all trials are symptomatic angina improvement and assessments of exercise capacity and radionuclide myocardial perfusion.

♥ Summary

Direct myocardial revascularization is a novel and provocative nonconventional option for patients with symptomatic coronary artery disease. Regardless of the mechanism or mechanisms of action, the preliminary clinical data from the surgical experiences are encouraging with regard to the safety and efficacy of this procedure. Catheter-based DMR is in its infancy. Further studies are needed to confirm its clinical benefit and mechanisms of action as an alternative form of nonconventional revascularization.

REFERENCES

1. Wearn JT, Mettier SR, Klumpp TG, Zschiesche LJ: The nature of the vascular communications between the coronary arteries and the chambers of the heart. *Am Heart J* 9:143, 1933.
2. Mirhoseini M, Muckerheide M, Cayton MM: Transventricular revascularization by laser. *Lasers Surg Med* 2:187, 1982.
3. Mirhoseini M, Fisher JC, Cayton MM: Myocardial revascularization by laser: A clinical report. *Lasers Surg Med* 3:241, 1983.
4. Mirhoseini M, Shelgikar S, Cayton MM: New concepts in revascularization of the myocardium. *Ann Thorac Surg* 45:415, 1988.
5. Mirhoseini M, Cayton MM, Shelgikar S, Fisher JC: Clinical report: Laser myocardial revascularization. *Lasers Surg Med* 6:459, 1986.
6. Frazier OH, Cooley DA, Kadipasaoglu KA, et al: Myocardial revascularization with laser. Preliminary findings. *Circulation* 92(Suppl):II-58, 1995.

7. Cooley DA, Frazier OH, Kadipasaoglu KA, et al: Transmyocardial laser revascularization: Clinical experience with twelve-month follow-up. *J Thorac Cardiovasc Surg* 111:791, 1996.
8. Horvath KA, Mannting F, Cummings N, et al: Transmyocardial laser revascularization: Operative techniques and clinical results at two years. *J Thorac Cardiovasc Surg* 111:1047, 1996.
9. Horvath KA, Cohn LH, Cooley DA, et al: Transmyocardial laser revascularization: Results of a multicenter trial with transmyocardial laser revascularization used as sole therapy for end-stage coronary artery disease. *J Thorac Cardiovasc Surg* 113:645, 1997.
10. Boyce SW, Cooke RH, Aranki S, et al: Quality of life following transmyocardial revascularization using the heart laser: Randomized study results. *J Am Coll Cardiol* 29(Suppl):105A, 1997.
11. Allen KB, Fudge TL, Selinger SL, Dowling RD: Prospective randomized multicenter trial of transmyocardial revascularization versus maximal medical management in patients with class IV angina. *Circulation* 96(Suppl):I-564, 1997.
12. Stoll H-P, Hutchins GD, Fain RL, et al: Transmyocardial laser revascularization (TMR) induces regional myocardial denervation (abstr). *Circulation* 98:I-349, 1998.
13. Lauer B, Junghans U, Diederich KW, et al: Percutaneous myocardial laser revascularization for patients with end-stage coronary artery disease and refractory angina pectoris (abstr). *Circulation* 98:I-349, 1998.
14. Burkhoff D, Fisher PE, Apfelbaum M, et al: Histologic appearance of transmyocardial laser channels after 4 1/2 weeks. *Ann Thorac Surg* 61:1532, 1996.
15. Gassler N, Wintzer HO, Stubbe HM, et al: Transmyocardial laser revascularization. Histologic features in human nonresponder myocardium. *Circulation* 95:371, 1997.
16. Kohmoto T, Fisher PE, DeRosa C, et al: Evidence of angiogenesis in regions treated with transmyocardial laser revascularization. *Circulation* 94(Suppl): I-294, 1996.
17. Almanza O, Wassmer P, Moreno CA, et al: Laser transmyocardial revascularization (LTMR) improves myocardial blood flow via collaterals. *J Am Coll Cardiol* 29(Suppl):99A, 1997.
18. Kim CB, Kasten R, Javier M, et al: Percutaneous methods of laser transmyocardial revascularization. *Cath Cardiovasc Diag* 40:223, 1997.
19. Oesterle S, Schuler G, Lauer B, Reifart N: Percutaneous myocardial laser revascularization: Initial human experience. *Circulation* 96(Suppl):I-218, 1997.
20. Kornowski R, Hong MH, Haudenschild CC, Leon MB: Potentially hazardous effects of high-power holmium:YAG lasers during direct myocardial revascularization in porcine hearts. *Am J Cardiol* 80(Suppl):14S, 1997.
21. Kornowski R, Hong MH, Moses JW, et al: Safety and feasibility of percutaneous direct myocardial revascularization guided by Biosense electromechanical left ventricular mapping (abstr). *Circulation* 98:I-349, 1998.

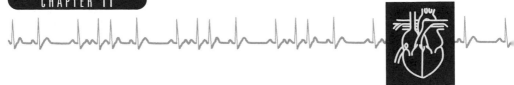

CHAPTER 11

Percutaneous Transluminal Angioplasty for the Treatment of Peripheral Vascular Disease

JOHN R. LAIRD, MD, FACC, FACP, AND ALEXANDRA J. LANSKY, MD

The concept of percutaneous transluminal angioplasty (PTA) can be credited to Charles Dotter, who in 1964 published his experience with a new technique to treat localized obstructions in the femoral and popliteal arteries.[1] He advanced catheters of increasing external diameter (up to 12 French [F]) through these femoropopliteal lesions to dilate the artery and improve the arterial lumen. Although there was little initial enthusiasm for this technique in the United States, a number of European Investigators including Porstmann, van Andel, and Staple contributed to the development of percutaneous dilatation catheters.[2–4]

After the development of a coaxial balloon catheter by Gruentzig and Hopff,[5] PTA became more practical, and enthusiasm for this technique increased. The Gruentzig balloon catheter was constructed of polyvinyl chloride and could be inflated to a fixed diameter to treat peripheral arterial obstructions. Gruentzig performed the first renal angioplasty in 1978 and went on to perform the first percutaneous transluminal coronary angioplasty (PTCA) shortly thereafter.[6,7] Subsequent advances in balloon catheter technology combined with improvements in technique allowed PTA to evolve from a novelty procedure to an established therapeutic modality for the treatment of peripheral arterial disease. By the mid 1980s, several studies had been published documenting the efficacy of PTA for occlusive disease of the iliac and femoropopliteal arteries.[8–10]

Despite advances in balloon catheter and guidewire technology, improvements in adjunct pharmacology, and refinements in operator technique, the effectiveness PTA remained somewhat limited by problems of failure to adequately dilate the lesion, dissection with acute vessel clo-sure, and restenosis. A number of new techniques such as atherectomy, laser, and stents were developed in an attempt to improve the results of PTA. Catheter-directed thrombolytic therapy became an established tech-nique to treat arterial occlusions. Newer imaging modalities such as angioscopy and intravascular ultrasound (IVUS) were developed and enhanced the understanding of the mechanisms of PTA as well as the mechanisms of restenosis. Modern endovascular therapy now encom-passes a wide array of complementary diagnostic and therapeutic modal-ities, which have greatly enhanced the ability to percutaneously treat arte-rial occlusive disease.

♥ Indications for Percutaneous Transluminal Angioplasty

Lower-extremity PTA is indicated for symptoms of claudication that are severe or lifestyle limiting. PTA is also commonly used in the set-ting of critical limb ischemia in which patients may suffer from ischemic rest pain, gangrene, or nonhealing ulcers. PTA may be per-formed in conjunction with a surgical bypass in the setting of multi-level arterial disease to improve inflow or outflow from the bypass graft. PTA may also be recommended for patients who are found to have a stenosis in a bypass graft during routine follow-up graft sur-veillance with duplex ultrasound. Intervention in this setting may help preserve patency of the graft. On occasion, iliac artery angioplasty or stenting may be required to facilitate vascular access for the perfor-mance of a coronary interventional procedure or to allow for safe placement of an intra-aortic balloon catheter during a high-risk inter-ventional procedure.

PTA may be indicated for symptoms of arm claudication or subclavian steal related to a severe stenosis of the proximal subclavian or brachio-cephalic artery. In addition, with the frequent use of the left and right internal mammary arteries as conduits during coronary artery bypass grafting (CABG), more and more patients are presenting with symptoms of myocardial ischemia due to subclavian artery narrowing proximal to the origin of the mammary artery. When this occurs, there may be reduced antegrade flow down the graft or actual coronary-subclavian steal, with retrograde flow up the mammary artery graft and "stealing" of blood away from the myocardium. A successful PTA can result in resolution of arm claudication symptoms and restoration of normal antegrade flow in the vertebral and mammary arteries.

Renal angioplasty (PTRA) or stent placement or both is indicated when there is severe unilateral or bilateral renal artery narrowing and when there is evidence of renovascular hypertension that is refractory to medical therapy. In addition, PTRA may improve or help preserve renal function when severe renovascular disease results in renal ischemia. There are anecdotal reports of patients with end-stage renal disease requiring dialysis due to renal artery stenosis, who were able to be removed from dialysis after successful PTRA.

Although controversial, carotid stenting is being investigated as an alternative to surgery for the prevention of stroke in patients with severe narrowing of the extracranial carotid artery (Fig. 11-1). The most generally accepted indication for this procedure is treatment of patients with severe carotid artery narrowing who are otherwise poor candidates for surgery due to inaccessibility of the stenosis (carotid bifurcation above the angle of the jaw), prior extensive neck surgery or radiation therapy, or severe medical or cardiac comorbidity. The early results with carotid stenting are promising. However, further study is required to determine whether this technique is a suitable alternative to carotid endarterectomy.

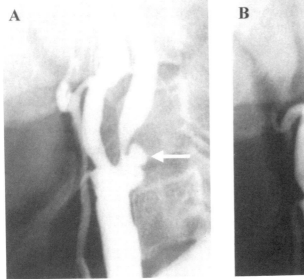
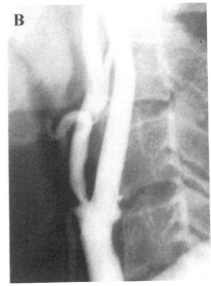

FIGURE 11–1 **(A)** Severe stenosis of the proximal internal carotid artery with ulceration (*arrow*) in a patient experiencing transient ischemic attacks. **(B)** After carotid angioplasty and stenting with a self-expanding Wallstent, the internal carotid artery is widely patent.

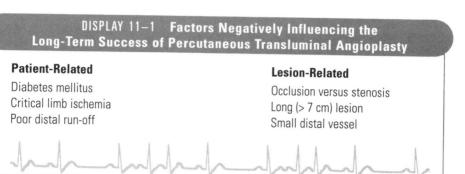

DISPLAY 11-1   Factors Negatively Influencing the
Long-Term Success of Percutaneous Transluminal Angioplasty

Patient-Related
Diabetes mellitus
Critical limb ischemia
Poor distal run-off

Lesion-Related
Occlusion versus stenosis
Long (> 7 cm) lesion
Small distal vessel

Results of Angioplasty

Several factors affect the long-term results of PTA (Display 11-1). Patient-related factors that influence patency include the presenting symptoms (claudication versus critical limb ischemia) and the presence or absence of diabetes. It has been well documented that patients who present with critical limb ischemia (rest pain, gangrene, nonhealing ulcers) have lower long-term patency rates than those who undergo angioplasty for claudication. In addition, diabetes has been consistently shown to negatively influence outcome. Lesion-related factors that are important include the size of the vessel being treated, the presence of stenosis or occlusion, the length of the lesion, and the status of the distal run-off vessels. Long-term patency rates are better when treating patients who have claudication and are found to have short-segment stenoses of the larger, more proximal vessels and good distal run-off.

Iliac Percutaneous Transluminal Angioplasty and Stenting

Patients with stenoses or occlusions of the iliac arteries often present with symptoms of buttock or thigh claudication (or both). If the lesion involves the common iliac artery or is associated with disease in the hypogastric arteries, the male patient may complain of impotence. When there is multilevel disease involving the iliac arteries, the femoropopliteal system, or below-knee vessels, the patient may present with rest pain, nonhealing ulcers, or gangrene.

TECHNIQUE

If a suitable lesion is present, angioplasty of the iliac arteries can be performed from the ipsilateral femoral artery using a retrograde approach or from the contralateral femoral artery using an iliac crossover approach. If the need arises, PTA can be performed from an axillary or brachial artery approach. The aortoiliac bifurcation is a common location for plaque formation, and if there is significant involvement of both common iliac arteries, a bilateral "kissing balloon" technique may be necessary (Fig. 11-2).

In the modern era, almost all iliac stenoses and most iliac occlusions can be successfully crossed with a guidewire and treated using endovascular techniques (Fig. 11-3). The development of hydrophilic guidewires (Terumo/Boston Scientific Vascular, Watertown, MA) has greatly increased the chances of successfully treating chronic iliac artery occlusions. After the lesion is crossed with a guidewire, dilatation can be performed with an appropriate-sized balloon catheter. The diameter of the common iliac artery ranges from 7 to 12 mm, with the most common size being 8 to 9 mm. The external iliac artery usually ranges from 6 to 8 mm in diameter.

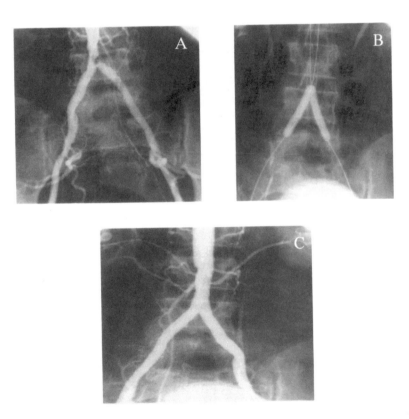

FIGURE 11—2 **(A)** Complex stenosis of the aortoiliac bifurcation. **(B)** Simultaneous inflation of balloons in the right and left common iliac arteries (*kissing balloons*). **(C)** Final result demonstrating no significant residual narrowing following implantation of Palmaz stents.

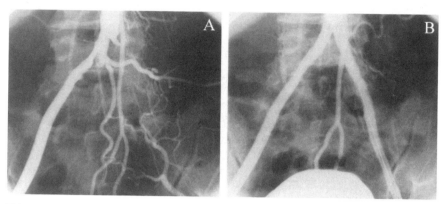

FIGURE 11–3 (A) Baseline angiogram demonstrating total occlusion of the left iliac artery. In addition, a significant stenosis of the right common iliac artery and occlusion of the internal iliac arteries are found. **(B)** Final result after angioplasty and stenting of the right and left common iliac arteries with Palmaz stents.

If a patient presents with acute or subacute occlusion of an iliac artery, a prolonged intra-arterial urokinase infusion may be necessary before PTA or stenting. A variety of infusion guidewires and catheters are available for this purpose. In most cases, a long occlusion can be successfully recanalized and converted to a short stenosis using thrombolytic therapy. The remaining stenosis can then be more safely and successfully treated with angioplasty.

RESULTS

Since the early years of angioplasty, a number of published studies have demonstrated the effectiveness of iliac artery PTA. Several investigators reported 2- to 4-year patency rates of 82% to 89%.[8,11,12] A review of the literature by Becker and associates[13] involving over 2500 procedures revealed an initial success rate of 92% with a 2-year patency rate of 81% and a 5-year patency rate of 75%. Tegtmeyer and associates[14] reported on 340 procedures in 200 patients. Patency at 4 years was 80% (including initial failures).

It is important to recognize that patients were selected carefully during the early years of angioplasty, and most of these early reports included only claudications with focal stenoses (rather than occlusions) of the iliac arteries. The results of balloon angioplasty in the setting of more diffuse disease, long stenoses, and occlusions are less favorable, and a number of investigators have reported somewhat lower long-term patency rates for iliac PTA. In addition, despite advances in equipment and technique, occasional procedural failures continue to occur as a result of vessel disruption with dissection and early vessel closure. The introduction of stents in the late 1980s offered the promise of improving upon the results of iliac PTA by providing a larger lumen than with balloon angioplasty alone, preventing/treating dissection, inhibiting elastic recoil, and thus potentially reducing the risk of restenosis.

The first iliac stent introduced for clinical use was the Palmaz stent (Johnson & Johnson, Warren, NJ). The Palmaz iliac stent is a stainless-steel balloon-expandable stent with a tubular slotted configuration. The initial design approved for iliac use was a 30-mm long stent that could be expanded from 8 to 12 mm in diameter.

A multicenter registry was established to evaluate the use of the Palmaz stent after suboptimal iliac angioplasty, and the results of this study were published in 1992.[15] A total of 587 procedures were performed on 486 patients. Two-hundred-and-one patients had angiographic follow-up at an average of 8.7 months. The angiographic patency rate (<50% stenosis) was 92%. Sustained clinical benefit was seen in 91% at 1 year, 84% at 2 years, and 67% at 43 months after angioplasty. A subsequent randomized trial was performed comparing the results of balloon angioplasty alone with stenting for iliac lesions. Stenting resulted in a better acute angiographic and hemodynamic result. At follow-up angiography, less restenosis was seen in the stent group. Most important, only 2% of the stent patients compared with 28% of the PTA patients required further intervention at 36 months after stenting.[16] This has led a number of interventionalists to recommend a strategy of primary stenting for all suitable lesions in the iliac arteries.

More recently, the Wallstent iliac prosthesis (Schneider/Boston Scientific Vascular, Watertown, MA) has been approved by the Food and Drug Administration (FDA) for iliac use. The Wallstent is a self-expanding mesh stent, which is available in a variety of diameters and lengths. The Wallstent has the advantage of flexibility and conforms well in tortuous anatomy. The stent can be easily advanced over the aortoiliac bifurcation and deployed from a contralateral femoral approach. In addition, because the Wallstent is nondeformable, it can be deployed at sites where a stent might be susceptible to external compression, such as below the inguinal ligament in the common femoral artery. The Wallstent is deployed by withdrawal of the protective sheath covering the stent. There is significant shortening of the Wallstent with expansion, and the degree of this shortening is often unpredictable. This unpredictable shortening of the stent sometimes precludes precise deployment of the stent.

The published experience with the Wallstent is not as extensive as with the Palmaz stent. The results of a Multicenter Registry involving the use of the Wallstent for iliac and femoropopliteal lesions was published in 1995. The 3-year primary patency with this stent was 77%. The secondary patency rate (patency with further intervention) was 92%.[17]

Newer stent designs are in the early phases of evaluation for iliac use. In addition, stent graft prostheses (stents covered with graft material) are also being evaluated as an alternative method to treat atherosclerotic as well as aneurysmal disease of the iliac arteries.

♥ Femoropopliteal Percutaneous Transluminal Angioplasty

Patients with stenosis or occlusion of the superficial femoral artery (SFA) or popliteal artery most often present with symptoms of calf claudication. The SFA is often a heavily diseased vessel and not infrequently is found to be totally occluded. In this setting, the profunda femoris artery is an important source of collaterals to the lower extremity. Several factors have been identified that clearly affect the long-term success of femoropopliteal PTA: the presence of occlusion versus stenosis, the length of the lesion, and the status of the below-knee run-off vessels.

TECHNIQUE

Lesions in the superficial femoral and popliteal arteries can be approached from a more direct antegrade femoral approach or from a contralateral femoral crossover approach. The SFA usually ranges from 5 to 7 mm in diameter. The popliteal artery ranges from 4 to 6 mm in diameter. After the stenosis or occlusion is successfully crossed with a guidewire, an appropriate-sized balloon catheter is used to dilate the lesion (Fig. 11-4). Balloon catheters in a variety of lengths (2 to 10 cm) and diameters are available. A variety of atherectomy catheters and laser systems have been evaluated as an alternative to balloon angioplasty for treating lesions in the femoropopliteal system. Despite initial enthusiasm for these devices, there have been no randomized trials demonstrating their superiority over plain old balloon angioplasty. Stents have been used for the treatment of femoropopliteal disease with variable success.[17-19] Ongoing studies help define the role of stents in this vascular bed.

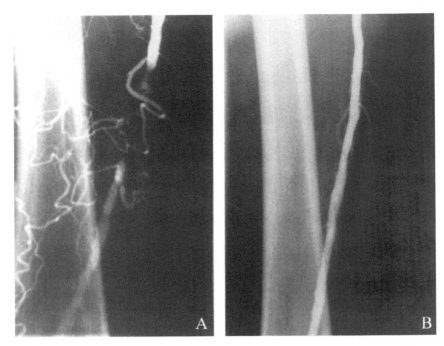

FIGURE 11–4 **(A)** Right lower-extremity angiogram demonstrating total occlusion of the distal right superficial femoral artery. **(B)** Final result after balloon angioplasty.

RESULTS

A wide disparity exists in the literature regarding long-term patency after femoropopliteal PTA. The reasons are many and include the different reporting standards used, whether initial procedural failures were included in the final patency numbers, the quality and completeness of patient follow-up, and the type of lesions/patients included. In the ideal setting (focal stenosis, good distal run-off), 3- to 5-year patency rates as high as 80% have been reported. In the worst-case scenario (i.e., long SFA occlusion, poor distal run-off), 3-year patency rates may be as low as 25%.[9,20,21] Most studies have demonstrated results that fall somewhere in between (Table 11-1).

In one of the largest and most often quoted studies, Johnston and colleagues[9] reported on 254 femoropopliteal PTA procedures in 236 patients. Procedural success was 96% with 1-month clinical success in 88.8%. Late success rates were 63% at 1 year, 51% at 3 years, and 38% at 5 years after PTA. Of note, initial failures were included in the analysis of late success. The predictors of late success in this study were the type of lesion (stenosis vs. occlusion) and distal runoff.

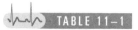
TABLE 11–1

Results of Femoropopliteal PTA

	Immediate Success (%)	3-Year Patency (%)
Overall	85	60
Ideal lesion	90	75
Worst case	70	20

♥ Tibioperoneal Percutaneous Transluminal Angioplasty

PTA of the below-knee tibioperoneal vessels is most often reserved for patients who have limb-threatening ischemia with either ischemic rest pain, gangrene, or nonhealing ulcers. The risk-to-benefit ratio of treating these small vessels does not favor the use of PTA for patients who present with only claudication or who are asymptomatic. If one were to attempt tibioperoneal PTA on a patient with claudication and if a complication were to occur, that patient's condition might be converted from stable claudication to limb-threatening ischemia.

TECHNIQUE

The equipment used for tibioperoneal PTA is similar to that used in coronary angioplasty. The tibioperoneal vessels usually range from 2 to 4 mm in diameter (similar to the coronary arteries). The antegrade approach is most often used to allow for access to the distal vessels. Heparin is administered to maintain an activated clotting time of at least 200 seconds, and nitroglycerin is often administered intra-arterially to prevent vessel spasm. Smaller 0.014-inch to 0.018-inch guidewires are used to cross the stenosis/occlusion, and lower-profile balloon catheters can then be used to dilate the lesions (Fig. 11-5). Rotational atherectomy can be used to treat heavily calcified lesions in the tibioperoneal vessels. There is limited experience with laser angioplasty and stenting for the treatment of diseased tibioperoneal vessels.

RESULTS

The success of tibioperoneal angioplasty is most often measured in terms of limb salvage rather than patency. Limb salvage is defined as freedom from amputation (or minimizing the extent of amputation) with healing of the ischemic ulcers. For successful limb salvage to occur,

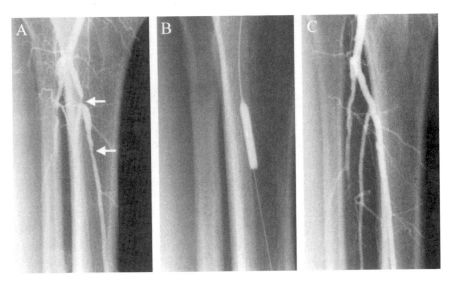

FIGURE 11−5 **(A)** Severe stenosis of the distal tibioperoneal trunk and proximal posterior tibial artery (*arrows*). The anterior tibial artery is totally occluded. **(B)** and **(C)** Final result after balloon dilatation of both lesions with a 3.5-mm balloon.

"straight line" flow to the foot through a patent femoropopliteal system is usually needed in addition to at least one patent tibioperoneal vessel (preferably the anterior or posterior tibial artery). The treated tibioperoneal vessel needs to remain patent only long enough to allow for healing of the foot. A number of studies have been published, demonstrating the effectiveness of PTA for limb salvage.[22,23] Success rates in these studies vary somewhat, but limb salvage rates in the 70% to 80% range can be expected.

♥ Renal Percutaneous Transluminal Angioplasty and Stenting

The primary indication for PTA or stenting of the renal arteries is treatment of renovascular hypertension or preservation of renal function in patients suffering from renal ischemia due to severe renal artery narrowing. The predominant cause of renal artery stenosis in the elderly patient is atherosclerosis. In up to 85% of these cases, the lesion is ostial in location and due to atherosclerotic plaque in the aorta encroaching on the lumen of the renal artery. These ostial stenoses often do not respond well to balloon angioplasty alone owing to difficulties effectively dilating aorto-ostial plaque. In addition, elastic recoil is common after balloon dilatation in this location. Stents achieve a better lumen than balloon angioplasty alone, and they resist elastic recoil. For this reason, stenting has evolved into the treatment of choice for ostial renal artery stenosis.

The predominant cause of renal artery narrowing in the younger patient is fibromuscular dysplasia, of which there are several types. Fibromuscular dysplasia more often involves the mid and distal segments of the renal artery and may involve the segmental and lobar renal branches. The most common type of fibromuscular dysplasia (medial fibroplasia) causes a "string-of-beads" appearance within the renal artery with alternating aneurysmal segments and stricture-like stenoses. Fibromuscular dysplasia responds well to balloon dilatation, and thus PTA remains the treatment of choice for this condition.

TECHNIQUE

The techniques applied for renal PTA and stenting can vary significantly from operator to operator and between specialists in different disciplines (interventional radiologists versus interventional cardiologists). The procedure can be performed from a femoral or brachial approach. A coaxial approach using a guiding catheter or long sheath is most commonly used. As with PTA in other vascular beds, the patient is pretreated with aspirin and given heparin to maintain an activated clotting time greater than 200 seconds. The lesion is crossed with a guidewire (usually 0.035 or 0.018 inch) and then dilated with an appropriate-sized balloon. The main renal artery usually ranges from 5 to 7 mm in diameter. If renal stenting is to be performed, the stent most often used is the Palmaz tubular slotted stent (Fig. 11-6). The Palmaz stent is hand crimped on a balloon that is the same size as the normal renal artery, and then it is advanced to the site of the lesion. The stent is then deployed with a high-pressure balloon dilatation. In the case of ostial renal artery stenosis, care must be taken to ensure that the ostium of the renal artery is completely covered by the stent with extension of the stent 1 to 2 mm into the aorta.

RESULTS

A number of published studies have demonstrated the effectiveness of renal PTA, particularly for the treatment of renal artery fibromuscular dysplasia and nonostial atherosclerotic narrowing.[24–29] The likelihood of cure of renovascular hypertension is greater in the young patient with fibromuscular dysplasia. Cure of hypertension in the elderly patient with atherosclerotic renal artery stenosis is infrequent. However, improvement in blood pressure control occurs in approximately two thirds to three

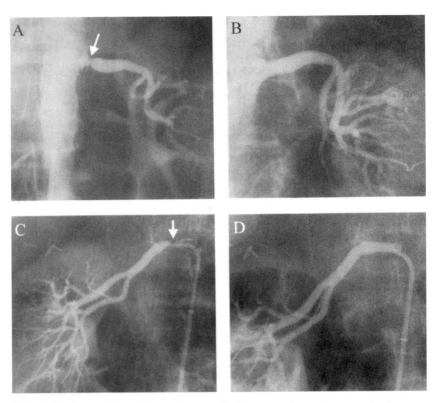

FIGURE 11–6 A patient with poorly controlled hypertension and recurrent pulmonary edema. Angiography demonstrated severe bilateral renal artery stenosis. **(A)** Complex stenosis of the proximal left renal artery (*arrow*). **(B)** Result after implantation of a Palmaz stent. **(C)** Severe, ostial stenosis of the right renal artery (*arrow*). **(D)** Result after successful implantation of a Palmaz stent.

fourths of patients. The incidence of restenosis after renal artery PTA, particularly for atherosclerotic renal artery stenosis, has not been well established because of the absence of prospective studies with angiographic follow-up.

Renal artery stenting is gaining acceptance as the treatment of choice for ostial renal artery stenosis. There is no FDA-approved stent for renal artery use, so biliary Palmaz stents are used in an "off label" manner for this procedure. Table 11-2 lists the results from a number of the published studies on renal artery stenting.[30–34]

With modern-day equipment and stenting techniques, restenosis rates of 10% to 20% can be expected. For the patient with renovascular hypertension, cure or improvement in blood pressure control occurs with a similar frequency to that seen after successful renal PTA.

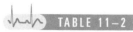 **TABLE 11-2**

Results of Renal Artery Stenting

Author (Year)	No. of Patients/Arteries	Hypertension Improved (%)	Restenosis Rate (%)
Saeed (1993)	50/65	75	36
Rees (1991)	263/296	64	33
Blum (1997)	68/74	78	11
Henry (1996)	138/151	83	10
White (1997)	100/133	76	19

♥ Subclavian and Brachiocephalic Percutaneous Transluminal Angioplasty and Stenting

Patients with stenosis or occlusion of the subclavian or brachiocephalic artery may present with arm claudication, digital ulceration, symptoms of subclavian steal, or symptoms of coronary subclavian steal.

TECHNIQUE

PTA can be performed from either a femoral or brachial approach using a guiding catheter or long sheath. The subclavian artery usually ranges from 7 to 9 mm in diameter. Stenoses and even occlusions can be successfully crossed with a guidewire and treated with balloon dilatation and stenting (Fig. 11-7). The risk of stroke is low (<1%) partly owing to reversal of flow in the vertebral artery that is commonly present in the setting of severe subclavian artery narrowing.

RESULTS

The first case of subclavian angioplasty was reported in 1980.[35] Since that time there have been a number of reports of PTA for the treatment of subclavian steal and coronary-subclavian steal syndrome.[36–41] Technical success rates of 86.5% to 100% have been reported with complication rates of 0% to 7.4%. Neurologic complications have been reported only rarely (<1%). Reversal of flow in the ipsilateral vertebral artery is commonly present in the setting of a severe subclavian stenosis and likely affords protection against embolism to the posterior circulation during the procedure. This reversed flow has been reported to persist 2 to 20 minutes after angioplasty.[42] Clinical follow-up after subclavian PTA suggests 80% to 95% patency rates at 2 to 4 years. This compares favorably with

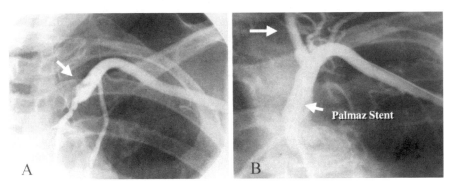

FIGURE 11–7 (A) Severe narrowing of the proximal left subclavian artery. There is a negative contrast jet as a result of retrograde flow from the vertebral artery (*arrow*). (B) Result after successful implantation of a Palmaz stent. There is normal antegrade flow in the vertebral artery (*arrow*).

surgery. Some evidence suggests, however, that late renarrowing of the subclavian artery may occur after PTA.[38,39] It is also likely that long-term patency rates will be lower for occlusions than for stenoses.

Improved results with stenting when applied in other vascular beds has led to the application of this technique for the treatment of subclavian and innominate stenoses and occlusions. Stenting has been shown to result in improved angiographic and hemodynamic results and reduced complications compared with balloon angioplasty alone. Early reports with subclavian artery stenting indicate high technical success rates (94% to 100%) with low complication rates. Long-term follow-up is lacking; however, experience with coronary, renal, and iliac stenting suggest that restenosis rates may be lower with subclavian stenting compared with balloon angioplasty alone.

Our experience at the Washington Hospital Center with subclavian or innominate artery stenting has been similar to the experience of others. Over a 2-year period from March of 1996 to March of 1998 we performed 36 procedures on 36 patients.[43] A femoral approach was used in 33 of 36 (91.7%), brachial approach in 2 (5.6%), and both in 1 (2.7%). The primary indication for revascularization was arm claudication in 6 of 36 (16.7%), subclavian steal in 11 (30.6%), myocardial ischemia in 18 (50%), and access for another procedure in 1 (2.8%). The lesions treated were in the left subclavian artery in 32 of 36 (88.9%), right subclavian artery in 2 (5.6%), and innominate artery in 2 (5.6%). Technical success was achieved in 35 of 36 (97%) patients. There was failure to cross a calcified chronic occlusion with the guidewire in one patient. Quantitative angiography was performed in all patients and demonstrated a reduction in the percent diameter stenosis from 69 ± 14% to 6 ± 11%. The hemodynamic result was excellent with abolishment of the translesional pressure gradient postprocedure and equalization of the right and left arm blood pressures. No deaths, myocardial infarctions, or strokes occurred. Complications consisted of one brachial artery repair (2.8%), and two hematomas (5.6%), one requiring transfusion (2.8%). Clinical follow-up is available on 35 of 36 patients at a mean of 11 months (range 1 to 24 months). Evidence of restenosis was present in 2 of 35 cases (5.6%).

♥ Summary

Minimally invasive endovascular therapies for peripheral vascular disease have evolved significantly since the early years of angioplasty. The term "PTA" now applies to a wide array of different modalities including balloon angioplasty, rotational atherectomy, directional atherectomy, laser, thrombolysis, and stenting. The addition of stents to the armamentarium of the interventionalist has improved the safety and results of this technique and greatly expanded the application of endovascular therapy. Research is now directed at reducing the restenosis rates after endovascular therapy and thus improving the long-term effectiveness of this technique. There will continue to be improvements in stent and balloon technology as well as adjunct pharmacology. Local drug delivery via coated stents will become a reality. Intra-arterial radiation therapy (brachytherapy) may prove beneficial for the prevention of restenosis after angioplasty and stenting. These and other innovative modalities will uphold the promise of a less invasive future for patients with peripheral vascular disease.

REFERENCES

1. Dotter CT, Judkins MP: Transluminal treatment of arteriosclerotic obstruction. Description of a new technique and a preliminary report of its application. *Circulation* 30:654, 1964.
2. Porstmann W: Ein neuer Korsett-Ballonkatheter zur transluminalen Rekanalisation nach Dotter unter besonderer Berucksichtigung von Obliterationen an den Beckenarterien. *Radiol Diagn (Berl)* 14:239, 1973.
3. van Andel GJ: *Percutaneous Transluminal Angioplasty—The Dotter Procedure: A Manual for the Radiologist.* Amsterdam, The Netherlands: Excerpta Medica, 1976.
4. Staple TW: Modified catheter for percutaneous transluminal treatment of arteriosclerotic obstructions. *Radiology* 91:1041, 1968.

5. Gruentzig A, Hopff H: Perkutane rekanalisation chronischer arterieller verschlusse mit einem neuen dilatationskatheter. *Dtsch Med Wochenschr* 99;2502, 1974.
6. Gruentzig A, Kuhlmann U, Lutolf U, et al: Treatment of renovascular hypertension with percutaneous transluminal dilation of a renal artery stenosis. *Lancet* 1:801, 1978.
7. Gruentzig A: Transluminal dilation of a coronary artery stenosis. *Lancet* 1:263, 1978.
8. Gallino A, Mahler F, Probst P, Nachbur B: Percutaneous transluminal angioplasty of the arteries of the lower limbs: A 5-year follow-up. *Circulation* 70:619, 1984.
9. Johnston KW, Rae M, Hogg-Johnston SA, et al: Five year results of a prospective study of percutaneous transluminal angioplasty. *Ann Surg* 206:403, 1987.
10. Hewes RC, White RI, Murray RR: Long-term results of superficial femoral artery angioplasty. *AJR* 146:1025, 1986.
11. Schwarten D: Percutaneous transluminal angioplasty of the iliac arteries: Intravenous digital subtraction angiography for follow-up. *Radiology* 150:363, 1984.
12. Spence R, Freiman D, Gatenby R, et al: Long-term results of transluminal angioplasty of the iliac and femoral arteries. *Arch Surg* 116:1377, 1981.
13. Becker G, Katzen B, Dake M: Noncoronary angioplasty. *Radiology* 170:921, 1989.
14. Tegtmeyer C, Hartwell G, Selby J, et al: Results and complications of angioplasty in aortoiliac disease. *Circulation* 83(Suppl):I-53, 1991.
15. Palmaz JC, Laborde JC, Rivera FJ, et al: Stenting of the iliac arteries with the Palmaz stent: experience from a multicenter trial. *Cardiovasc Intervent Radiol* 15:291, 1992.
16. Richter GM, Roeren TH, Noeldge G, et al: Superior clinical results of iliac stent placement versus percutaneous transluminal angioplasty: four-year success rates of a randomized study (abstr). *Radiology* 181:161, 1991.
17. Martin EC, Katzen BT, Benenati JF, et al: Multicenter trial of the Wallstent in the iliac and femoral arteries. *J Vasc Interv Radiol* 6:843, 1995.
18. Henry M, Amor M, Ethevenot G, et al: Palmaz stent placement in the iliac and femoropopliteal arteries: Primary and secondary patency in 310 patients with 2–4 year follow-up. *Radiology* 197:167, 1995.
19. Gray BH, Sullivan TM, Childs M, et al: High incidence of restenosis/reocclusion of stents in the percutaneous treatment of long-segment superficial femoral artery disease after suboptimal angioplasty. *J Vasc Surg* 2:74, 1997.
20. Capek P, McLean GK, Berkowitz HD: Femoropopliteal angioplasty: factors influencing long-term success. *Circulation* 83(Suppl):I-70, 1991.
21. Jeans WD, Armstrong S, Cole SE, et al: Fate of patients undergoing transluminal angioplasty for lower-limb ischemia. *Radiology* 177:559, 1990.
22. Schwarten DE, Cutcliff WB: Arterial occlusive disease below the knee: Treatment with percutaneous transluminal angioplasty performed with low-profile catheters and steerable guide wires. *Radiology* 169:71, 1988.
23. Bakal CW, Sprayregen S, Scheinbaum K, et al: Percutaneous transluminal angioplasty of the infrapopliteal arteries: results in 52 patients. *AJR* 154:171, 1990.

24. Canzanello V, Millan M, Spiegel J, et al: Percutaneous transluminal renal angioplasty in management of atherosclerotic renovascular hypertension: results in 100 patients. *Hypertension* 13:163, 1989.
25. Greminger P, Steiner A, Schneider E, et al: Cure and improvement of renovascular hypertension after percutaneous transluminal angioplasty of renal artery stenosis. *Nephron* 51:362, 1989.
26. Klinge J, Mali W, Puijlaert C, et al: Percutaneous transluminal renal angioplasty: Initial and long-term results. *Radiology* 171:501, 1989.
27. Martin L, Price R, Casarella, et al: Percutaneous angioplasty in clinical management of renovascular hypertension: Initial and long-term results. *Radiology* 155:629, 1985.
28. Sos T, Pickering T, Sniderman K, et al: Percutaneous transluminal renal angioplasty in renovascular hypertension due to atheroma or fibromuscular dysplasia *N Engl J Med* 309:274, 1983.
29. Tegtmeyer C, Kellum C, Ayers C: Percutaneous transluminal angioplasty of the renal artery. Results and long-term follow-up. *Radiology* 153:77, 1984.
30. Saeed M, Knowles HJ, Schatz RA: Stent placement in renal artery stenoses. SCVIR 18th Annual Scientific Meeting Program. Fairfax, VA: Society of Cardiovascular and Interventional Radiology 47:1993.
31. Rees C, Palmaz J, Becker G, et al: Palmaz stent in atherosclerotic stenoses involving the ostia of the renal arteries: preliminary report of a multicenter study. *Radiology* 181:507, 1991.
32. Blum U, Krumme B, Flugel P, et al: Treatment of ostial renal-artery stenoses with vascular endoprostheses after unsuccessful balloon angioplasty. *N Engl J Med* 336:459, 1997.
33. White CJ, Ramee SR, Collins TJ, et al: Renal artery stent placement: Utility in lesions difficult to treat with balloon angioplasty. *J Am Coll Cardiol* 15:1445, 1997.
34. Henry M, Amor M, Henry I, et al: Stent placement in the renal artery: Three-year experience with the Palmaz stent. *J Vasc Interv Radiol* 7:343, 1996.
35. Bachman D, Kim R: Transluminal dilation for subclavian steal syndrome. *AJR* 135:995, 1980.
36. Dorros G, Lewin R, Jamnadas P, Mathiak L: Peripheral transluminal angioplasty of the subclavian and innominate arteries utilizing the brachial approach: Acute outcome and follow-up. *Cathet Cardiovasc Diagn* 19:71, 1990.
37. Erbstein R, Wholey M, Smoot S: Subclavian artery steal syndrome: Treatment by percutaneous transluminal angioplasty. *AJR* 151:291, 1988.
38. Farina C, Mingoli A, Schultz R, et al: Percutaneous transluminal angioplasty versus surgery for subclavian artery occlusive disease. *Am J Surg* 158:511, 1989.
39. Hebrang A, Maskovic J, Tomac B: Percutaneous transluminal angioplasty of the subclavian arteries: Long-term results in 52 patients. *AJR* 156:1091, 1991.
40. Millaire A, Trinca M, Marache P, et al: Subclavian angioplasty: Immediate and late results in 50 patients. *Cathet Cardiovasc Diagn* 29:8, 1993.
41. Motarjeme A, Keifer J, Zuska A, Nabawi M: Percutaneous transluminal angioplasty for treatment of subclavian steal. *Radiology* 155:611, 1985.

42. Ringlestein E, Zeumer H: Delayed reversal of vertebral artery blood flow following percutaneous transluminal angioplasty for subclavian steal syndrome. *Neuroradiology* 26:189, 1984.
43. Laird JR, Mehran R, Satler LF, et al: Primary stent deployment for obstructive lesions of the subclavian or innominate artery (abstr). *J Am Coll Cardiol* 31:46A, 1998.

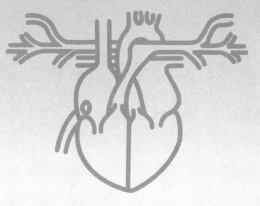

SECTION III

Clinical
Issues

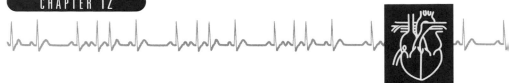

CHAPTER 12

Restenosis

RON WAKSMAN, MD

Restenosis is the term applied to renarrowing or closure of the vessel lumen after vascular interventions such as angioplasty or bypass surgery.

Simply defined, restenosis is wound healing that reduces the vessel lumen diameter by scar tissue formation. It is considered significant when the amount of stenosis compromises hemodynamics.

Restenosis is defined angiographically as renarrowing of the lumen of the vessel after coronary intervention to more than 50% of the "normal" lumen diameter measured in the adjacent arterial segments. Clinically, restenosis is defined as recurrence of symptoms that require medical therapy or repeat revascularization at the lesion site.

Twenty-two years after the first balloon angioplasty in coronary arteries, restenosis still remains the Achilles' heel of the procedure. Despite the introduction of new procedural techniques, devices, and pharmaceutical agents, the overall restenosis rate is still reported in the range of 25% to 50% within 6 to 12 months after the procedure.[1-4] The rate of restenosis is influenced by clinical and morphologic characteristics, such as the type of vessel treated, the location of the lesion or lesions, the vessel size, the amount of residual stenosis following the procedure, the lesion length, and so on. Among the clinical risk factors that influence restenosis are diabetes, hyperlipidemia, smoking, and impaired renal function.[4-8]

Restenosis can be detected on angiography or by a stress test in an asymptomatic patient. It often produces recurrent angina,[9] but rarely is restenosis associated directly with acute myocardial infarction or death.[10] Restenosis usually necessitates repeat revascularization, which may be associated with an increase in morbidity, subsequent recurrence of stenosis and the need for repeat revascularization, and additional cost. The estimated cost of restenosis is $2 billion annually in the United States alone and is targeted intensively by scientists and clinicians for a definitive panacea.[11] To prevent restenois, it is essential to understand the pathophysiology and the mechanisms that contribute to this phenomenon. This chapter presents the current understanding of the pathophysiology of restenosis, as well as the clinical attempts to control it.

♥ Mechanisms and Pathophysiology

Although the cause of restenosis is multifactorial (Fig. 12-1),[1–10,12,13] several components of restenosis had been clearly identified. Among them are early recoil, thrombus formation, proliferation, and late vascular contraction.

RECOIL

Early recoil occurs immediately after opening the obstruction, and is primarily seen after balloon angioplasty.[14] Early recoil can be eliminated by stent placement.[9]

THROMBUS FORMATION

Thrombus deposition is seen immediately after the procedure, its presence is usually related to the degree of injury. The use of devices such as

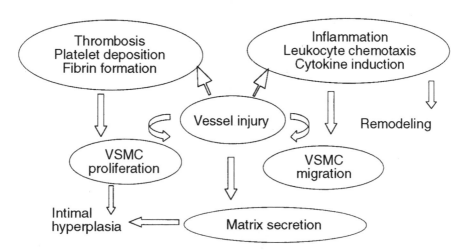

FIGURE 12–1 Mechanisms of restenosis. (VSMC, vascular smooth muscle cell.)

atherectomy, laser angioplasty, and stents are associated with even further damage to the endothelial wall, to the intimal layer, and to the medial cells, resulting in disruption of the media and frequently damaging the adventitia. These injuries stimulate subsequent recruitment of platelets and inflammatory cells, which then migrate into the thrombus within the first week after the injury.[15] The platelets release growth factors and cytokines such as transforming growth factor-β (TGF-β), vascular endothelial growth factor (VEGF), and platelet-derived growth factor (PDGF), which contribute to the proliferative state of the myofibroblasts and matrix formation.

Macrophages and smooth muscle cells also migrate and penetrate into the thrombus as part of a process of digestion and absorption of the thrombus. The by-product of this is neointimal formation, which continues until healing is completed. So far, neither inhibition of thrombus formation nor complete deactivation of platelets after revascularization procedures has shown a significant reduction in the hyperplastic proliferative response.

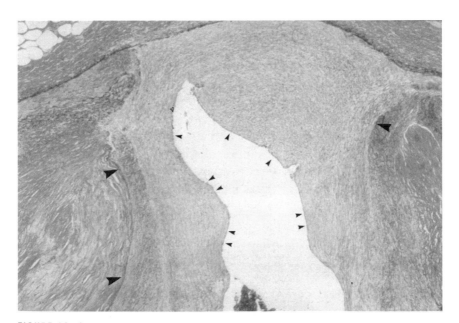

FIGURE 12–2 Intimal proliferation 3 months after balloon angioplasty. The accumulation of neointimal tissue (*small arrows*), composed of smooth muscle cells and matrix formation, is located between the disrupted media (*large arrows*), compromising the vessel lumen.

THE PROLIFERATIVE RESPONSE

The proliferative phase, which consists of myofibroblasts and matrix formation, is completed within 3 to 6 months after the revascularization procedure (Fig. 12-2).[16] Recent animal experiments suggest that myofibroblasts from the adventitia proliferate after angioplasty and migrate into the neointima, where they appear as actin-containing smooth muscle cells.[17] Cell proliferation begins 24 to 48 hours after injury in the porcine model. However, in this model the greatest number of proliferating cells are found at the adventitia surrounding the injured artery and not in the medial wall. Later proliferating adventitial cells extend circumferentially around the entire vessel, even opposite the medial tear.

Scott and colleagues[17] reported that the adventitia was also the site of the greatest PDGF-A and PDGF receptor expression, as determined by in situ hybridization. These studies suggested that the adventitia plays an important role with respect to the first wave of growth after angioplasty of the coronary arteries and later growth of the lesion occurring in the neointima. In addition, immunohistochemistry identified the proliferating cells as myofibroblasts. Further studies showed that removal of the adventitia or injury of the vasa vasorum might cause further stimulation of the proliferation of adventitial myofibroblasts. Therefore, to control restenosis, therapy should be targeted to the adventitial layer.

Neointimal thickening is critical, especially in smaller arteries where the minimal luminal diameter obtained after the intervention is less than 2.5 mm. Any success in reduction of tissue formation in these vessels will contribute to the reduction of restenosis.

The classic animal model to show the effect of therapy on proliferation is the porcine overstretch or coronary stent implantation model.[18] An exuberant proliferative response composed of myofibroblasts matrix formation and vascular contraction is seen within 1 month after the injury. The porcine model was used extensively to study different therapeutic approaches, agents, or devices targeting the neointimal formation. Because the degree of injury either by balloon or stent is related to the amount of tissue proliferation,[19] it is essential to match the injury score among the treated groups when the effectiveness of an agent is tested.

VASCULAR REMODELING

Changes in vessel size and lumen size, which occur after injury, are considered to be the vascular or geometric remodeling component of restenosis. Glagov and associates[20] introduced the concept of vascular remodeling in relation to response of the vessel to formation of athero-

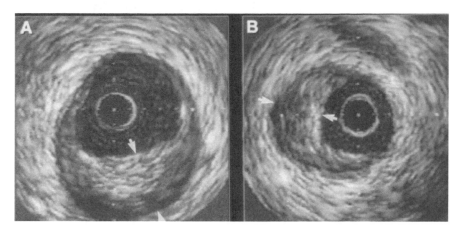

FIGURE 12–3 Intravascular ultrasound study of a patient immediately after directional atherectomy **(A)** and at follow-up **(B)**. Most late lumen loss is from a decrease in the external elastic membrane cross-sectional area. There is no difference in the volume of tissue at follow-up.

sclerotic lesions. Remodeling due to restenosis is primarily related to vascular contraction resulting from adventitial fibrosis.

Mintz and colleagues[21,22] performed serial intravascular measurements on patients undergoing coronary angioplasty and found that intimal thickening in restenotic lesions, as measured by the intima–media cross-sectional area, was responsible for only 24% of the loss in the lumen cross-sectional area. More important, Mintz and associates[22] found that arterial contraction in restenotic lesions, as measured by the area circumscribed by the external elastic lamina, was responsible for 76% of the loss in lumen area. Arteries that did not undergo restenosis had significantly less arterial contraction ("negative remodeling") (Fig. 12-3).

At present, the basis of the differences in remodeling between the restenotic and nonrestenotic arteries is unclear. One explanation is the failure of the restenotic arteries to have normal reendothelialization; therefore, they undergo endothelium-mediated remodeling. Another mechanism could be the lack of arterial expansion or arterial shrinkage owing to excessive adventitial fibrosis.

Recent studies suggested that the adventitia also plays a major role in remodeling and collagen formation, which provides the external forces that result in late contraction. Nitric oxide and antioxidants may minimize the effect of vascular contraction through reduction of factors promoting reendothelialization.

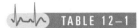 **TABLE 12-1**

Pharmacologic Agents Examined in Various Trials to Reduce Restenosis

Drug	Mode of Therapy	Study Model	Results	Reference
Trapidil	Systemic	Patients	Reduction in angiographic restenosis	STARC study: *Circulation* 88(Suppl 40):595J, 1993
Probucol	Systemic	Patients post-PTCA	Restenosis rate 23% vs 58% in the control	Reference 56
Angiopeptin (somatostatin analogue)	Systemic (continuous subcutaneous)	Rabbit aorta	61% reduction in neointimal volume	Hong et al: *Circulation* 88:638–648, 1993
Angiopeptin (somatostatin analogue)	Systemic (slow release intramuscular)	Porcine coronary	45% reduction in neointimal volume	Hong et al: *Coron Artery Dis* 8:101–104, 1997
αvβ3 integrin antagonist	Systemic (intravenous)	Porcine coronary	43% reduction in neointimal area	Srivatsa et al: *Circulation* 94:I–41, 1996
Anti-CD11b blocking Mab	Systemic (intravenous)	Rabbit iliac	38% reduction in neointimal growth	Rogers et al: *Circulation* 96:I–667, 1997
Cilostazol (antiplatelet agent)	Systemic (oral)	Patients	64% reduction in late loss	Hara et al: *Circulation* 94:I–91, 1996
Tranilast (anti-allergic and anti-keloid drug)	Systemic (oral)	Patients	44% vs 19% restenosis rates	Hsu et al: *Circulation* 94:I–620, 1996
Estrogen	Systemic	Patients	44% vs 19% repeat revascularization	Singh et al: *J Am Coll Cardiol* 29(Suppl):454A, 1997
VEGF	Local delivery (channel balloon)	Rabbit iliac	41% reduction in neointimal area	Van Belle et al: *J Am Coll Cardiol* 29(Suppl):77A, 1997
Ribozymes	Local delivery InfusaSleeve)	Porcine coronary	42% reduction in diameter stenosis	Frimerman et al: *Circulation* 96:I–87, 1997
Alcohol	Local delivery (dispatch catheter)	Patients	No final results	Liu et al: *J Am Coll Cardiol* 27(Suppl):112A, 1996
Low molecular weight heparin	Local delivery (infiltrator)	Patients	No final results	Pavlides et al: *Circulation* 94:I–615, 1996
Low molecular weight heparin	Local delivery (transport catheter)	Patients	Late loss of 0.19	Deutsch et al: *Circulation* 96:I–710, 1997
Heparin	Local delivery (InfusaSleeve)	Patients	No final results	Wilensky et al: *Circulation* 96:I–710, 1997
Nitric oxide donor	Stent coating	Porcine carotid	Significantly less thrombus and neointima	Folts et al: *J Am Coll Cardiol* 27(Suppl):86A, 1996
Hirudin/Prostacyclin	Stent coating	Porcine coronary	24–30% reduction in restenosis	Prietzel et al: *Circulation* 94:I–260, 1996
Tyrosine kinase inhibitor	Biodegradable stent	Porcine coronary	47% reduction in diameter stenosis	Yamawaki et al: *Circulation* 96:I–608, 1997
Paclitaxel	Stent immersion	Porcine coronary	35% reduction in neointimal area	Heldman et al: *Circulation* 96:I–288, 1997
Paclitaxel	Stent coating	Porcine coronary	40% reduction in neointima thickness	Kornowski et al: *Circulation* 96:I–341, 1997
Paclitaxel	Stent coating	Rabbit iliac	50% reduction in neointima thickness	Farb et al: *Circulation* 96:I–608, 1997

Mab, monoclonal antibody; PTCA, percutaneous transluminal coronary angioplasty; VEGF, vascular endothelial growth factor.

Recently, for the first time intracoronary radiation therapy (brachytherapy) was shown to eliminate the vascular contraction component of restenosis with some evidence of increasing in the vessel size of irradiated arteries. This suggests a possibility of favorable remodeling.[23]

❤ Pharmaceutical Approaches to Prevent Restenosis

Over 40 different pharmacologic agents with various therapeutic targets and strategies were tried in an attempt to control restenosis, with overall disappointing results (Table 12-1).

Antiplatelet agents such as aspirin,[22,24] dipyridamole,[22] ticlopidine, and dextran were administered under the premise that inhibition of antiplatelet activity will control restenosis. Most of these agents were compared with aspirin alone, but at most they showed the importance of aspirin to prevent acute thrombosis.

Anticoagulation agents included warfarin, heparin, and antithromboxane synthase inhibitors. These agents were compared with aspirin alone for the prevention of platelet aggregation and thrombus formation.[25] Heparin did not change the restenosis rate, regardless of the length or time (before or after angioplasty) of administration.[26] Finally, low molecular weight heparin did not reduce the rate of clinical events and restenosis rate in placebo-controlled trials.[27,28]

The direct thrombin inhibitors, hirudin[29] and Hirulog, were associated with increased bleeding without any improvement of the incidence of restenosis. These comparison studies discounted the hypothesis that elimination of thrombus may have a beneficial effect on restenosis.

Platelet glycoprotein (GP IIb/IIIa) receptor inhibitors such as abciximab, tirofiban, and eptifibatide clearly show benefit in reduction of acute clinical events in patients with unstable angina and in patients after angioplasty.[30–33] Unfortunately, reduction in restenosis has not been demonstrated. Although in one study abciximab showed a reduction of target vessel revascularization without angiographic documentation of restenosis,[30] most recent trials using these agents showed no difference in the 6-month clinical and angiographic restenosis rate.[34–37]

The calcium channel blockers, nifedipine,[38] verapamil,[39] and diltiazem,[40,41] all claimed to have an antiplatelet effect. These agents may also have an antiproliferative effect on neointimal formation in animal studies. However, they did not show benefit in five clinical human trials, although a meta-analysis of three trials showed some reduction in the angiographic restenosis rate.[42]

Lipid-lowering agents such as lovastatin[43] and pravastatin[44,45] are used to control the atherosclerotic process. Although improvement in endothelial function was shown with high doses of lovastatin, these effects were not translated to reduction in angiographic restenosis at 6 months.

Fish oil supplements, the omega-3 fatty acids, may have an antiatherogenic effect, but failed to show antirestenotic effect in controlled trials.[46–54]

The antiproliferative agent colchicine was associated with aneurysm formation when used in clinical trials.[52,53]

Anti-inflammatory agents (corticosteroids) were not clinically effective at various doses.[54]

The angiotensin-converting enzymes, cilazapril and fosinopril, showed effect in small animal models, but failed to show effectiveness in the pig model and in clinical trials.[53]

Several agents have been reported to have the potential to reduce restenosis. Among them were trapidil[37] (a platelet-derived growth factor inhibitor). Despite the positive results from a large clinical study, this agent is not in clinical use.

Angiopeptin is a somatostatin analogue that works by preventing an increase in the potent insulin growth factor (IGF-1) in the vascular wall after balloon angioplasty. This agent had initial positive reports, but results from larger multicenter clinical trial were disappointing.[55,56]

Antioxidants such as multivitamins and probucol demonstrated effect primarily on arterial remodeling. Probucol, which has strong antioxidant properties, also showed reduction of neointima formation in animal studies.[57] The Probucol Angioplasty Restenosis Trial (PART) was associated with a reduction of restenosis from 58% in the control group to 23% in the probucol group, with clinical results sustained at 1 and 3 years.[58] However, the necessity of pretreatment with probucol for 30 days before angioplasty limits the practicality of this approach.

♥ Mechanical Devices

With the failure of the pharmacologic approach to combat restenosis, a variety of devices have been suggested. Among them were atheroablative devices, such as laser angioplasty and directional atherectomy, and the scaffolding prostheses, stents.

Laser angioplasty was not tested in a randomized fashion and showed benefit only as an ablative device or to facilitate optimal result for balloon angioplasty.[59] However, it was associated with an increase in the restenosis rate, explained by an excess of trauma to the vessel wall.[60,61]

Great expectations were held out for directional atherectomy, based on the hypothesis that plaque removal will contribute to a reduction of restenosis and based on the ability to obtain a larger lumen with this device—the "bigger is better concept." However, randomized trials did not show the benefit of directional atherectomy over balloon angioplasty.[62–64] The increase in clinical events with this device did reduce the enthusiasm of its use to less than 3% of all interventional procedures, despite improvement of the results with optimal directional atherectomy in the Balloon Versus Optimal Atherectomy Trial (BOAT)[65] and guided atherectomy in the Optimal Atherectomy Restenosis Study (OARS) trials.[66]

Rotational atherectomy was involved with higher complication rates and higher restenosis rates compared with balloon angioplasty as evaluated in the Excimer Laser, Rotational Atherectomy, and Balloon Angioplasty Comparison (ERBAC) Trial.[61] Different strategies of multiple burrs and larger burrs did not affect the restenosis rate (>50%). Today, the use of the rotational atherectomy device is limited to an ablative tool to obtain a smooth angiographic result in calcified and diffuse lesions that are unfavorable for balloon angioplasty.

Stents are the only devices that have obtained a better acute result and have reduced the clinical and angiographic restenosis rates. The landmark studies to prove the superiority of stents over balloons were the two multicenter trials, the Stent Restenosis Study (STRESS)[67] and the Belgium Netherlands Stent Study Group (BENESTENT),[68] with a reduction of the restenosis rate from 42% to 32% and from 32% to 22%, respectively, in the balloon versus the stent arm.

IN-STENT RESTENOSIS

In-stent restenosis has become a clinical problem, and its presence after stent implantation is estimated in more than 100,000 patients annually in the United States alone. The efforts to prevent in-stent restenosis were targeted toward coated stents with antiplatelet and antiproliferative agents. Some of these agents, such as paclitaxel (Taxol), are showing encouraging results in porcine coronaries. A list of several of the examined coating agents are included in Table 12-1. The clinical trial BENESTENT II using heparin-coated stents demonstrated a lower rate of subacute thrombosis, with favorable results in reduction of clinical events at 6 months in the heparin-coated group compared with the control without significant reduction in the angiographic restenosis rate.[69]

♥ Gene Therapy

Gene therapy has enormous potential to reduce restenosis by targeting the proliferating cell cycle at the DNA level and by maintaining the smooth muscle cells in the resting phase.[70] A number of different approaches are being tested for the prevention of neointima formation. Among these are transferring the gene directly into the smooth muscle cell.[71] Genes can be encoded for cell cycle inhibitory proteins, angiogenic proteins, or vasodilatory antithrombotic antiproliferative proteins. These altered smooth muscle cells affect the restenosis pattern.

A different method is to deliver the genes that code for cytotoxic products using adenovirus or others viruses as a vector and transfecting the smooth muscle cells. Introduction of gene coding for nitric oxide synthase (NOS) has also been shown to reduce restenosis in a rat carotid model.

Another approach is the antisense technology. Antisense oligonucleotides are short pieces of DNA with sequences that are complementary to specific regions of messenger RNA. Antisense sequences can target specific mediators of the cell cycle, such as c-*myc* and c-*myb*; this approach has also shown positive but not consistent results in animal models. Once completely understood, molecular intervention has the potential to control the process of restenosis.[70]

♥ Vascular Brachytherapy

Endovascular radiation therapy—vascular brachytherapy—is the most promising approach to prevent restenosis and to treat in-stent restenosis. Animal trials using the porcine model showed profound effects in reduction of neointima formation after arterial wall injury.[72–77]

Initial clinical registry trials have shown significant lower late loss and late loss indices and suggested favorable remodeling as well as reduction of neointima formation.[76,77] Lower rates of target lesion revascularization were reported when radiation was applied as adjunct therapy to stenting in the SCRIPPS investigation.[78] The Washington Radiation for In-Stent Restenosis Trial (WRIST)[23] demonstrated a reduction of more than 60% in recurrence of restenosis in the radiation arm compared with placebo. Other large controlled trials are on their way; the late outcome (3 to 5 years) of patients who were treated with endovascular radiation is pending.

❤ Conclusions

Despite ongoing improvements and progression in the field of interventional cardiology the incidence of restenosis is high and limits the results of a successful intervention. Over the years, pharmacologic agents, new devices, and techniques were recruited to the combat to reduce restenosis by altering the response of the arterial wall to injury. The main accomplishment in the past few years was in better understanding the mechanisms of restenosis and identifying targets for therapies. Reduction in restenosis was achieved in part with the introduction of stents but created a new challenge, in-stent restenosis.

Vascular brachytherapy is a breakthrough in terms of prevention of late loss and intimal hyperplasia. With the encouraging reports of vascular brachytherapy and the future potential of gene therapy and new pharmacologic agents, it is conceivable that the restenosis problem following intervention will be nearly cured within the next 5 years.

REFERENCES

1. Aora RR, Konrad K, Badhwar K, Hollman J: Restenosis after transluminal coronary angioplasty: A risk factor analysis. *Cathet Cardiovasc Diagn* 19:17, 1990.
2. Nobuyoshi M, Kimura T, Nosaka H, et al: Restenosis after successful percutaneous transluminal coronary angioplasty: Serial angiographic follow-up of 229 patients. *J Am Coll Cardiol* 12:616, 1988.
3. Popma JJ, Califf RM, Topol EJ: Clinical trials of restenosis after coronary angioplasty. *Circulation* 84:1426, 1991.
4. Kuntz RE, Gibson CM, Nobuyoshi M, Baim DS: Generalized model of restenosis after conventional balloon angioplasty, stenting and directional atherectomy. *J Am Coll Cardiol* 21:15, 1993.
5. Aronson D, Bloomgarden Z, Rayfield EJ: Potential mechanisms promoting restenosis in diabetic patients. *J Am Coll Cardiol* 27:528, 1996.
6. Carrozza JP, Kuntz RE, Fishman RF, Baim DS: Restenosis after arterial injury caused by coronary stenting in patients with diabetes mellitus. *Ann Intern Med* 118:344, 1993.
7. Van Belle E, Bauters C, Hubert E, et al: Restenosis rates in diabetic patients. A comparison of coronary stenting and balloon angioplasty in native coronary vessels. *Circulation* 96:1454, 1997.
8. Kornowski R, Mintz GS, Kent KM, et al: Increased restenosis in diabetes mellitus after coronary interventions is due to exaggerated intimal hyperplasia: A serial intravascular ultrasound study. *Circulation* 95:1366, 1997.
9. Foley JB, Chisholm RJ, Common AA, et al: Aggressive clinical pattern of angina at restenosis following coronary angioplasty in unstable angina. *Am Heart J* 124:1174, 1992.
10. Weintraub WS, Ghazzal ZM, Douglas JS Jr, et al: Usefulness of the substitution of nonangiographic endpoints (death, acute myocardial infarction, coro-

nary bypass and/or repeat angioplasty) for follow-up coronary angiography in evaluating the success of coronary angioplasty in-patients with angina pectoris. *Am J Cardiol* 81:382, 1998.

11. Weintraub WS: The economics of restenosis: Implications for brachytherapy. In Waksman R (ed): *Vascular Brachytherapy,* 2nd ed, pp. 601–611. Armonk, NY, Futura Publishing, 1998.

12. Forrester JS, Fishbein M, Helfant R, Fagin J: A paradigm for restenosis based on cell biology: Clues for the development of new preventive therapies. *J Am Coll Cardiol* 17:758, 1991.

13. Liu MW, Roubin GS, King SB III: Restenosis after coronary angioplasty. Potential biologic determinants and role of intimal hyperplasia. *Circulation* 79:1374, 1989.

14. Haude M, Erbel R, Hassan I, Meyer J: Quantitative analysis of elastic recoil after balloon angioplasty and after intracoronary implantation of balloon-expandable Palmaz-Schatz stents. *J Am Coll Cardiol* 21:26, 1993.

15. Schwartz R: The vessel wall reaction in restenosis. *Semin Intervent Cardiol* 2:83, 1997.

16. Austin GE, Ratliff MB, Hollman J: Intimal proliferation of smooth muscle cells as an explanation for recurrent coronary artery stenosis after percutaneous transluminal coronary angioplasty. *J Am Coll Cardiol* 6:369, 1985.

17. Scott, NA, Cipolla GD, Ross CE, et al: Identification of potential role for the adventitia in vascular lesion formation after balloon overstretch injury of porcine coronary arteries. *Circulation* 93:2178, 1996.

18. Karas SP, Gravanis MB, Santoian EC, et al: Coronary intimal proliferation after balloon injury and stenting in swine: An animal model of restenosis. *J Am Coll Cardiol* 20:467, 1992.

19. Schwartz R, Huber K, Murphy J, et al: Restenosis and the proportional neointima response to coronary artery injury results in the porcine model. *J Am Coll Cardiol* 19:267, 1992.

20. Glagov S, Weisenberg G, Zarins CK, et al: Compensatory enlargement of human atherosclerotic coronary arteries. *N Engl J Med* 316:1371, 1987.

21. Mintz GS, Popma JJ, Pichard AD, et al: Arterial remodeling after coronary angioplasty: A serial intravascular ultrasound study. *Circulation* 94:35, 1996.

22. Mintz GS, Popma JJ, Pichard AD, et al: Intravascular ultrasound predictors of restenosis after percutaneous transcatheter coronary revascularization. *J Am Coll Cardiol* 27:1678, 1996.

23. Waksman R, White LR, Chan RC, et al: Intracoronary radiation therapy for patients with in-stent restenosis: Six month follow-up of a randomized clinical study (WRIST) (abstr). *Circulation* 98:I-651, 1998.

24. Schwartz L, Bourassa MG, Lesperance J, et al: Aspirin and dipyridamole in the prevention of restenosis after percutaneous transluminal coronary angioplasty. *N Engl J Med* 318:1714, 1988.

25. Taylor RR, Gibbons FA, Cope GD, et al: Effects of low-dose aspirin on restenosis after coronary angioplasty. *Am J Cardiol* 68:874, 1991.

26. Serruys PW, Rutsch W, Heyndrickx GR, et al: Prevention of restenosis after percutaneous transluminal coronary angioplasty with thromboxane A-2 receptor blockade. A randomized, double blind, placebo-controlled trial. Coronary Artery Restenosis Prevention on Repeated Thromboxane-Antagonism Study (CARPORT). *Circulation* 84:1568, 1991.

27. Brack MJ, Ray S, Chauhan A, et al: The Subcutaneous Heparin and Angioplasty Restenosis Prevention (SHARP) Trial: Results of a multicenter-randomized trial investigating the effects of high dose unfractionated heparin on angiographic restenosis and clinical outcome. *J Am Coll Cardiol* 26:947, 1995.

28. Faxon DP, Spiro TE, Minor S, et al: Low-molecular-weight heparin in prevention of restenosis after angioplasty. Results of Enoxaparin Restenosis (ERA) Trial. *Circulation* 90:908, 1994.

29. Serruys PW, Herrman JP, Simon R, et al: A comparison of hirudin with heparin in the prevention of restenosis after coronary angioplasty. Helvetica investigators. *N Engl J Med* 333:757, 1995.

30. Topol EJ, Califf RM, Weisman HF, et al: Randomized trial of coronary intervention with antibody against platelet IIb/IIIa integrin for reduction of clinical restenosis: Results at six months. The EPIC investigators. *Lancet* 343:881, 1994.

31. Lefkovits J, Ivanhoe RF, Califf RM, et al: Effects of platelet glycoprotein IIb/IIIa receptor blockade by a chimeric monoclonal antibody (abciximab) on acute and six-month outcomes after percutaneous transluminal coronary angioplasty for acute myocardial infarction. EPIC investigators. *Am J Cardiol* 77:1045, 1996.

32. Tcheng JE: Glycoprotein IIb/IIIa receptor inhibitors: Putting the EPIC, IMPACT II, RESTORE, and EPILOG trials into perspective. *Am J Cardiol* 78:35, 1996.

33. The EPIC Investigators: Use of monoclonal antibody directed against the platelet glycoprotein IIB/IIIa receptor in high-risk coronary angioplasty. *N Engl J Med* 330:956, 1994.

34. The IMPACT-II investigators: Randomized placebo-controlled trial of effect of eptifibatide on complications of percutaneous coronary intervention: IMPACT-II. Integrilin to Minimize Platelet Aggregation and Coronary Thrombosis-II. *Lancet* 349:1422, 1997.

35. The RESTORE investigators: Effects of platelet glycoprotein IIb/IIIa blockade with tirofiban on adverse cardiac events in patients with unstable angina or acute myocardial infarction undergoing coronary angioplasty. Randomized Efficacy Study of Tirofiban for Outcomes and Restenosis. *Circulation* 96:1445, 1997.

36. The EPILOG investigators: Platelet glycoprotein IIb/IIIa receptor blockade and low-dose heparin during percutaneous coronary revascularization. *N Engl J Med* 336:1689, 1997.

37. Maresta A, Balducelli M, Cantini L, et al: Trapidil (triazolopyridine), a platelet-derived growth factor antagonist, reduces restenosis after percutaneous transluminal coronary angioplasty. Results of the randomized, double blind STARC study. *Circulation* 90:2710, 1994.

38. Whitworth HB, Roubin GS, Hollman J, et al: Effect of nifedipine on recurrent stenosis after percutaneous transluminal coronary angioplasty. *J Am Coll Cardiol* 8:1271, 1986.

39. Hoberg E, Dietz R, Frees U, et al: Verapamil treatment after coronary angioplasty in patients at high risk of recurrent stenosis. *Br Heart J* 71:254, 1994.

40. O'Keefe JH Jr, Giorgi LV, Hartzler GO, et al: Effects of diltiazem on complications and restenosis after coronary angioplasty. *Am J Cardiol* 67:373, 1991.

41. Corcos T, David PR, Val PG, et al: Failure of diltiazem to prevent restenosis after percutaneous transluminal coronary angioplasty. *Am Heart J* 109:926, 1985.
42. Hillegass WB, Ohman EM, Leimberger JD, Califf RM: A meta-analysis of randomized trials of calcium antagonists to reduce restenosis after coronary angioplasty. *Am J Cardiol* 73:835, 1994.
43. Bertrand ME, McFadden EP, Fruchart JC, et al: Effect of pravastatin on angiographic restenosis after coronary balloon angioplasty. The PREDICT Trial investigators. Prevention of Restenosis by Elisor after Transluminal Coronary Angioplasty. *J Am Coll Cardiol* 30:863, 1997.
44. O'Keefe JH Jr, Stone GW, McCallister BD Jr, et al: Lovastatin plus probucol for prevention of restenosis after percutaneous transluminal coronary angioplasty. *Am J Cardiol* 77:649, 1996.
45. Weintraub WS, Boccuzzi SJ, Klein JL, et al: Lack of effect of lovastatin on restenosis after coronary angioplasty. Lovastatin Restenosis Trial Study Group. *N Engl J Med* 331:1331, 1994.
46. Cairns JA, Gill J, Morton B, et al: Fish oils and low-molecular-weight heparin for the reduction of restenosis after percutaneous transluminal coronary angioplasty. The EMPAR Study. *Circulation* 94:1553, 1996.
47. Leaf A, Jorgensen MB, Jacobs AK, et al: Do fish oils prevent restenosis after coronary angioplasty? *Circulation* 90:2248, 1994.
48. Bairati I, Roy L, Meyer F: Double blind, randomized, controlled trial of fish oil supplements in prevention of recurrence of stenosis after coronary angioplasty. *Circulation* 85:950, 1992.
49. Grigg LE, Kay TW, Valentine PA, et al: Determinants of restenosis and lack of effect of dietary supplementation with eicosapentaenoic acid on the incidence of coronary artery restenosis after angioplasty. *J Am Coll Cardiol* 13:665, 1989.
50. Reis GJ, Boucher TM, Sipperly ME, et al: Randomized trial of fish oil for prevention of restenosis after coronary angioplasty. *Lancet* 2:177, 1989.
51. Dehmer GJ, Popma JJ, van den Berg EK, et al: Reduction in the rate of early restenosis after coronary angioplasty by a diet supplemented with omega-3 fatty acids. *N Engl J Med* 319:733, 1988.
52. O'Keefe JH Jr, McCallister BD, Bateman TM, et al: Ineffectiveness of colchicine for the prevention of restenosis after coronary angioplasty. *J Am Coll Cardiol* 19:1597, 1992.
53. Freed M, Safian RD, O'Neill WW, et al: Combination of lovastatin, enalapril, and colchicine does not prevent restenosis after percutaneous transluminal coronary angioplasty. *Am J Cardiol* 76:1185, 1995.
54. Pepine CJ, Hirshfeld JW, MacDonald RG, et al: The M-Heart Group. A controlled trial of corticosteroids to prevent restenosis after coronary angioplasty. *Circulation* 81:1753, 1990.
55. Schneider JE, Berk BC, Gravanis MB, et al: Probucol decreases neointimal formation in a swine model of coronary artery balloon injury. A possible role for antioxidants in restenosis. *Circulation* 88:628, 1993.
56. Tardif JC, Cote G, Lesperance J, et al: Probucol and multivitamins in the prevention of restenosis after coronary angioplasty. Multivitamins and Probucol Study Group. *N Engl J Med* 337:365, 1997.
57. Rodes J, Cote G, Lesperance J, et al: Prevention of restenosis after angioplasty in small coronary arteries with probucol. *Circulation* 97:429, 1998.

58. Yokoi H, Daida H, Kuwabara Y, et al: Effectiveness of an antioxidant in preventing restenosis after percutaneous transluminal coronary angioplasty: The Probucol Angioplasty Restenosis Trial. *J Am Coll Cardiol* 30:855, 1997.

59. Bittl JA, Kuntz RE, Estella P, et al: Analysis of late lumen narrowing after excimer laser facilitate coronary angioplasty. *J Am Coll Cardiol* 23:1314, 1994.

60. Mehran R, Mintz GS, Satler LF, et al: Treatment of in-stent restenosis with excimer laser coronary angioplasty. Mechanisms and results compared to PTCA alone. *Circulation* 96:2183, 1997.

61. Reifart N, Vandormael M, Krajcar M, et al: Randomized comparison of angioplasty of complex coronary lesions at a single center. Excimer Laser, Rotational Atherectomy and Balloon Angioplasty Comparison (ERBAC) study. *Circulation* 96:91, 1997.

62. Topol EJ, Leya F, Pinkerton CA, et al: A comparison of directional atherectomy with coronary angioplasty in patients with coronary artery disease (CAVEAT -I). *N Engl J Med* 329:221, 1993.

63. Adelman AG, Cohen EA, Kimball BP, et al: A comparison of directional atherectomy with balloon angioplasty for lesions in the left anterior descending coronary artery (CCAT). *N Engl J Med* 329:228, 1993.

64. Holmes DR Jr, Topol EJ, Califf RM, et al: The CAVEAT-II investigators. A multicenter randomized trial of coronary angioplasty versus directional atherectomy for patients with saphenous vein bypass grafts. *Circulation* 91:1966, 1995.

65. Baim DS, Cutlip DE, Sharma SK, et al: Final results of the Balloon versus Optimal Atherectomy Trial (BOAT). *Circulation* 97:322, 1998.

66. Simonton CA, Martin MB, Baim DS, et al: "Optimal" directional coronary atherectomy: Final results of the Optimal Atherectomy Restenosis Study (OARS). *Circulation* 97:332, 1998.

67. Serruys PW, de Jaegere P, Kiemeneij F, et al: A comparison of balloon-expandable-stent implantation with balloon angioplasty in patients with coronary artery disease. *N Engl J Med* 331:489, 1994.

68. Fischman DL, Leon MB, Baim DS, et al: A randomized comparison of coronary-stent placement and balloon angioplasty in the treatment of coronary artery disease. *N Engl J Med* 331:496, 1994.

69. Serruys PW, Emanuelsson H, van der Giessen W, et al: Heparin-coated Palmaz-Schatz stents in human coronaries. Early outcome of the Benestent-II pilot study. *Circulation* 93:412, 1996.

70. Kutryk MJB, Serruys PW: Antirestenosis alternatives for the next millennium. In Waksman R (ed): *Vascular Brachytherapy*, 2nd ed, pp. 53–60. Armonk, NY, Futura Publishing, 1998.

71. Nabel EG, Plautz G, Nabel GJ: Gene transfer into the vascular cells. *J Am Coll Cardiol* 17(Suppl):189B, 1991.

72. Wiedermann JG, Marboe C, Amols H, et al: Intracoronary irradiation markedly reduces restenosis after balloon angioplasty in a porcine model. *J Am Coll Cardiol* 23:1491, 1994.

73. Wiedermann IG, Marboe C, Amols H, et al: Intracoronary irradiation markedly reduces neointimal proliferation after balloon angioplasty in swine: Persistent benefit at 6-month follow-up. *J Am Coll Cardiol* 25:1451, 1995.

74. Waksman R, Robinson KA, Crocker IR, et al: Endovascular low-dose irradiation inhibits neointima formation after coronary artery balloon

injury in swine: A possible role for radiation therapy in restenosis prevention. *Circulation* 91:1533, 1995.

75. Waksman R, Robinson KA, Crocker IR, et al: Intracoronary radiation before stent implantation inhibits neointima formation in stented porcine coronary arteries. *Circulation* 92:1383, 1995.

76. Condado JA, Waksman R, Gurdiel O, et al: Long-term angiographic and clinical outcome after percutaneous transluminal coronary angioplasty and intracoronary radiation therapy in humans. *Circulation* 96:727, 1997.

77. King SB III, Williams DO, Chougule P, et al: Endovascular beta-radiation to reduce restenosis after coronary balloon angioplasty: Results of the beta energy restenosis trial (B.E.R.T.). *Circulation* 97:2025, 1998.

78. Teirstein PS, Massullo V, Jani S, et al: Catheter-based radiotherapy to inhibit restenosis after coronary stenting. *N Engl J Med* 336:1697, 1997.

CHAPTER 13

Interdisciplinary Management of the Interventional Patient

SUE APPLE, RN, DNSc, CCRN

Since the first percutaneous transluminal coronary angioplasty (PTCA) performed by Andreas Gruentzig in 1977[1], technologic changes in the field of interventional cardiology have advanced at an ever-increasing rate. In the mid 1980s, PTCA procedures, limited to hemodynamically stable patients with good ventricular function and single-vessel coronary disease, were performed with the operating room on standby. After "plain old balloon angioplasty," patients were transferred to the coronary intensive care unit for a recovery period of 1 to 2 days, followed by several more days of care on a general nursing unit.[2–4] Patients were kept almost flat in bed with arterial and venous sheaths left in place until at least the morning after the procedure. Anticoagulation regimens were extensive. Manual compression was the only method of achieving hemostasis of the access site.

Patients with multiple atherosclerotic lesions in native coronary arteries and saphenous vein grafts are presently treated with a variety of balloons, atherectomy devices, and stents. The use of "bail-out" procedures to treat patients with unstable angina or acute myocardial infarction has become routine in most large centers. Cardiac catheterization laboratory and nursing unit personnel have had to expand their clinical expertise because interventional procedures performed in the catheterization laboratory now include treatment of lesions in the cerebral and peripheral circulation.

Even with the rapid changes taking place in the field of interventional cardiology, the principles of patient management have not changed greatly since those early days. Patients still require a period of bed rest until sheaths are removed, although for a much shorter time. Anticoagulation and medication regimens remain crucial to a successful outcome. Management of access site complications continues to evolve. This chapter reviews the current principles and practice of clinical management of the interventional patient from admission through hospital discharge.

❤ Preparation for the Procedure

Changes in technology and advances in patient management have combined with directives from managed care providers to produce a dramatically shortened hospitalization for most patients. The end result is that most preparation for elective procedures in the catheterization laboratory must take place before the patient enters the hospital. Time allotted for patient assessment and teaching must be sandwiched between admission paperwork, laboratory tests, and the schedule of the catheterization laboratory. Incorporating preprocedure standards of care for the interventional patient ensures that the patient and family will be thoroughly and safely prepared for the scheduled procedure (Display 13-1). These standards can be incorporated into a clinical pathway that allows all members of the health care team to monitor the patient's progress throughout the hospitalization[5] (Exhibit 13-1). The clinical pathway can be "translated" for use by patients and their families to assist them during the hospitalization (Exhibit 13-2).

For elective procedures, the patient should be contacted by the tertiary hospital, ideally 2 days before the scheduled procedure. This contact serves both as a method of verifying the scheduled date and time of the procedure and as an opportunity to review patient instructions, such as refraining from eating or drinking after midnight the night before the test. Patients should also be questioned about medications, including the use of oral anticoagulants and oral hypoglycemics, especially metformin. Patients who are taking warfarin need to be admitted before the procedure to make a transition from the oral agent to heparin.

Patients may have to stop taking metformin before their procedure. The biguanides have been associated with severe and even fatal lactic acidosis.[6,7] This risk is increased in the presence of renal impairment (plasma creatinine > 1.4 mg/dL), which is a complication after the use of contrast materials.[8]

❤ Laboratory Tests

Screening laboratory tests are necessary to obtain baseline values before the procedure and to confirm that it is safe for the patient to proceed with

DISPLAY 13–1   Nursing Standard of Care Preprocedure

In the care of the patient undergoing a cardiac interventional procedure in the catheterization laboratory, the nursing standard of care involves the following.

Assessment

1. Assess patient/family's understanding of the procedure.
2. Obtain baseline vital signs including 12-lead electrocardiogram.
3. Place telemetry monitor; verify transmission of heart rhythm to the central station.
4. Perform a complete nursing history and physical assessment with emphasis on the cardiovascular and peripheral vascular systems.
5. Screen the patient for any potential problems, including:
    a. History of contrast agent allergies or blood dyscrasias
    b. Medications taken today, including warfarin, metformin, diuretic, or insulin
    c. Prothrombin time >16 sec.
    d. Creatinine >1.4 mg/dL
    e. Potassium <3.0 or >6.0 mEq/L
    f. Hematocrit <30%
    g. White blood cell count $>10,500 \times 10^3/mm^3$

Intervention

1. Review the proposed procedure, including postprocedure care; answer any questions.
2. Notify the physician of patient/family concerns before any sedation is administered to the patient.
3. Verify that informed consent and any other necessary paperwork are completed.
4. Insert a saline lock in patients' left arm if not already present.
5. Notify the physician/catheterization laboratory personnel of any abnormal vital signs, physical findings, laboratory results, contrast allergies, or potential medication problems before patient is prepped for the procedure.
6. Have the patient void on call to the catheterization laboratory.

Documentation

1. Informed consent
2. Medical and nursing history and physical forms
3. Precatheterization checklist

Patient Outcomes

The patient will be able to undergo the scheduled procedure.

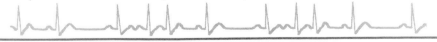

the scheduled test (Display 13-2). All patients should have a complete blood count, serum chemistries, and coagulation times measured before the procedure. Other tests may be included as warranted by the patient's condition.

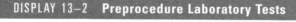

DISPLAY 13–2   **Preprocedure Laboratory Tests**

Tests for all patients
    Complete blood count (CBC)
    Serum glucose, blood urea nitrogen (BUN), creatinine, and electrolytes
Optional Tests
    Coagulation studies
        Platelet count
        Prothrombin time (PT)
        International normalized ratio (INR)
        Activated partial thromboplastin time (aPTT)
        Fibrinogen level
    Cardiac enzymes
        Creatine kinase-MB (CK-MB)
        Troponin
    Serum chemistries
    Lipid profile, homocysteine
Other tests
    Electrocardiogram (ECG)
Consider chest x-ray

♥ History and Physical Assessment

A thorough evaluation of the patient begins with a history and physical examination. Different members of the heath care team focus on different aspects of the medical history and physical examination, but all members should be required to review and assimilate this essential information into their care of the patient.[9] The use of standardized forms ensures that all important areas of the history are covered. They also serve as a method of organizing the data (Exhibits 13-3 and 13-4). A complete patient history includes:

- Chief complaint
- History of the present illness
- Past medical history, including allergies
- Family and social history
- Functional status

The physical examination should be as thorough as time permits, with emphasis on the cardiovascular and peripheral vascular systems. Patients undergoing investigational neurologic procedures such as placement of carotid stents need a more detailed neurologic assessment before the procedure. This includes examination by a neurologist[10] in addition to an evaluation using the National Institute of Health Stroke Scale (NIHSS).[11]

PATIENT AND FAMILY TEACHING

Undergoing any procedure in the catheterization laboratory is a stressful event for patients and their family members.[12–15] Patients are typically admitted the morning of the procedure, further increasing their anxiety. Therefore, instructions given before the procedure need to be brief and concise while at the same time reviewing important information with the patient and family.[16] The focus should be on the anticipated procedure, the sights, sounds, and other sensations encountered in the laboratory, as well as care of the patient after the procedure is completed (Display 13-3). Written descriptions are helpful for the family members, who often have time to review this material while waiting for the procedure to be completed.

FINAL PREPARATION

A checklist ensures that the patient and family are fully prepared for the scheduled procedure (Exhibit 13-5). Shortly before the procedure is scheduled to start, the patient is typically moved into a holding area to

---

DISPLAY 13–3   Topics for Patient/Family Education Preprocedure

Informed consent
Advanced directives
NPO
Blood work
Review planned interventional procedure
    Conscious sedation
    Preparation of the access site
    Catheterization laboratory personnel
    Cine camera
Estimated length of the procedure
Family waiting area
Introduction to the patient care unit

allow final preparation to begin. Because they are separated from their family members and waiting for the transfer into the catheterization laboratory, this period can be a trying time for the patient.

Conventional management calls for the use of preprocedure sedation at this point, such as a benzodiazepine. Alternative methods of relaxation that do not rely on medications have recently been introduced.[17–19] An example is guided imagery. Imagery is the technique of accessing internal or stored memories to achieve a goal, typically relaxation from a stressful situation.[20] *Guided imagery* implies accessing these memories with the help of a structured program or guide.[21] Reported physical benefits of guided imagery include relaxed breathing, slower heart rate, lower breathing rate, and a decreased sensation of pain.[17,19] Guided imagery using prerecorded audiocassette tapes has been used at the Washington Hospital Center catheterization laboratory since 1997 as an adjunct to preprocedure sedation. Preliminary findings indicate a high level of patient satisfaction, as well as a decrease in the amount of sedation necessary to relax the patient during the procedure.

❤ Management of the Patient After the Procedure

Patients returning from the interventional laboratory require a level of care not usually found on a general nursing unit, but less than is available in a critical care unit. This has led to the development of specialized patient units that can safely meet the needs of this patient population.[22] This level is reflected in the postprocedure standards of nursing care (Display 13-4).

CLINICAL ASSESSMENT

Assessment of the patient begins with a physical examination, including the vascular access site (VAS) and the arterial and venous sheaths. Sheaths are left in place after the procedure to allow rapid access in the event of complications, such as abrupt closure or subacute thrombosis, and to allow gradual reversal of any heparin administered during the procedure. Heparin activity is monitored through the use of the activated clotting time (ACT). ACT, a bedside measurement of the clotting time, is widely used to monitor heparin therapy during and after interventional procedures.[23,24] Using a reliable bedside test prevents delay in removing sheaths. The ACT is measured 4 hours after the heparin is stopped. If the value is 150 seconds or less, the sheaths can be removed (Display 13-5). If

---

DISPLAY 13–4   Nursing Standard of Care: Postprocedure

In the care of the patient who has undergone a cardiac interventional procedure in the catheterization laboratory, the nurse will do the following:

Assessment

1. Assess patient/family's understanding of the completed procedure.
2. Obtain baseline vital signs, including 12-lead electrocardiogram (ECG).
3. Perform a complete assessment, including vascular access site for evidence of adequate perfusion, bleeding, or hematoma formation.
4. Evaluate the patient for any ischemic cardiac pain.
5. Examine the patient for any other potential complications related to the procedure.

Intervention

1. Obtain vital signs and peripheral pulses every 15 minutes 4 times or until stable, every 30 minutes two times, every hour four times, and then routine.
2. Connect patient to bedside ECG; verify that ECG rhythm is transmitting to the central monitoring station.
3. Review the patient record for a summary of the procedure, noting type of intervention device, target lesion(s) and outcome, last activated clotting time, and plan for arterial/venous sheath removal.
4. Obtain a 12-lead ECG; review with nurse practitioner/MD
5. Review planned care with patient and family.
6. If patient is unable to tolerate liquids, start intravenous infusion according to standing orders.

Documentation

1. Vital signs, access site, and peripheral pulses on the nursing critical care flowsheet.
2. Nursing notes in the general progress notes.

Patient Outcome

The patient will have an uneventful recovery from the procedure.

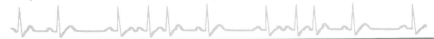

---

the ACT is above 150, the test is repeated hourly until the desired clotting time is reached.

The patient requires frequent assessment after the procedure to detect any potential complications and initiate prompt treatment.

COMPLICATIONS

Complications after interventional procedures include any of the problems that may occur with a diagnostic cardiac catheterization (Table 13-1), as well as complications specific to interventional procedures as a

DISPLAY 13–5 *Procedure for Sheath Removal*

Before the procedure
    Review procedure with the patient.
    Assess need for analgesic or sedative.
    Verify activated clotting time <150, or at ordered value.
    Verify adequate peripheral intravenous access site.
    Obtain bedside electrocardiograph monitor.
    Gather supplies for sheath removal.
        Gloves
        Goggles
        Suture removal set
        4 × 4 sterile gauze
        Material for dressing
        Sandbag or compression device, if ordered
    Gather equipment to treat any side effects or complications.
        Intravenous normal saline
        Atropine
During the procedure
    If patient is in a private room, two qualified personnel must be in attendance during
        actual removal of sheaths and for first 15 minutes after sheaths are removed.
    Obtain baseline vital signs; assess pulses in affected limb.
    Maintain manual compression of the site until hemostasis is attained.
    Apply sterile dressing with sandbag or compression device, if ordered.
    If adequate hemostasis is not obtained within 20 minutes after removal, place com-
        pression device, check activated partial thromboplastin time (aPTT) immediately.
    Treat any vagal response (symptomatic bradycardia, hypotension, nausea) immediately
        with intravenous fluids and atropine, if necessary, according to standard orders.
Following femoral sheath removal
    Take vital signs with pulse checks every 15 minutes four times or until stable, every 30
        minutes two times, every hour four times, then every 4 hours. If compression device
        in place, pulse checks in affected limb every hour until device removed.
    Assess access site with vital signs. Notify MD/nurse practitioner of any bleeding or
        hematoma formation.
    Treat any vagal response immediately with intravenous fluids and atropine according to
        standard orders.

result of device manipulation within the coronary artery.[25–27] Incidence is related to several factors, including the specific patient characteristics (especially gender and age), the type of cardiac disease, the clinical presentation of the patient (i.e., stable versus acute myocardial infarction), and the type of procedure being performed.[27,28]

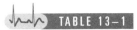 **TABLE 13-1**

Complications After Cardiac Catheterization

Complication	Percent (Low-Risk Population)	Percent (High-Risk Population)*
Death	<0.1	0.3–2.5
Myocardial infarction	0.05	0.08–0.17
Cerebrovascular events	0.07	
Vascular access site complications	0.5–0.6	
Arrhythmias or conduction disturbances	0.4	
Perforation of the heart or great vessels	<0.1	
Infection or pyrogenic reactions	Femoral: 0.06	
	Brachial: 0.62	
Allergic and anaphylactoid reactions	0.1	
Contrast-induced renal failure	5.0	≥26

*High-risk patients: age >60, New York Heart Functional Class IV, left ventricular ejection fraction <30%, left main disease, severe valvular disease, severe noncardiac disease.
Adapted from Baim D, Grossman W: Complications of cardiac catheterization. In Baim DS, Grossman W (eds): *Cardiac Catheterization, Angiography, and Intervention,* 5th ed, pp. 17–38. Baltimore, Williams & Wilkins, 1996.

MAJOR

Major complications after interventional procedures include death, Q-wave myocardial infarction, and the need for emergency bypass surgery (Table 13-2). These outcomes can be the result of extensive coronary artery dissection resulting in abrupt closure, or thrombus formation in the target vessel.

Abrupt closure of the coronary artery can lead to catastrophic outcomes if not recognized and treated immediately (Fig. 13-1). Patients should be assessed for the presence of angina or anginal equivalents, such as shortness of breath. However, the clinician cannot rely on symptoms alone to diag-

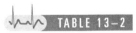 **TABLE 13-2**

In Hospital Complications After Interventional Procedures

Major Complications	POBA* (%)	Early New Device* (%)	Stent Era New Device† (%)
Death	1.0	1.8	0.4–1.0
Q-wave MI	3.3	1.5	0.3–0.5
Emergency CABG	5.8	3.5	0.5–1.0

CABG, coronary artery bypass graft; MI, myocardial infarction; POBA, plain old balloon angioplasty.
*King SB, et al: Balloon angioplasty versus new device intervention: Clinical outcomes. *J Am Coll Cardiol* 31:558, 1998.
†Lindsay J, Pinnow EE, Pichard AD: New devices enhance hospital results of coronary angioplasty. *Cathet Cardiovasc Diagn* 43:1, 1998.

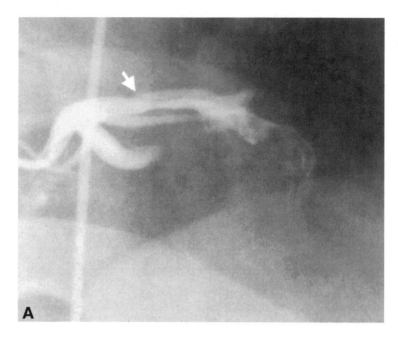

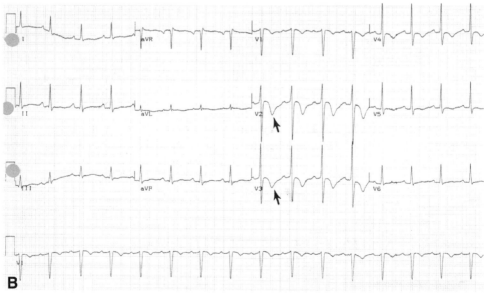

FIGURE 13–1 **(A)** Coronary angiogram demonstrating abrupt closure of the left anterior descending artery. Arrow indicates dissection flap. **(B)** Electrocardiogram recorded shortly before angiogram shown in **A**. Note symmetric T-wave inversion in the anterior leads. Patient was hemodynamically stable and was not experiencing chest pain.

nose abrupt closure.[29] Diabetics and elderly persons often do not experience typical anginal pain. Patients may still be under the influence of the conscious sedation administered during the procedure and therefore may not notice the chest pain. Further chest pain can be related to the procedure itself ("bruise pain") rather than to true ischemia. The 12-lead electrocardiogram (ECG) should be reviewed with attention to the leads reflecting the coronary anatomy that was treated during the procedure (see Fig. 13-1). After abrupt closure is identified, patients are usually returned to the catheterization laboratory for urgent repeat revascularization.

VASCULAR

VAS complications continue to be the most common problem encountered in the clinical management of interventional patients.[30-32] These include groin hematomas, pseudoaneurysms, arteriovenous fistulas, retroperitoneal hematomas, infection, and acute thrombosis. VAS complications involving the brachial artery are more typically arterial thromboses.[33]

The reported overall incidence of VAS complications ranges from 1.0%[33] to approximately 6.0%[34,35] to as high as 9%.[36] Studies report VAS complications after PTCA of 1.0% to 6.0 %.[31,33,34,37-39] VAS complications in new device angioplasty are significantly higher—from 6.6% with directional coronary atherectomy[40] to as high as 14% with intracoronary stenting.[34]

To date, little agreement exists regarding the identification of patients at risk for VAS complications. Some of the difficulty is related to the different definitions of what constitutes a VAS complication, as well as different methods of screening patients after interventional procedures to diagnose these clinical problems. Being elderly (age > 65 years), female, and having peripheral vascular disease have been identified as consistent risk factors for VAS complications in a number of studies.[31,32] The amount and length of anticoagulation during and after the procedure have also been predictors of complications in several investigations.[33-35,39]

Diagnosis of suspected arterial injuries is made through a careful physical assessment and confirmed through noninvasive vascular studies and arteriography where indicated.[37] Physical examination of the femoral site should be performed assessing for the presence of localized tenderness, a hematoma, femoral bruit, or pulsatile mass.[41] Groin hematomas are recognized by the presence of swelling at the site of the arterial puncture. Hematomas have been described as major or minor by size (in centimeters of diameter) as well as by the amount of decrease in the hematocrit or the need for blood transfusion or surgical repair. Large hematomas need to be assessed by ultrasound to rule out pseudoaneurysms or arteriovenous fistulas.

A femoral pseudoaneurysm is an extravascular cavity communicating with the femoral artery by a channel or neck at the needle puncture site[31,42,43] (Fig. 13-2). Physical examination of the site reveals localized tenderness and a palpable, pulsatile mass, often associated with a bruit. Large pseudoaneurysms can compress the adjacent nerves, causing significant discomfort for the patient. Diagnosis of femoral pseudoaneurysm is confirmed through the use of ultrasound with Doppler color flow imaging, which will demonstrate a cavity that communicates with the artery as well as the to-and-fro movement of blood through the neck. The reported incidence of pseudoaneurysms is between 0.5% and 6.3%—the higher rates occurring with new device angioplasty.[31,34,35,40]

Treatment depends on the size of the pseudoaneurysm and the clinical assessment of the patient. Asymptomatic patients with a well-defined pseudoaneurysm with a lumen less than 2.0 cm in diameter can initially

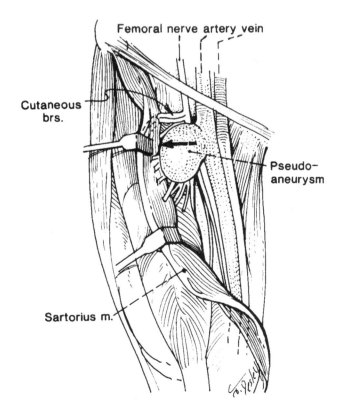

FIGURE 13–2 Illustration of a femoral pseudoaneurysm. (Adapted from Hallett JW Jr, et al: The femoral neuralgia syndrome after arterial catheter trauma. *J Vasc Surg* 11:702, 1990. Used with permission.)

be managed conservatively, with observation for spontaneous thrombosis.[44] Pseudoaneurysms larger than 2.0 cm are best treated with ultrasound-guided direct compression[42] (Fig. 13-3).

External compression is becoming the standard of treatment for femoral artery pseudoaneurysms.[43–45] Success rates higher than 90% are reported in patients who are not on anticoagulants at the time of compression.[43,46] Pseudoaneurysms associated with a rapidly expanding hematoma should be considered for urgent operative repair. Delay could expose the patient to the risks of infection, compression neuropathy, or rupture of the pseudoaneurysm.

An arteriovenous (AV) fistula is a direct communication between the artery and vein, resulting in a high-velocity jet from the artery into the lumen of the vein (Fig. 13-4). Occurrence after interventional procedures ranges from 0.2% to 2.1%[31] to as high as 15.0%.[39] AV fistulas are detected clinically by the presence of a bruit over the access site. Unrepaired, they can lead to venous thrombosis, painful lower extremity, or even congestive heart failure. Diagnosis is confirmed through Doppler ultrasound, demonstrating increased diastolic flow in the supplying artery and pronounced turbulence within the receiving vein.[43]

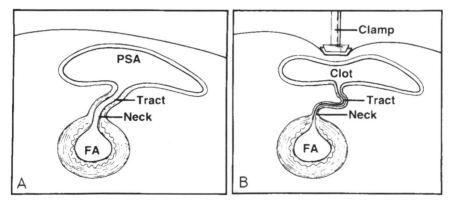

FIGURE 13–3 Noninvasive closure of a femoral artery (FA) pseudoaneurysm (PSA) by ultrasound-guided compression. **(A)** The pseudoaneurysm with its neck and tract arising from the femoral artery. **(B)** External application of a vascular clamp obliterates the neck and tract, resulting in clot formation in the pseudoaneurysm. (Adapted from Agarwal R, et al: Clinically guided closure of femoral arterial pseudoaneurysms complicating cardiac catheterization and coronary angioplasty. *Cathet Cardiovasc Diagn* 30:96, 1993, copyright Wiley-Liss, Inc. Reprinted by permission of Wiley-Liss, Inc, a subsidiary of John Wiley & Sons, Inc)

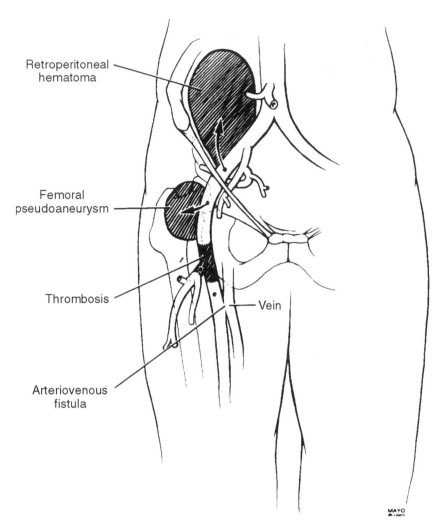

Retroperitoneal
hematoma

Femoral
pseudoaneurysm

Thrombosis

Vein

Arteriovenous
fistula

FIGURE 13–4 Types of iatrogenic vascular complications. (From Hallett JW: Iatrogenic complications of arterial and venous catheterizations. In Rutherford RB (ed): *Vascular Surgery*, 4th ed. Philadelphia, WB Saunders, 1995. By permission of Mayo Foundation.)

As with pseudoaneurysms, clinically asymptomatic patients with AV fistulas without evidence of expansion may be followed up conservatively for evidence of spontaneous thrombosis. When treatment is indicated, ultrasound-guided compression should be attempted first. In situations in which compression fails or there is evidence of clinical deterioration, the patient should be referred for surgical repair.[31,44,45]

Retroperitoneal hematomas are a rare but potentially fatal VAS complication (see Fig. 13-4). Studies report occurrence between 0.5%[34] and 0.44%.[47] Nevertheless, retroperitoneal hematomas account for significant morbidity, involving the need for blood transfusions and surgical repair.[37,39,48] Bleeding into the retroperitoneal space can be difficult to detect until there has been significant blood loss.[39] Early symptoms include flank or back pain, as well nausea and vomiting, often associated with a vagal reaction (hypotension and bradycardia). Diagnosis is confirmed through an abdominopelvic computed tomography scan. Small retroperitoneal hematomas in clinically stable patients may be managed conservatively. However, at the first sign of an expanding hematoma or deterioration in the patient's condition, urgent surgical repair should be performed.

Infections at the VAS occur only in less than 1.0% of cases.[31,34] Infections are related to length of sheath insertion time, the need for repeat procedures,[49,50] and the need for surgical repair.[34] Organisms are usually gram-positive cocci, most often *Staphylococcus aureus*. Treatment may require several weeks of appropriate antibiotic therapy.

Although the femoral approach is preferred in most patients, the brachial artery is reported to be a safe alternative.[47] Arterial thrombosis is the complication usually associated with this site.[33] Thrombosis of the radial artery is readily recognized through physical examination. Treatment includes immediate removal of the sheaths. Surgery may be indicated if this does not result in prompt restoration of blood flow.[31,38,47]

CONTRAST-INDUCED RENAL FAILURE

Contrast-induced nephropathy remains a major cause of hospital-acquired acute renal failure.[32,51,52] Reported incidence ranges from 0% to 44%, the higher percentage in patients with preexisting renal dysfunction (serum creatinine >1.5 mg/dL).[32,53] The wide variation in incidence is partly due to differences in the definition of contrast-induced renal failure. Most authors define a rise in the serum creatinine within 48 hours after injection of the contrast material, but the amount of increase necessary varies from 0.5 mg/dL[52] to at least a 50% increase in the baseline serum creatinine level.[51]

Regardless of the definition, it is widely accepted that contrast-induced renal failure is a very rare occurrence in patients with normal renal function.[8] In addition to preexisting renal dysfunction, risk factors for the development of this complication include advanced age, diabetes, and amount of contrast agent, not the type of agent.[8,30] Formulas have been proposed to limit the amount of contrast agent[54]; however, interventional patients must frequently undergo more than one procedure, increasing the contrast load.

Several treatments have been studied in an attempt to reduce the incidence of contrast-induced renal failure, including hydration, dopamine for renal perfusion, adenosine antagonists, calcium channel blockers, furosemide, and mannitol.[8,32,52] To date, the only effective preventive measure has proved to be adequate hydration before the procedure.[30,52] Patients with preexisting renal failure or who have an increased risk for developing renal failure should be hydrated for at least 12 hours before the contrast procedure with intravenous 0.45% saline at a rate of 1 mL per kilogram of body weight per hour. Hydration may have to be reduced in patients with decreased left ventricular function.

When contrast-induced renal failure does develop, serum creatinine levels return to normal in most patients within 7 days. Hemodialysis is rarely needed in this population.

NON–Q-WAVE MYOCARDIAL INFARCTION

Patients who experience a non–Q-wave myocardial infarction, as evidenced by an increase in the creatine kinase MB (CK-MB) isoform, have been identified as also having an increased risk for late complications related to the interventional procedure.[30,55] Minor elevations of CK-MB (one to three times the upper limit of normal) occur frequently and are probably not clinically significant. However, CK-MB levels greater than 50 IL/L after interventional procedures are rare but are associated with adverse long-term outcomes.[30,55]

CLINICAL MANAGEMENT

Knowledge of the potential complications after any interventional procedure is the basis for clinical management of the patient. Nurses must be skilled in assessing ischemic chest pain and must be able to differentiate procedural pain from true anginal pain. They must be able to obtain a 12-lead ECG whenever they suspect a problem, and they must posses the ability to interpret significant changes. Abrupt closure of the target vessel must be treated immediately. When detected, the nurse must immediately notify the physician and the catheterization laboratory. The patient requires immediate treatment for ischemia, including supplemental oxygen, nitrates, heparin, and possibly morphine. As soon as the catheterization laboratory is ready, the patient must be transported back for urgent revascularization.

Other potentially catastrophic situations that the nursing staff must be prepared to identify and initiate treatment for include cardiac tamponade, major bleeding, and loss of distal pulses. Cardiac tamponade can be recognized by the triad of muffled heart sounds, pulsus paradoxus, and distended neck veins.[56] Major bleeding requires direct pressure where possible, rapid volume replacement, and preparation for an urgent trip to the operating room. Loss of distal pulses may be the result of an arterial occlusion, recognized by the classic symptoms of pain, paralysis, paresthesias, pulselessness, and pallor.[31,57] These and other situations require early identification and treatment to decrease morbidity and mortality and to improve patient outcomes.

In addition to careful monitoring for any potential complications, clinical management of the patient involves comfort, pain relief, nutrition, and postprocedural medications.

Bed rest with arterial and venous sheaths in place is the standard until the anticoagulation administered during the procedure has dissipated. Even after the sheaths are removed, patients are still required to remain in bed with the affected limb straight for several hours. Studies designed to improve patient comfort during this time have examined the use of special mattresses, exercises, and the use of flexible sheaths.[58–60] There have been no consistent findings regarding methods to ease patient discomfort, which is assumed to be directly related to the length of bed rest and relative immobility during this time.

At the Washington Hospital Center, padded mattresses are routinely placed on all beds. This has significantly reduced the number of complaints concerning back pain after the procedure. Foam egg crates also ease the strain of prolonged bed rest. The head of the bed can be elevated 45 degrees if desired. Analgesics are included in the standard postprocedure orders to be administered as needed.

Nutrition is always a concern after the interventional procedure is complete. Even though the patient and family may request a regular meal, the first meal after the procedure is a full liquid diet. Doing so eliminates most of the nausea and vomiting that used to be a part of postprocedural care. If the patient tolerates liquids, the diet is advanced to an American Heart Association (AHA) diet, which is low in saturated fats. Intravenous fluids are administered if the patient's oral intake is not adequate.

Medications after a cardiac interventional procedure include antiplatelet agents, usually both aspirin and clopidogrel or ticlopidine to prevent thrombosis in the target vessel. To control the gastrointestinal side effects of these medications, a gastric acid suppressant such as omeprazole is given. Calcium channel blockers are prescribed to prevent spasm in the coronary arteries. Antioxidants such as vitamins E and A may also be included; however, their role at this time is controversial.

After sheath removal, patients remain in bed for another 6 hours with a mechanical compression device in place. The use of these devices, such as the Femostop (USCI, CR Bard, Inc, Billerica, MA) have improved patient comfort with no significant change in patient outcomes.[61]

♥ Discharge

Patients are usually released the day after their procedure. Serum laboratory values are obtained that morning to verify that the hemoglobin and hematocrit are within acceptable values, as well as CK-MB and troponin I level. If the cardiac enzymes are abnormally elevated, discharge is delayed until the levels have returned to normal. The ECG is also examined.

Physical examination includes the cardiovascular system, as well as auscultation and palpation of the VAS. The presence of a hematoma, tenderness, or bruit require further workup before the patient can be safely released.

Discharge instructions include pictures, diagrams, and written instructions. Pictures of the target lesion or lesions before and after the intervention are given to the family members at the conclusion of the procedure. Any devices placed in the coronary arteries are added to diagrams included in the discharge packet. All medications that the patient is to take are listed. This avoids confusion regarding medications from the referring physician and medications ordered after the interventional procedure. Without this medication list, patients could unknowingly take two calcium channel blockers or two different forms of aspirin.

Individual assessment of cardiovascular risk factors, including the results of the lipid profile and homocysteine levels, are reviewed at this time.[62,63] Smoking cessation, control of high blood pressure, and a heart healthy diet are discussed. A list of available community resources is included with the discharge packet.

Finally, written instructions concerning activity, follow-up appointments with referring physicians, return to work or usual activities, and a phone number to call with questions are included. Because VAS complications can occur days to weeks after the intervention,[39] clinical follow-up is very important. In addition, patients need additional laboratory tests, such as a complete blood cell count and platelet count if they are taking ticlopidine.

Patients and family members are relieved that the procedure is over and anxious to return home. It is not realistic in this setting to expect patients to remember all the instructions they are given before leaving the hospital. Instructions can be included on a standard form that requires the physician, nurse, and patient/family member to sign (Exhibit 13-6). The original stays with the hospital record; a copy is given to the patient.

❤ Conclusion

Management of complex patients undergoing percutaneous interventions in the coronary and peripheral vascular tree has evolved rapidly since 1977. It will continue to evolve as new technologies and advances in the basic sciences expand the indications and treatment options. All members of the health care team must continue to deliver expert care at the bedside, while participating in the research that will define our practice in the future.

REFERENCES

1. Gruentzig AR: Transluminal dilation of coronary artery stenosis (letter). *Lancet* 1:263, 1978.
2. Cimini DM, Goldfarb J: Standard of care for the patient with percutaneous transluminal coronary angioplasty. *Crit Care Nurse* 3:77, 1983.
3. Partridge SA: The nurse's role in percutaneous transluminal coronary angioplasty. *Heart Lung* 11:505, 1982.
4. Purcell JA, Giffin PA: Percutaneous transluminal coronary angioplasty. *Am J Nurs* 81:1620, 1981.
5. Doran K, Sampson B, Staus R, et al: Clinical pathway across tertiary and community care after an interventional cardiology procedure. *J Cardiovasc Nurs* 11:1, 1997.
6. DeFronzo RA, Goodman AM: The Multicenter Metformin Study Group. *N Engl J Med* 333:541, 1995.
7. Stumvoll M, Nurjhan N, Perriello G, Dailey G, Gerich JE: Metabolic effects of metformin in non-insulin dependent diabetes mellitus. *N Engl J Med* 333:550, 1995.
8. Tommaso CL: Contrast-induced nephrotoxicity in patients undergoing cardiac catheterization. *Cathet Cardiovasc Diagn* 31:316, 1994.
9. Skov P, Underhill Motzer S: History taking and physical examination. In Woods S, Sivarajan Froelicher ES, et al (eds): *Cardiac Nursing*, 3rd ed, pp. 226–258. Philadelphia, JB Lippincott, 1995.
10. Yadav JS, Roubin GS, Iyer S, et al: Elective stenting of the extracranial carotid arteries. *Circulation* 95:376, 1997.
11. Goldstein LB, Samsa GP: Reliability of the National Institutes of Health Stroke Scale. Extension to non-neurologists in the context of a clinical trial. *Stroke* 28:307, 1997.

12. Beckerman A, Grossman D, Marquez L: Cardiac catheterization: The patients' perspective. *Heart Lung* 24:213, 1995.
13. Grossman W: Current practice standards. In Baim DS, Grossman W (eds): *Cardiac Catheterization, Angiography, and Intervention,* 5th ed, pp. 9–16. Baltimore, Williams & Wilkins, 1996.
14. Gulanick M, Bliley A, Perino B, et al: Patients' responses to the angioplasty experience: A qualitative study. *Am J Crit Care* 6:25, 1997.
15. Newton KM: Cardiac catheterization. In Woods S, Sivarajan Froelicher ES, et al (eds): *Cardiac Nursing,* 3rd ed, pp 407–423. Philadelphia, JB Lippincott, 1995.
16. Weld L: Developing a cardiac catheterization education program. *J Cardiovasc Nurs* 11:47, 1997.
17. Good M: Relaxation techniques for surgical patients. *Am J Nurs* 95:39, 1995.
18. Houston S, Eagen M, Freeborg S, Dougherty D: A comparison of structured versus guided preheart catheterization information on mood states and coping resources. *Appl Nurs Res* 9:189, 1996.
19. Mandle CL, Jacobs SC, Arcari PM, Domar AD: The efficacy of relaxation response interventions with adult patients: A review of the literature. *J Cardiovasc Nurs* 10:4, 1996.
20. Stephens R: Imagery: A strategic intervention to empower clients. Part I—Review of the literature. *Clin Nurs Spec* 7:170, 1993.
21. Vines SW: The therapeutics of guided imagery. *Holistic Nurs Pract* 2:34, 1988.
22. Sullivan J, Howland-Gradman J, Schell M, Goldsmith J: Reducing costs and improving processes for the interventional cardiology patient. *J Cardiovasc Nurs* 11:22, 1997.
23. Baim DS: Coronary angioplasty. In Baim DS, Grossman W (eds): *Cardiac Catheterization, Angiography, and Intervention,* 5th ed, pp. 537–579. Baltimore, Williams & Wilkins, 1996.
24. Noureddine SN: Research review: Use of activated clotting time to monitor heparin therapy in coronary patients. *Am J Crit Care* 4:272, 1995.
25. Baim DS, Kent KM, King SB, et al: Evaluating new devices. Acute (in-hospital) results from the New Approaches to Coronary Intervention Registry. *Circulation* 89:471, 1994.
26. Landau C, Lange RA, Hillis LD: Percutaneous transluminal coronary angioplasty. *N Engl J Med* 330:981, 1994.
27. Lincoff AM, Topol EJ: Interventional catheterization techniques. In Braunwald E (ed): *Heart Disease,* 5th ed, pp. 1366–1391. Philadelphia, WB Saunders, 1997.
28. King SB, Yeh W, Holubkov R, et al. The National Heart, Lung, and Blood Institute Percutaneous Transluminal Coronary Angioplasty and The New Approaches to Coronary Intervention Investigators. Balloon angioplasty versus new device intervention: Clinical Outcomes. *J Am Coll Cardiol* 31:558, 1998.
29. Caldwell MA, Pelter MM, Drew BJ: Chest pain is an unreliable measure of ischemia in men and women during PTCA. *Heart Lung* 25:423, 1996.
30. Baim DS, Grossman W: Complications of cardiac catheterization. In Baim DS, Grossman W (eds): *Cardiac Catheterization, Angiography, and Intervention,* 5th ed, pp. 17–38. Baltimore, Williams & Wilkins, 1996.

31. Nasser TK, Mohler ER, Wilensky RL, Hathaway DR: Peripheral vascular complications following coronary interventional procedures. *Clin Cardiol* 18:609, 1995.
32. O'Meara JJ, Dehmer GJ: Care of the patient and management of complications after percutaneous coronary artery interventions. *Ann Intern Med* 127:458, 1997.
33. Khoury M, Batra S, Berg R, et al: Influence of arterial access sites and interventional procedures on vascular complications after cardiac catheterizations. *Am J Surg* 164:205, 1992.
34. Popma JJ, Satler LF, Pichard AD: Vascular complications after new device angioplasty. *Circulation* 88(Part 1):1569, 1993.
35. Waksman R, King SB, Douglas JS, et al: Predictors of groin complications after balloon and new-device coronary intervention. *Am J Cardiol* 75:886, 1995.
36. Kresowik TF, Khoury MD, Miller BV, et al: A prospective study of the incidence and natural history of femoral vascular complications after percutaneous transluminal coronary angioplasty. *J Vasc Surg* 13:328, 1991.
37. Franco CD, Goldsmith J, Veith FJ, et al: Management of arterial injuries produced by percutaneous femoral procedures. *Surgery* 113:419, 1993.
38. Muller DWM, Shamir KJ, Ellis SG, Topol EJ: Peripheral vascular complications after conventional and complex percutaneous coronary interventional procedures. *Am J Cardiol* 69:63, 1992.
39. Oweida SW, Roubin GS, Smith RB, Salam A: Post catheterization vascular complications associated with percutaneous transluminal coronary angioplasty. *J Vasc Surg* 12:310, 1990.
40. Omoigui NA, Califf RM, Pieper K, et al: Peripheral vascular complications in the coronary angioplasty versus excisional atherectomy trial (CAVEAT-I). *J Am Coll Cardiol* 26:922, 1995.
41. Davis C, VanRiper S, Longstreet J: Vascular complications of coronary interventions. *Heart Lung* 26:118, 1997.
42. Agarwal R, Agrawal SK, Roubin GS, et al: Clinically guided closure of femoral arterial pseudoaneurysms complicating cardiac catheterization and coronary angioplasty. *Cathet Cardiovasc Diagn* 30:96, 1993.
43. Schaub F, Theiss W, Zagel M, Schömig A: New aspects in ultrasound-guided compression repair of postcatheterization femoral artery injuries. *Circulation* 90:1861, 1994.
44. Kent KC, McArdle CR, Kennedy B, et al: A prospective study of the clinical outcome of femoral pseudoaneurysms and arteriovenous fistulas induced by arterial puncture. *J Vasc Surg* 17:125, 1993.
45. Feld R, Patton GM, Carabasi A, et al: Treatment of iatrogenic femoral artery injuries with ultrasound-guided compression. *J Vasc Surg* 16:832, 1992.
46. Johnson LW, Esente P, Giambartolomei A, et al: Peripheral vascular complications of coronary angioplasty by the femoral and brachial techniques. *Cathet Cardiov Diagn* 31:165, 1994.
47. Agrawal SK, Pinheiro L, Roubin GS, et al: Nonsurgical closure of femoral pseudoaneurysms complicating cardiac catheterization and percutaneous transluminal coronary angioplasty. *J Am Coll Cardiol* 20:610, 1992.
48. Lumsden AB, Miller JM, Kosinski AS, et al: A prospective evaluation of surgically treated groin complications following percutaneous cardiac procedures. *Am Surg* 60:132, 1994.

49. Cleveland KO, Gelfand MS: Invasive staphylococcal infections complicating percutaneous transluminal coronary angioplasty: Three cases and review. *Clin Infect Dis* 21:93, 1995.
50. Malanoski GJ, Samore MH, Pefanis A, Karchmer AW: *Staphylococcus aureus* catheter-associated bacteremia. *Arch Intern Med* 155:1161, 1995.
51. Parfrey PS, Griffiths SM, Barrett BJ, et al: Contrast material-induced renal failure in patients with diabetes mellitus, renal insufficiency, or both. *N Engl J Med* 320:143, 1989.
52. Solomon R, Werner C, Mann D, et al: Effects of saline, mannitol, and furosemide on acute decreases in renal function induced by radiocontrast agents. *N Engl J Med* 331:1416, 1994.
53. Byrd L, Sherman RL: Radiocontrast-induced acute renal failure: A clinical and pathophysiologic review. *Medicine* 58:270, 1979.
54. Cigarroa RG, Lange RA, Williams RH, Hillis LD: Dosing of contrast material to prevent contrast nephropathy in patients with renal disease. *Am J Med* 86:649, 1989.
55. Kegelmass AD, Cohen DJ, Moscucci M, et al: Elevation of the creatinine kinase myocardial isoform following otherwise successful directional coronary atherectomy. *Am J Cardiol* 74:748, 1994.
56. Lorell BH: Pericardial diseases. In Braunwald E (ed): *Heart Disease*, 5th ed, pp. 1478–1534. Philadelphia, WB Saunders, 1997.
57. Moravec CK: Hematopoiesis, coagulation, and bleeding. In Woods S, Sivarajan Froelicher ES, Halpenny CJ, et al (eds): *Cardiac Nursing*, 3rd ed, pp. 101–120. Philadelphia, JB Lippincott, 1995.
58. Mayer DM, Hendricks L: Comfort and bleeding after percutaneous transluminal coronary angioplasty: Comparison of a flexible sheath and a standard sheath. *Am J Crit Care* 6:341, 1997.
59. Scriver V, Crowe J, Wilkinson A, Medowcroft C: A randomized controlled trial of the effectiveness of exercise and/or alternating air mattress in the control of back pain after percutaneous transluminal coronary angioplasty. *Heart Lung* 23:308, 1994.
60. Waksman R, Scott N, Ghazzal ZMB, et al: A randomized comparison of flexible vs. non-flexible femoral sheaths on patient comfort after angioplasty. *Am Heart J* 131:1076, 1996.
61. Rudisill PT, Williams LB, Craig S, Schopp P: Study of mechanical versus manual/mechanical compression following various interventional cardiology procedures. *J Cardiovasc Nurs* 11:15, 1997.
62. Dolman S: PTCA: The role of the angioplasty program nurse. *Can J Cardiovasc Nurs* 5:25, 1995.
63. McKenna KT, Maas F, McEniery PT: Coronary risk factor status after percutaneous transluminal coronary angioplasty. *Heart Lung* 24:207, 1995.

Washington Hospital Center Clinical Pathway: PTCA

	DATE: Preprocedure	DATE: Postprocedure First Hour	DATE: Postprocedure Next 24 Hours	DATE: Day 2	DATE: Discharge Day
Assessment	♥ Complete nursing assessment ♥ Preprocedure checklist complete ♥ Informed consent ♥ Guided imagery	♥ Type of procedure, device(s) used location (coronary or peripheral, artery vein, SVG, LIMA, RIMA, other ♥ Complete nursing assessment ♥ Vascular access site(s)	♥ AV sheaths removed ♥ Access site(s ♥ I&O (if patient has not voided, consider Foley)	♥ Complete nursing assessment ♥ Vascular access site(s) ♥ Bruit? ♥ Hematoma? ♥ I&O	♥ Nursing assessment—Patient at preprocedure levels? ♥ Vascular access site ♥ Final labs, ECG
Diagnostic Tests/Evaluations	♥ Pro B, CBC, Coags ♥ Lipids? ♥ Homocysteine ♥ 12-Lead ECG ♥ Telemetry	♥ 12-lead ECG ♥ Last ACT ♥ Telemetry	♥ H&H, K^+, Coags, Pro Hrt ♥ 12-Lead ECG ♥ ACT 4 hours after heparin stopped and every 1 hour until ≤ 150	♥ H&H, Pro B, Coags, Pro Hrt ♥ 12-Lead ECG ♥ Lipids	♥ Appointments for follow-up labs
Treatments/Medications	♥ Patient taking own meds? ♥ Saline lock in L arm ♥ Heparin infusion? ♥ Sedation ♥ ? Dye allergy (if yes, appropriate meds ordered?) ♥ Aspirin given ♥ Plavix or Ticlid? ♥ Prilosec?	♥ Nitroglycerin ♥ Heparin ♥ Analgesics ♥ IV Ds 1/2 NS @75 mL c/hr for 6 hours if not tolerating PO ♥ O_2 @ 2 l nasal cannula PRN	♥ Nitroglycerin ♥ Heparin ♥ Plavix/Ticlid ♥ Ca^{++} blockers ♥ Vitamins ♥ Lipid-lowering agent ♥ Femostop after AV sheaths removed ♥ Heparin restart?	♥ Aspirin ♥ Plavix/Ticlid ♥ Ca^+ blockers ♥ Vitamins ♥ Lipid-lowering agent	♥ Discharge prescriptions given to patient and reviewed

(continued)

EXHIBIT 13–1 Clinical Pathway for Patients Undergoing Percutaneous Transluminal Coronary Angioplasty. (Copyright Washington Hospital Center.)

Washington Hospital Center Clinical Pathway: PTCA—*Continued*

	DATE: Preprocedure	DATE: Postprocedure First Hour	DATE: Postprocedure Next 24 Hours	DATE: Day 2	DATE: Discharge Day
Consults	▼	▼	▼	▼ Dietary ▼ Social Service ▼ GI	▼ All consults finished
Diet/Fluid Balance	▼ NPO	▼ AHA Full liquids ▼ NPO (if yes, IV fluids indicated)	▼ AHA1 ▼ Other	▼ AHA1 ▼ Other	▼ AHA Diet reviewed
Activity/Safety	▼ BRP	▼ Bed rest, may have HOB ↑ 30° with affected limb straight ▼ Siderails up, bed in low position	▼ Bed rest for 4 hours after sheaths removed ▼ Siderails up, bed in low position	▼ Up ad lib	▼ Activity ad lib
Discharge Planning	▼ Patient Interdisciplinary Care Map	▼ Anticipated discharge next day	▼	▼	
Patient Education	▼ Explanation of intended procedure ▼ Guided Imagery ▼ Post Procedure care	▼ Notify RN of any chest pain, back pain, or discomfort at access site ▼ Affected limb(s) immobile ▼ Need for clear liquids only ▼ Anticipated length of BR	▼ Notify RN of any chest pain, back pain, or discomfort at access site ▼ Affected limb(s) immobile ▼ Anticipated length of bed rest	▼ Notify RN of any chest pain, back pain, or discomfort at access site	▼ Written discharge instructions ▼ Meds ▼ Follow-up MD ▼ Activity

(continued)

EXHIBIT 13–1 CONTINUED

Washington Hospital Center Clinical Pathway: Outcomes Assessment—*Continued*

DATE: Preprocedure	DATE: Postprocedure First Hour	DATE: Postprocedure Next 24 Hours	DATE: Day 2	DATE: Discharge Day
Are there any other deviations from the pathway?	Are there any other deviations from the pathway?	Are there any other deviations from the pathway?	Are there any other deviations from the pathway?	Are there any other deviations from the pathway?
Yes ☐ No ☐	Yes ☐ No ☐	Yes ☐ No ☐	Yes ☐ No ☐	Yes ☐ No ☐
Can patient progress to next 12 hours?	Can patient progress to next day?	Can patient progress to next day?	Can patient progress to next day or be discharged?	Is patient ready for discharge?
Yes ☐ No ☐	Yes ☐ No ☐	Yes ☐ No ☐	Yes ☐ No ☐	Yes ☐ No ☐
Variance	Variance	Variance	Variance	Variance
Signatures	Signatures	Signatures	Signatures	Signatures
D ____	D ____	D ____	D ____	D ____
E ____	E ____	E ____	E ____	E ____
N ____	N ____	N ____	N ____	N ____

Disclaimer: This pathway and guidelines do not purport to reflect all relevant medical considerations and are not intended to replace clinical judgment.
ACT, activated clotting time; AHA, American Heart Association (diet); AV, arteriovenous; BRP, bathroom privileges; CBC, complete blood count; Coags, coagulation blood tests; H&H, hematocrit and hemoglobin; HOB, head of bed; LIMA, left internal mammary artery; Pro B, serum chemistries; Pro Hrt, cardiac enzymes; RIMA, right internal mammary artery; SVG, saphenous vein graft.

EXHIBIT 13–1 CONTINUED

Patient/Family Edition Washington Hospital Center Clinical Pathway: PTCA

	DATE: Preprocedure	DATE: Postprocedure First Hour	DATE: Postprocedure Next 24 Hours	DATE: Postprocedure Day 2	DATE: Discharge Day
Assessment	You may receive a: ♥ Review of your medical history and a physical examination by a member of the health care team, usually a nurse practitioner ♥ Review of your scheduled procedure and any research trials in which you may be eligible to participate ♥ Review to make sure all consent forms are signed ♥ Review to make sure all necessary tests are complete	♥ You will be checked by your nurse frequently, especially the site where your procedure was done, usually your leg. ♥ Tell your nurse immediately if you have any chest pain or pain in the procedure site.	♥ When it is time to remove the sheaths, your nurse and a cardiovascular (CV) tech will work together to quickly and safely complete this procedure. Follow their instructions.	♥ Your nurse will check you at least every 4 hours. ♥ Let us know if you are having any chest pain, pain at the procedure site, or any other discomfort.	♥ More than one member of the health care team will ask to examine your procedure site. We want to make sure there are no problems, so we need to look at the site, feel the site, and listen to the site with a stethoscope.
Diagnostic Tests/Evaluations	♥ You may have blood taken. ♥ You may have an electrocardiogram (ECG)	♥ A small amount of blood will be taken from the catheters (sheaths) for tests. Once your blood is able to clot, we will remove the sheaths from your leg. ♥ You will have at least one more ECG.	♥ Blood will be drawn from a vein in your arm for tests. ♥ You may have another ECG.	♥ You will have some additional blood tests performed the morning after the procedure.	♥ We will review the results of your blood tests, including your cholesterol and other lipids. You will not be discharged until we have reviewed your morning laboratory tests.

(continued)

EXHIBIT 13–2 Clinical Pathway for Patients and Families. (Copyright Washington Hospital Center.)

Patient/Family Edition Washington Hospital Center Clinical Pathway: PTCA—*Continued*

	DATE: Preprocedure	DATE: Postprocedure First Hour	DATE: Postprocedure Next 24 Hours	DATE: Postprocedure Day 2	DATE: Discharge Day
Treatments/Medications	Important questions: ♥ Are you allergic to shellfish or contrast dye? Are you allergic to any medications? ♥ Are you currently taking a blood thinner? ♥ Are you currently taking Glucophage (metformin)? ♥ Are you taking insulin? ♥ You will have a needle inserted in your left arm. This needle (IV) will be used to administer medications. ♥ You may receive some medication to relax you during your procedure.	♥ You will receive IV nitroglycerin until the next morning. ♥ You will be started on your usual medications when you are able to eat regular food. ♥ We will also give you medicine for pain or to relax you if you need these. ♥ Still anxious? Try guided imagery.	♥ You are still receiving IV nitroglycerin. ♥ You should be taking your other medication by mouth. ♥ We may add some new medications; ask if you don't recognize some of the pills you are taking.	♥ The nitroglycerin will be stopped in the morning.	♥ We will give you a written list of all medications that you need to take; we will review this list with you and your family.
Consults	♥ These are specialists that some patients or families may need, such as the dietitian or the social worker.				

EXHIBIT 13–2 CONTINUED

(continued)

255

Patient/Family Edition Washington Hospital Center Clinical Pathway: PTCA—*Continued*

	DATE: Preprocedure	DATE: Postprocedure First Hour	DATE: Postprocedure Next 24 Hours	DATE: Postprocedure Day 2	DATE: Discharge Day
Diet/Fluid Balance	▼ You should have had nothing to eat or drink for at least 12 hours before your procedure. ▼ Let us know if you have any special food requests.	▼ Your first meal after your procedure will be clear liquids. Even though you may feel very hungry, your stomach knows you have been through a stressful procedure. ▼ You need to take plenty of liquids to help flush the dye used during your procedure out of your body. If you are having trouble with this, your nurse may give you extra fluids by vein (IV).	▼ If you have taken liquids with no problem, we will give you a heart-healthy meal.	▼ You should be eating regular heart-healthy meals.	▼ We will review a heart-healthy menu with you and your family.
Activity/Safety	▼ You will be asked to stay in bed after your procedure for at least several hours.	▼ You must stay in bed with your leg straight. The sheaths in your leg may cause pain or bleeding if you move around too much. Your nurse will help you get comfortable.	▼ You must stay in bed for several hours after your sheaths are removed. The puncture site needs time to heal.	▼ The first time you get out of bed, ask for help. You may be a little unsteady on your feet.	▼ You may be a little sore, but we need to make sure that you can walk in the halls and go to the bathroom without any difficulty before we can let you go home.
Discharge Planning	▼	▼ Most patients can return home the day after their procedure. Your doctor will discuss this with you and your family.	▼	▼ The exact time you can go home will depend on the results of your blood tests. We need to make sure there were no problems with your procedure.	▼ Make sure to take all of the written information we have given you to review when you are finally home.

(continued)

EXHIBIT 13–2 CONTINUED

Patient/Family Edition Washington Hospital Center Clinical Pathway: PTCA—*Continued*

	DATE: Preprocedure	DATE: Postprocedure First Hour	DATE: Postprocedure Next 24 Hours	DATE: Postprocedure Day 2	DATE: Discharge Day
Patient Education	♥ We will review the procedure and ith you and your family. ♥ To help relax, try guided imagery. We will explain this special therapy to you.	♥ We will review the procedure and usual hospital care with you and your family. ♥ To help relax, try guided imagery. We will explain this special therapy to you.		♥ Your doctor will need to review your blood tests and your ECG before you can be released.	♥ Make sure you know when to visit your regular doctor, any follow-up tests that need to be done, and when you can return to your usual activity. This information should be written down for you to take home.

This pathway is designed to help you understand the usual procedures and laboratory tests that you may experience when you have a procedure in the catheterization laboratory. However, all patients are unique. This pathway is intended only as a guide. Your physician will determine what procedures and tests are right for you. You may not need all the procedures or tests that are on this pathway.

EXHIBIT 13–2 CONTINUED

WASHINGTON HOSPITAL CENTER

Date/Time: _____ Height: _____ Weight : _____ TPR: _____ BP: _____

General Description: | d = deferred |

Head: *Eyes:* PUPILS _____ WNL   EOM _____ WNL   *Mouth:* DENTITION _____ WNL

Neck: NECK _____ WNL

CV: _____ S1S2 RRR ABNORMAL: _____

MURMURS _____

ECG: _____
_____
_____
_____

PULSES   **1-4 Scale**   **B = Bruits**

Lungs: _____ WNL

	Carotids	Radial	Femoral	P.T.	D.P.
R					
L					

Thorax and Abdomen: _____ WNL   *Skin:* _____ WNL

Gross *Musculo:* _____ WNL   *Gross Neuro:* _____ WNL

Extremities: _____ WNL Abnormal: _____
IMPRESSION: _____
_____
_____

PLAN: _____
_____

Signature:

**PHYSICAL
EXAMINATION**   Labs:

EXHIBIT 13–3 Standard Medical History and Physical Form. (Copyright Washington Hospital Center.)

WASHINGTON HOSPITAL CENTER

Date/Time: _____ DOB: _____ Cardiologist: _____   Dye Allergy: Yes/No Premed: Yes/No

Allergies: _____

Age: _____ Sex: ___ Male ___ Female   Marital Status: ___ S ___ M ___ W ___ D ___ Sep   Race: _____

Social: _____

Chief Complaint/History of Present Illness: _____

_____

_____

_____

Cardiovascular tests: _____

Risk Factors: ____ HTN ____ DM. ____ Ʌ CHOL/TRI ____ + Family Hx	Drug	Dosage	Freq
____ Menopausal ____ ERT ____ Sedentary lifestyle			
Tobacco: ___ Current : _____ Cig/pk/day Cigars/day Chew/pk/day			
_____ Quit/Date _____ Pk/Yrs or ____ pk/day x __ yrs			
Past Medical/Surgical Hx: _____			
_____			
_____			
_____			
_____			
Recent Hospitalization: _____			

Systems Review: General: ____ Weight Changes _____ Fevers _____ Malignancies

HEENT: ____ Cataracts _____ Glaucoma _____ Glasses _____ Hearing _____ Dysphagia _____ Rheumatic fever

Resp: ____ DOE ____ Asthma _____ Emphysema _____ TB Hx _____ Pulm. Embolus _____ Chronic Cough _____ Pneumonia

CV: ____ Orthopnea _____ CHF _____ Edema _____ Syncope _____ PVD _____ Claudication _____ Murmur Hx

_____ Arrhythmia   _____ Other:
I:

GI: ____ Ulcer Hx _____ Hiatal Hernia/GERD _____ Gallbladder _____ Liver Abn. _____ Constipation _____ Bleeding

GU: ____ Urinary Dysfunction _____ BPH LMP: _____ Renal Disease: _____ CRI _____ CRF _____ Dialysis

Musculoskeletal: _____ DJD / Rheumatoid Arthritis / Osteoarthritis _____ Gout **Endocrine:** _____ Thyroid Dysfunction

Hematologic: _____ Anemia **Neuro:** _____ Carotid DX _____ CVA _____ TIAs _____ Seizure Disorder

Psych: **Skin:**

ETOH: Signature:

HISTORY

EXHIBIT 13—3 CONTINUED

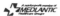

Doctor Notified of Admission:			Date:		Time:	
Reason for Admission:						
Mode of Admission:			Accompanied by:			
History of:	**Patient**	**Family**	**History of:**	**Patient**	**Family**	
Diabetes			Bleeding Disorders			
Hypertension			IV Dye Reactions			
Heart Disease			GU/Renal Disease			
Hypercholesteremia			Allergy			
Smoking						

Previous Illnesses/Hospitalizations:

Current Medications:

☐ With Patient: ☐ Taken by Nurse

Chief Complaint/History Present Illness:

Chest Pains/Shortness of Breath/Syncope/Other *(Describe)*:

Onset:	Precipitating/Alleviating Factors:
Location:	
Radiation:	
Duration:	Associated Symptoms:
Intensity: 0 1 2 3 4 5 6 7 8 9 10	
(None) (Severe)	

DATE   ADDRESSOGRAPH

CARDIAC
48-HOUR ADMISSION DATA BASE

EXHIBIT 13—4 Standard Nursing History and Physical Form. (Copyright Washington Hospital Center.)

PHYSICAL ASSESSMENT

A. Vital Signs

1. BP: Right Arm_____ Left Arm_____

   ☐ Audible   ☐ Palpable   ☐ Doppler

2. Temperature: _____

   ☐ Oral   ☐ Rectal

3. Apical Pulse: _____

4. Respirations: _____

5. Height: _____ Weight: _____

B. **a.** Heart Sounds:

b. ARP: ☐ Regular   ☐ With Deficit
             ☐ Irregular   ☐ Without Deficit

c. Pulses:

	Right	Left	
	☐	☐	Carotid
	☐	☐	Brachial
	☐	☐	Radial
	☐	☐	Femoral
	☐	☐	Popliteal
	☐	☐	Pedal

Key: 0 = Absent   1+ = Weak   3+ = Strong
        D = Doppler   2+ = Normal

C. Respiratory System

1. Character Respirations: ☐ Regular   ☐ Irregular   ☐ Short of Breath

2. Assessment *(Identify prescence of rales, rhonchi, wheezes):*

   RUL _____   LUL _____

   RML _____

   RLL _____   LLL _____

TELEMETRY

PATIENT INFORMATION

Diet:	Call System:	Roomlights:
Bathroom:	I.D. Band	Siderails:
Introduction to Room Mate:	Telephone, TV	Visiting Hours
Patient Education Booklet Given: Hot / Cath / PTCA / Device		
Valuables: ☐ With Patient	☐ Family	☐ Security
Prosthetic Devices: ☐ Dentures	☐ Glasses	☐ Contact Lens
☐ Hearing Aid	☐ Limb Prosthesis:	
Discharge ☐ Home	☐ Other *(describe)*:	
Person to Notify for Transportation:	Phone:	
Signature >	Date:	

EXHIBIT 13–4 CONTINUED

WASHINGTON HOSPITAL CENTER

MEDLANTIC
A not-for-profit member of
Healthcare Group

PTCA Checkpoint	Yes	No*	*All Negatives Require Explanation
Permit Signed			
H&P Completed			
12 Lead ECG Done			
Patient Voided on Call			
Valuables Removed			
NPO Since midnight or: *(indicate time)*			
Contrast Allergy†			† If yes, allergy meds must be ordered.
° Benadryl ° Steroids			
Aspirin			Most patients must receive an aspirin prior to going to the Cath Lab. *Call the NP or MD for orders if not given.*
TICLID/PLAVIX			
Sedation			

Date / Time:	Lab Values (Normal)	Normal	Abnormal	Comments
Height:	Hgb (12 – 16 F) (14 – 18 M) Hct 37 – 47 F) (42 – 52 M)			
Weight:	Platelet Count (150 – 400)			
Temp:	WBC (4.8 – 10.8)			
Pulse:	PT < 16			
Resp:	BUN (6 – 25)			
BP:	Cr (0.5 – 1.4)			
	K (3.5 – 5.5)			
	Glucose (70 – 115) < 50 Yrs 85 – 125 > 50 Yrs			

Additional Comments:

Signature>   Date:

PRECARDIAC CATH
PTCA
CHECKLIST

EXHIBIT 13–5 Preprocedure Checklist. (Copyright Washington Hospital Center.)

WASHINGTON HOSPITAL CENTER

DATES: Admission :   Discharge:

Date Ent	MAJOR ACTIVE PROBLEMS **	CONSULTS: ** Service/Name (see chart for indications)	Date Completed

PROCEDURES DURING HOSPITALIZATION **	ADDITIONAL DOCUMENTATION USED*
	CLINICAL PATHWAY:
	SPECIALTY DISCHARGE PLAN:

DISCHARGE MEDICATIONS: Name/Dose/Instructions **	DISCHARGE CONDITION:	ACTIVITY:
	FOLLOWUP APPOINTMENTS:	DIET:
		SPECIAL INSTRUCTIONS:
	FOR HELP AFTER DISCHARGE CALL:	

SIGNATURES:

Patient >_____   Nurse >_____   Physician>_____

★ Attach Documentation
★★□ Check here if additional pages required

ADDRESSOGRAPH

PATIENT INTERDISCIPLINARY CARE MAP

EXHIBIT 13–6   Patient Interdisciplinary Care Map. (Copyright Washington Hospital Center.)

CHAPTER 14

Management of Acute Myocardial Infarction

LUCY VAN VOORHEES, MD

President Dwight Eisenhower suffered a myocardial infarction in 1955. He was treated with the standard therapy of the day, which included oxygen, morphine, sedatives and prolonged bed rest. After several weeks, he was gradually permitted to resume his normal activities. There were no tests available to assess the extent of his coronary atherosclerosis or to determine the amount of myocardial damage that he had sustained.

Management of patients with myocardial infarction has changed radically in the forty years since President Eisenhower had his heart attack. Most deaths from myocardial infarction were thought to occur in the first hour; they were attributed to malignant ventricular arrhythmias.[1] The mortality of patients who survived their myocardial infarction long enough to reach the hospital was significantly reduced by the recognition and treatment of ventricular tachycardia and ventricular fibrillation.[2] Treatment shifted from provision of analgesia and prolonged bed rest to active monitoring of arrhythmias, hemodynamic assessment and the treatment of heart failure resulting from extensive myocardial damage. With the advent of coronary care units, the in-hospital mortality of patients with a myocardial infarction was decreased from 30%, to 15% to 20 % by the mid 1970's.[3]

♥ Role of Intracoronary Thrombus

Changes in the treatment of myocardial infarction have evolved from the knowledge that thrombosis of coronary arteries heralds the onset of myocardial ischemia, and if persistent, myocardial cell necrosis. Occlu-

265

sion of coronary arteries by thrombus has been shown to occur in 86% of patients angiographically studied within six hours of onset of symptoms of a transmural myocardial infarction.[4] Sixty-seven per cent of patients studied between 6 and 24 hours of symptom development were found to have total occlusion of the infarct vessel.

The extent of myocardial infarction is determined by the amount of myocardium perfused by the occluded vessel and the time course of the occlusion. Reimer and his colleagues first described the timing of myocardial infarction in dogs when they occluded canine coronary arteries and found a "wave front" of cell injury which spread from endocardium to epicardium in the territory of an occluded coronary artery. If the occlusion was relieved within an hour, the cell damage was reversible. If occlusion lasted one to two hours, a variable amount of the myocardial cells could be salvaged by reperfusion. After more than 2 hours of coronary occlusion, most of the myocardial cells were irreparably damaged and could not be salvaged even if the coronary artery was reopened.[5]

Reimer and Jennings determined in further canine studies that the amount of myocardium perfused by the coronary artery and the extent of collateral flow were also important determinants of the extent of myocardial damage inflicted by acute coronary occlusion.[6] Studies in humans using thallium scintigraphy to measure myocardial perfusion have corroborated Reimer's findings that amount of muscle perfused and extent of collateral flow may be as important as the time of coronary occlusion in the development of myocardial necrosis.[7]

♥ Current Treatment Strategies

The recognition of the role of thrombus in the development of myocardial infarction, and the knowledge that the time course of coronary artery occlusion and the presence of collateral flow could alter the extent of myocardial cell damage, has led to the evolution of current treatment strategies for patients with acute myocardial infarction. Bergmann, et al., studied the evolution of coronary thrombosis in the canine model and the effect of thrombolytic therapy on myocardial necrosis. Their studies emphasized the time dependence of ischemic cells on reperfusion.[8]

STREPTOKINASE

During the 1970s, a number of trials were carried out in Europe and the United States investigating the safety and effectiveness of streptokinase in patients with acute myocardial infarctions. Verstraete and associates[9] summarize the European trials in a paper published in 1981.[9] Patients who presented to the hospital with infarctions less than 24 hours old were treated with long infusions of streptokinase. Effects on mortality were promising, but the patients encountered significant bleeding complications. The National Institutes of Health also sponsored a pilot trial in this country. The trial utilized a continuous infusion of streptokinase, but was stopped by the Safety Monitoring Board before completion due to excess mortality from bleeding complications.[10]

Rentrop and associates[11] rekindled enthusiasm for the use of thrombolytic agents when he successfully recanalized coronary arteries during acute myocardial infarction with the use of intracoronary streptokinase. The Western Washington Intracoronary Streptokinase Study randomized 250 patients to receive either intracoronary streptokinase or conventional therapy. Time to reperfusion was 6 hours or more in the majority of patients. In spite of this delay, a significant decrease in mortality (3.7% compared with 11.2%, $P = 0.02$) was observed.[12]

Further study soon determined that intravenous streptokinase was just as effective as intracoronary streptokinase therapy in the reduction of mortality from myocardial infarction.[13] Given the success of these trials, two large international trials, GISSI (Gruppo Italiano per lo Studio della Streptochinasi nell'Infarto Miocardico)[14] and ISIS-2 (Second International Study of Infarct Survival Collaborative Group) were begun.[15] The GISSI trial enrolled 11,806 patients presenting within 12 hours of symptoms. The 21-day mortality of patients treated with streptokinase was 18% less than patients treated with more conservative therapy. The ISIS trial involved 17,189 patients, randomizing them to receive aspirin, streptokinase, both or neither. The patients treated with both aspirin and streptokinase demonstrated a 42% decrease in 5-week mortality when compared with the placebo-treated patients. This difference was maintained over a follow-up period of 15 months.

Thrombolytic therapy with streptokinase is not free of problems. If infused too rapidly, it may cause significant hypotension further compromising coronary blood flow and myocardial function. Because streptokinase is a foreign bacterial protein, it is antigenic and frequently associated with allergic reactions. Although the usual allergic reactions are mild (fever, rash, and nausea), more life-threatening anaphylactic reactions may also occur. Recent streptococcal infection may render a patient more likely to be resistant to the therapeutic action of streptokinase and more likely to experience an allergic reaction.

The infusion of streptokinase induces a systemic lytic state. Minor bleeding complications are common. Central venous or arterial punctures are contraindicated in patients who have recently received thrombolytic therapy. Patients who have had arterial blood gas studies done before or soon after the administration of lytic therapy may develop significant hematomas at the site of arterial puncture, sometimes severe enough to require fasciotomy for relief.

Streptokinase is contraindicated in patients who are at risk for bleeding from recent surgery, malignancies or recent cardiopulmonary resuscitation, and so on. Patients with a history of gastrointestinal bleeding may also develop significant bleeding after thrombolytic therapy. Intracranial hemorrhage—a devastating complication—may occur in as many as 1% of patients after the administration of thrombolytic therapy.[16]

TISSUE PLASMINOGEN ACTIVATOR

Although streptokinase therapy decreased mortality in patients with acute myocardial infarction, the incidence of significant side effects as well as a desire to reperfuse starved myocardium more rapidly led to the development of other thrombolytic agents.

Tissue plasminogen activator (t-PA) is a genetically engineered substance, which acts more rapidly than the endogenous substance to convert plasminogen to plasmin. t-PA is rapidly cleared by the liver and has a much shorter half-life than streptokinase, properties that were thought to enhance its value as a thrombolytic agent.

After encouraging dosing studies, Collen and colleagues[17] compared recombinant t-PA (rt-PA) with placebo in 33 patients with acute myocardial infarction and found 75% of the patients to have angiographically patent arteries within 90 minutes after the start of therapy. The Thrombolysis in Myocardial Infarction (TIMI) trial was the first trial to compare therapy with either t-PA or streptokinase. A group of 214 patients underwent baseline angiography to assess for presence of occluded infarct arteries before receiving either intravenous streptokinase or t-PA. Angiograms were repeated at 90 minutes, demonstrating a 60% patency rate for patients treated with t-PA compared with a 35% patency rate for patients treated with streptokinase. Despite the presumed clot specificity of t-PA, patients in both treatment groups had the same rate of bleeding complications.[18]

MORTALITY TRIALS

Determination of the effect of t-PA therapy on mortality in patients suffering an acute myocardial infarction has been the focus of many large multicenter international trials. The Anglo-Scandinavian Study of Early Thrombolysis (ASSET) randomized 5011 patients with symptoms of myocardial infarction to either t-PA therapy or placebo. They demonstrated a significant reduction in mortality. Within 30 days, 9.7% of the patients in the placebo group had died compared with 7.2% of patients in the t-PA group.[19] The Gruppo Italiano per lo Studio della Sopravivenza nell' Infarto Miocardico (GISSI - 2) randomized 12,490 patients to receive either intravenous t-PA or streptokinase. All patients received aspirin and a regimen of subcutaneous heparin or no-heparin therapy. Most of the patients received thrombolytic therapy within 6 hours of onset of symptoms, and many patients in the trial were older than 70 years. The GISSI trial produced similar results to the ASSET trial. Patients who received t-PA had an 8.7% mortality rate compared with 9.0% in patients who received streptokinase.[20]

The GUSTO (Global Utilization of Streptokinase and Tissue Plasminogen Activator for Occluded Coronary Arteries) trial was the first large-scale international trial to demonstrate a significant decrease in mortality for patients treated with t-PA. GUSTO randomized 41,021 patients to receive streptokinase and subcutaneous heparin, streptokinase and intravenous heparin, t-PA and intravenous heparin or streptokinase, t-PA and intravenous heparin. Thirty-day mortality rates were 7.2%, 7.4%, 6.3% and 7.0%, respectively. All patients received oral aspirin in the trial. The combination of t-PA, intravenous heparin and aspirin produced a significant decrease in acute myocardial infarction mortality when compared to the other regimens.[21]

A substudy of this trial studied infarct patency in all of the treatment groups at four times after the initiation of thrombolytic therapy (90 minutes, 180 minutes, 24 hours and 5 to 7 days). At 90 minutes, 81% of the 246 patients who received t-PA and intravenous heparin were found to have a patent infarct-related artery. Only 60% of the 231 patients receiving streptokinase and intravenous heparin had an open infarct-related artery at the 90-minute angiogram. Complete reperfusion was noted in 54% of the t-PA and intravenous heparin group at 90 minutes. Only 34% of the streptokinase and heparin group demonstrated complete reperfusion at 90 minutes. Mortality rate (4.4%) at 30 days was lowest in patients who had complete reperfusion and highest (8.9%) in patients who did not achieve reperfusion with thrombolytic therapy.[22]

The same substudy of the GUSTO trial also examined left ventricular function after treatment for myocardial infarction with the thrombolytic therapies offered in the trial. Patients with an ejection fraction greater than 45% at the 90-minute angiogram had a 30-day survival rate of 95%, whereas patients who had ejection fractions of less than 45% at 90 minutes had only an 85% chance of surviving for 30 days.

The latter trials and many others conducted during the same years came to similar conclusions. Treatment of patients with thrombolytic therapy early in the course of their acute myocardial infarction saved lives and preserved ventricular function. However, the thrombolytic agents have not proved to a perfect therapy. Complete reperfusion occurs in about 50% of the patients treated with an accelerated t-PA and intravenous heparin regimen. Other regimens may induce complete reperfusion in only one third of the infarct-related arteries. Residual thrombus is left in many of the infarct vessels, and in many cases, a significant residual stenosis is also present. Additionally, a percentage of infarct vessels initially opened with thrombolytic therapy reocclude during the early postinfarction period. Aside from therapeutic problems, thrombolytic therapy confers a significant risk of systemic bleeding complications, particularly in elderly patients. For these reasons, many investigators have been interested in the technique of primary angioplasty for patients with acute myocardial infarction.

♥ Primary Angioplasty

In 1993, the results of four trials comparing the treatment of acute myocardial infarction with acute angioplasty or thrombolysis were published (three in the same issue of the New England Journal of Medicine). The PAMI (Primary Angioplasty in Myocardial Infarction) trial randomized 395 patients to treatment with either t-PA (administered over 3 hours) or primary angioplasty. Patients who were found to have left main coronary artery disease on their initial angiogram were referred immediately to coronary artery bypass surgery and did not receive either intervention. Successful angioplasty was performed in 99% of the patients in the angioplasty arm of the trial. Time to infarct patency was similar in the two groups. In-hospital mortality was slightly better in the angioplasty group, but the difference was not statistically significant. Fewer patients who received primary angioplasty developed recurrent ischemia in the early postinfarction period prior to hospital discharge. Left ventricular function assessed by ventriculogram at the time of angiography demonstrated better myocardial preservation in the patients treated with primary angioplasty.[23]

A similar trial at the Mayo Clinic randomized 103 patients to receive either t-PA or primary angioplasty. Angioplasty success rate was comparable to the PAMI trial. In-hospital mortality in the t-PA treated group was only 3.6% whereas patients who underwent primary angioplasty had a 4.3% mortality rate during their hospitalization. These differences were not statistically significant.[24]

The Netherlands Trial randomized 302 patients to receive either primary angioplasty or streptokinase with intravenous heparin and aspirin. Investigators found impressive results in the angioplasty group, with only 2% in-hospital mortality, whereas the group treated with streptokinase had a 7.4% mortality rate.[25]

Ribiero and associates[26] randomized a smaller group of patients to receive either streptokinase or primary angioplasty, reaching the opposite conclusion to the Netherlands Trial. The streptokinase group had only 2% in-hospital mortality compared with the primary angioplasty group who had a 6% mortality rate while in the hospital.

All of the above-mentioned trials enrolled small groups of patients in either the thrombolytic or primary angioplasty groups. Although there is a trend toward superiority of primary angioplasty in decreasing inpatient mortality from acute myocardial infarction, this trend is not statistically significant. Some investigators have also found that the trend toward superiority of primary angioplasty fades with the passage of time.

The Alabama Registry found a 1-year survival rate of 88% in patients treated with immediate angioplasty for myocardial infarction. The patients treated with thrombolytic therapy had a 91% survival rate in the first year following their myocardial infarction. Reinfarction rates within the first year were also similar.[27]

The Myocardial Infarction Triage and Intervention Project Registry presented data on three-year survival in patients who were treated either with primary angioplasty or thrombolytic therapy. Over 12,000 consecutive patients with myocardial infarction were entered in their database; 1272 received angioplasty and 2664 received thrombolytic therapy. After 3 years, there was no difference in survival between the two groups.[28]

The Netherlands Trial and the Mayo Clinic Trial also attempted to assess the effect of their treatments on myocardial salvage. The Netherlands Trial found a significantly increased ejection fraction in patients who received primary angioplasty, $51 \pm 11\%$, compared with $45 \pm 12\%$ for the patients who received streptokinase. The Mayo Clinic Trial performed technetium-99 sestamibi scans to assess myocardial perfusion. They measured the size of the perfusion defect in tomographic scans performed before and after reperfusion. No significant differences were found in the size or change in perfusion defects between the angioplasty and the thrombolytic groups.

STENTS IN ACUTE MYOCARDIAL INFARCTION

Angioplasty of coronary arteries has been performed for more than 15 years. Despite changes in equipment and techniques, a substantial number of patients develop restenosis at the site of the angioplasty within 6 months after treatment. A significant number of patients who undergo immediate angioplasty of an infarct-related coronary artery also experience recurrent signs of ischemia.

Treatment of stenotic coronary arteries with the placement of intracoronary stents evolved in an effort to decrease the rate of restenosis after coronary angioplasty. Stents were found to be particularly effective when placed in coronary arteries dissected or suboptimally dilated with traditional balloon techniques. However, early in the experience with stent placement, many investigators recognized that the presence of thrombus in the coronary artery undergoing stent placement predisposed the patient to early stent closure or restenosis. For this reason, interventional cardiologists were hesitant to place stents in patients undergoing angioplasty as the treatment for acute myocardial infarction.

During the process of primary angioplasty, suboptimal balloon dilatation or dissections have occurred, necessitating the stent placement. Small studies and pilot trials to date suggest that stent placement in the setting of acute myocardial infarction is technically feasible despite the presence of thrombus. In fact, the placement of stents during primary angioplasty may decrease mortality and improve long-term outcome.[29,30]

The largest trial to date, Stent PAMI, enrolled patients within 10 hours of onset of symptoms to primary angioplasty or primary stent placement in infarct-related vessels that were angiographically amenable to stent placement. Acute angiographic success was similar between the stent and percutaneous transluminal coronary angioplasty groups. Outcomes at 30 days were also similar although the stent group was less likely to undergo symptom-mediated target vessel revascularization.[31]

Stent placement for patients in cardiogenic shock from their myocardial infarction may be particularly advantageous. Antoniucci and associates found a 26% in-hospital mortality rate in patients with cardiogenic shock who were successfully revascularized with stent placement compared with a 36% to 61% mortality rate found in other studies.[32,33]

♥ Conclusion

Treatment for patients with acute myocardial infarctions has evolved significantly over the almost 50 years since President Eisenhower suffered his heart attack. We now understand that rapid revascularization is crucially important in the preservation of life and myocardial function. Optimal methods for revascularization are still in the process of investigation.

REFERENCES

1. Bainton C, Peterson D: Deaths from coronary heart disease in persons fifty years and younger. *N Engl J Med* 268:569, 1963.
2. MacMillan R, Brown K: Comparison of the treatment of acute myocardial infarction in a coronary care unit and on a general medical ward. *Can Med Assn J* 105:1037, 1971.
3. Levenstein J: Myocardial infarction and the evolution of the intensive coronary care unit. *S Afr Med J* 50:918, 1976.
4. DeWood M, Spores J, Notske R, et al: Prevalence of total coronary occlusion during the early hours of a transmural myocardial infarction. *N Engl J Med* 303:897, 1980.
5. Reimer K, Lowe J, Rasmussen M, Jennings R: The wave-front phenomenon of ischemic cell death: Myocardial infarct size versus duration of coronary occlusion in dogs. *Circulation* 56:786, 1977.
6. Reimer K, Jennings R: The "wavefront" phenomenon of myocardial ischemic cell death. *Lab Invest* 40:633, 1979.
7. Christian T, Schwartz R, Gibbons R: Determinants of infarct size in reperfusion therapy for acute myocardial infarction. *Coron Artery Dis* 3:481, 1992.
8. Bergmann S, Lerch R, Fox K, et al: Temporal dependence of beneficial effects of coronary thrombolysis characterized by positron tomography. *Am J Med* 73:573, 1981.
9. Verstraete M, Van de Loo I, Jesdinsky H: Streptokinase in acute myocardial infarction. *Acta Med Scand Suppl* 648:1, 1981.
10. Ness P, Simon T, Cole C, et al: A pilot study of SK therapy in acute myocardial infarction: Observation on complication and relation to trial design. *Am Heart J* 88:705, 1974.
11. Rentrop K, Blanke H, Karsch K, et al: Initial experience with transluminal recanalization of the recently occluded infarct-related coronary artery in acute myocardial infarction: Comparison with conventionally treated patients. *Clin Cardiol* 2:92, 1979.
12. Kennedy J, Ritchie J, Davis K, et al: The western Washington randomized trial of intracoronary streptokinase in acute myocardial infarction. *N Engl J Med* 312:1073, 1985.
13. Simoons M, Brand M, de Zwaan C, et al: Improved survival after early thrombolysis in acute myocardial infarction. *Lancet* 2:578, 1985.
14. Gruppo Italiano per lo Studio della Streptokinasi Nell'Infarto Miocardico (GISSI): Effectiveness of intravenous thrombolytic treatment in acute myocardial infarction. *Lancet* 1:397, 1986.
15. ISIS-2 Collaborative Group: Randomized trial of intravenous streptokinase, oral aspirin, both or neither among 17,187 cases of suspected acute myocardial infarction: ISIS-2. *Lancet* 2:349, 1988.
16. DeJaegere P, Arnold A, Balk A, et al: Intracranial hemorrhage in association with thrombolytic therapy: Incidence and clinical predictive factors. *J Am Coll Cardiol* 19:289, 1992.

17. Collen D, Topol E, Tiefenbrunn A, et al: Coronary thrombolysis with recombinant tissue-type plasminogen activator: A prospective, randomized, placebo-controlled trial. *Circulation* 70:1012, 1984.

18. Chesebro J, Knatterud G, Roberts R, et al: Thrombolysis in myocardial infarction (TIMI) trial, Phase I: A comparison between intravenous tissue-type plasminogen activator and intravenous streptokinase. *Circulation* 76:142, 1987.

19. Wilcox R, Olsson C, Skene A, et al: The ASSET Study Group. Trial of tissue plasminogen activator for mortality reduction in acute myocardial infarction: Anglo-Scandinavian Study of Early Thrombolysis (ASSET). *Lancet* 2:525, 1988.

20. Gruppo Italiano per lo Studio della Sopravivenza nell'Infarto Miocardico. GISSI-2: A factorial randomized trial of alteplase versus streptokinase and heparin versus no heparin among 12,490 patients with acute myocardial infarction. *Lancet* 336:65, 1990.

21. The GUSTO Investigators: An international randomized trial comparing four thrombolytic strategies for acute myocardial infarction. *N Engl J Med* 329:673, 1993.

22. The GUSTO Angiographic Investigators: The effects of tissue plasminogen activator, streptokinase or both on coronary-artery patency, ventricular function and survival after acute myocardial infarction. *N Engl J Med* 329:1615, 1993.

23. Grines C, Browne K, Marco J, et al: A comparison of primary angioplasty with thrombolytic therapy in acute myocardial infarction. *N Engl J Med* 328: 623, 1993.

24. Gibbons R, Holmes D, Reeder G, et al: Immediate angioplasty compared with the administration of a thrombolytic agent followed by conservative treatment for myocardial infarction. *N Engl J Med* 328:685, 1993.

25. Zijlstra F, Jan de Boer M, Hoorntje J, et al: A comparison of immediate coronary angioplasty with intravenous streptokinase in acute myocardial infarction. *N Engl J Med* 328:680, 1993.

26. Ribiero E, Silva L, Carneiro R, et al: Randomized trial of direct coronary angioplasty versus intravenous streptokinase in acute myocardial infarction. *J Am Coll Cardiol* 22:376, 1993.

27. Rogers W, Dean L, Moore P, et al: Comparison of primary angioplasty versus thrombolytic therapy for acute myocardial infarction. *Am J Cardiol* 74:111, 1994.

28. Every NR, Parsons LS, Hlatky M, et al: A comparison of thrombolytic therapy with primary coronary angioplasty for acute myocardial infarction. *N Engl J Med* 335:1253, 1996.

29. Rodriguez A, Bernardi V, Santaera O, et al: Coronary stents improve outcome in acute myocardial infarction: Immediate and long-term results of the GRAMI trial (abstr). *J Am Coll Cardiol* 31(Suppl):64A, 1998.

30. Jacksch R, Niehues R, Knobloch W, et al: PTCA vs. stenting in acute myocardial infarction. *Circulation* 98(Suppl):307, 1998.

31. Grines C, Cox D, Garcia E, et al: Stent PAMI: Primary Endpoint Results of a Multicenter Randomized Trial of Heparin Coated Stenting vs. Primary PTCA for AMI. *Circulation* 98(Suppl):22, 1998.

32. Antoniucci D, Valenti R, Santoro G, et al: Systematic direct angioplasty and stent-supported direct angioplasty therapy for cardiogenic shock complicating acute myocardial infarction: In-hospital and long-term survival. *J Am Coll Cardiol* 31:294, 1998.
33. Hochman J, Boland J, Sleeper LA, et al: Current spectrum of cardiogenic shock and effect of early revascularization on mortality: Results of an international registry. *Circulation* 91:873, 1995.

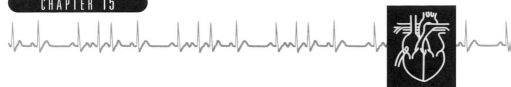

CHAPTER 15

Outcomes of Percutaneous Transluminal Coronary Revascularization

JOSEPH LINDSAY, Jr, MD, AND ELLEN E. PINNOW, RN, MS

This book has provided a snapshot of the state of the art in percutaneous transluminal coronary revascularization (PTCR) in the late 1990s. Introduced only 20 years ago, PTCR has evolved more rapidly than could have been imagined by the pioneers who embraced Andreas Gruentzig's work and set out to increase its effectiveness. PTCR will surely continue to evolve and assume increasing importance in the management of patients with coronary heart disease.

Previous chapters have emphasized a specific PTCR tool or strategy. This final chapter reviews broadly the results of the application of this technology to the care of patients. First, the improvement that has occurred in hospital outcomes over the past 20 years is presented. Then, the comparatively limited information describing the long-term results of PTCR is reviewed, using the available controlled clinical trials comparing PTCR with alternative treatment strategies.

♥ Hospital Outcomes

The immediate consequences of PTCR, both favorable and unfavorable, manifest during hospitalization for the procedure. Because symptom relief may be evident only in some unstable patients, the immediate angiographic result is usually taken as evidence of benefit to the patient.

277

ANGIOGRAPHIC SUCCESS

The goal of PTCR is the reduction or elimination of one or more targeted coronary artery stenoses. This result, termed "angiographic success," has traditionally been defined as improvement in the narrowing of the artery at the target lesion by at least 20% to less than 50% luminal diameter stenosis.[1] A more stringent definition could be justified because the incidence of restenosis is clearly inversely related to the final luminal diameter at the close of the procedure.[2] However, because this review compares current and older data, the traditional definition is used.

The percentage of angiographic success has steadily increased. Initially, approximately a 70% success rate was reported.[1] Presently, 95% of targeted stenoses are successfully treated (Table 15-1).[3,4] This improvement has been achieved despite the fact that far more complex lesions are now targeted for treatment. The earliest experience was limited to the simplest stenoses: single, discrete, and concentric narrowings. Chronic total occlusions, a particularly difficult problem, were seldom targeted.

In contrast, 54.3% of lesions treated at the Washington Hospital Center in 1995 were assigned to the most complex (type C) of the American Heart Association/American College of Cardiology (AHA/ACC) categories.[5] *Type C lesions* include long, eccentric, and calcified lesions and those located in difficult-to-reach sites in the artery. Chronic total occlusions are also included in type C. Increased operator experience, improved

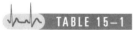 **TABLE 15-1**

In-Hospital Results After Percutaneous Transluminal Coronary Revascularization

	NHLBI 1977–81[1] (N = 1155)	NHLBI 1985–86[1] (N = 1802)	WHC 1991–92[3] (N = 3725)	WHC 1995[4] (N = 3113)
Angiographic Success*	68.6%	89.0%	93.4%	96.2%
Death	1.0%	1.2%	0.9%	0.9%
Q-wave MI	4.3%	4.9%	0.5%	0.3%
Emergency CABG	5.8%	3.5%	2.7%	0.8%
Major complications†	8.8%	7.2%	3.8%	1.7%
Procedural success‡	63.6%	84.3%	88.5%	92.4%

NHLBI, National Heart, Lung, and Blood Institute; WHC, Washington Hospital Center; MI, myocardial infarction; CABG, coronary artery bypass grafting.
*Post-treatment stenosis <50%.
†Death, emergency CABG, or Q-wave MI.
‡Post-treatment stenosis <50% in all target lesions and no major complications.

guiding catheters and wires, and the introduction of new devices all have contributed to this remarkable improvement.

ADVERSE EVENTS

Adverse outcomes include direct complications of the PTCR procedure, such as abrupt closure, death, and myocardial infarction, and the need for additional revascularization.

ABRUPT CLOSURE

Abrupt closure of the target artery at the site of treatment is the most common cause of an ischemic complication of PTCR. Reclosure during the attempt or within a few hours of initial treatment was encountered in 4% to 8% of attempts in the early experience.[6,7]

Dissection of the arterial wall is thought to be the precipitating factor in this complication, but thrombosis and vasospasm also contribute. As might be imagined, such events require either additional transcatheter treatment (prolonged balloon inflation or "bail-out" coronary stenting) or emergency coronary bypass surgery. Despite prompt restoration of flow, myocardial infarction, sometimes fatal, often results.

Stents are associated with their own abrupt closure problem, subacute thrombosis. Unlike abrupt closure after balloon angioplasty or atherectomy, subacute thrombosis often appears several days after the procedure.[8] Because the patient typically has left the hospital, reperfusion may be delayed. As a consequence of this delay, myocardial infarction, sometimes fatal, nearly always accompanies subacute thrombosis. Fortunately, high-pressure balloon inflation to deploy the stent fully and a change from warfarin anticoagulation to antiplatelet therapy have reduced the incidence of this complication from 3% to 4% to about 1%.[9,10]

DEATH

Mortality after PTCR has changed very little from the early experience. When patients with acute myocardial infarction are excluded, the mortality rate has remained at about 1% (see Table 15-1). The age of the patient, the severity of the underlying disease, and the frequency of comorbid conditions all contribute to mortality. The older and more ill the patient, the less able he or she is to tolerate an unsuccessful PTCR or a complication.[3]

Not all deaths after PTCR are a direct consequence of a procedural complication. Often, death occurs in a patient with a life-threatening clinical condition that was not reversed by the procedure, as in the patient treated during an evolving myocardial infarction, particularly one with cardiogenic shock.

MYOCARDIAL INFARCTION

Certain events subsequent to angioplasty are easy to enumerate (e.g., death or coronary artery bypass surgery). Others are more difficult to define. For example, how is postprocedure myocardial infarction defined? If the development of an electrocardiographic Q wave is required, the incidence is low. On the other hand, if only a rise in the cardiac enzymes is counted (non–Q-wave myocardial infarction), the incidence is much greater and varies according to whether, in addition to an enzyme rise, symptoms or electrocardiogram (ECG) changes are required for the diagnosis.

Unfortunately, reports of myocardial infarction after PTCR have not consistently defined the term. The National Heart, Lung, and Blood Institutes (NHLBI) Registries of 1978–81 and 1985–86 reported non-fatal Q-wave myocardial infarction. In both trials, the rate was about 4.5%.[11] Most recently, perhaps because of the availability of better means to treat abrupt closure, the rates of Q-wave myocardial infarction have declined to less than 1% (see Table 15-1).[3,4]

On the other hand, several recent reports indicate that when serum levels of cardiac enzymes are routinely measured, abnormal levels may be present in 10% or more of patients, often without symptoms or ECG changes. Abnormal serum levels appear to be more common when atherectomy devices or stents have been used.[12] Furthermore, some studies suggest that patients with such enzyme elevations appear to have a less favorable long-term prognosis than patients who do not. Investigators debate whether the reduced survival observed in patients with such postprocedural enzyme increases is attributable to the procedural complication or whether it is merely a marker of more severe underlying atherosclerotic disease.

EMERGENCY CORONARY ARTERY BYPASS GRAFT

The need for emergency coronary artery bypass grafting (CABG) after an attempted PTCR most often reflects inability to restore blood flow after abrupt closure by means of catheter-based therapy. The incidence of this complication has declined markedly since the introduction of coronary stents, the deployment of which (bail-out stenting) can often correct an occlusion triggered by dissection of the coronary arterial wall.[7,13] In the early experience, represented by the 1978–81 NHLBI Registry, emergency

CABG was required in 5.8%; in the 1985–86 Registry, it was 3.5%.[11] By 1995, emergency CABG had declined to 0.8% (see Table 15-1).[4]

MAJOR COMPLICATIONS

Many authors have reported a combined variable consisting of any of the following: death, Q-wave myocardial infarction, or emergency CABG. One or more of these events was recorded in 8.8% in the NHLBI Registry of 1978–81 and in 7.2% in the registry of 1985–86.[11] By 1995, the major complication rate had declined to 1.7%, largely as a result of the declines both in the need for emergency CABG and in the occurrence of Q-wave myocardial infarction (see Table 15-1).[4,13]

REPEAT OR ADDITIONAL REVASCULARIZATION

Even an uncomplicated PTCR procedure cannot be regarded as completely successful if an additional catheter-based revascularization of the same lesion is needed during the initial hospitalization or if elective CABG is needed because of an unsuccessful treatment of the stenosis. The need for repeat revascularization was observed in 2.2% of patients at the Washington Hospital Center during 1995.

It is important to recognize that not all revascularization procedures subsequent to a PTCR indicate failure of the initial effort. Some are planned as staged procedures. For example, the cardiologist may perform PTCR of a right coronary or left circumflex narrowing, planning to complete the revascularization by having a surgeon implant an internal mammary artery by means of one of the limited thoracotomy approaches.

CLINICAL SUCCESS

Three possible in-hospital outcomes of PTCR may be envisioned. A patient may have (a) successful dilatation of all targeted lesions and no postprocedural adverse events, (b) successful dilatation of the most important of several targeted lesions and no adverse events, or (c) an adverse postprocedural event (mortality, nonfatal myocardial infarction, CABG, or repeat PTCR).

In the Washington Hospital Center's 1995 experience, 89% of patients had all targeted lesions successfully dilated with no adverse events, and 92% had at least one targeted lesion successfully dilated with no reported adverse events. Of these patients, 5.3% had an adverse outcome, including 1.7% who sustained a major complication (mortality, Q-wave myocardial infarction, or emergency CABG).[4]

♥ Long-Term Outcomes

Initial in-hospital outcomes are important, but before any treatment strategy can be accepted for clinical application, it should demonstrably enhance survival or improve symptoms in at least some identifiable patient categories compared with existing therapies. At present, PTCR is clearly not appropriate in certain patient subsets. For example, those with left main coronary disease are best managed with CABG, whereas medical management is preferable to PTCR or CABG in many mildly symptomatic patients with single-vessel stenosis.

In other patients, cardiologists may legitimately disagree regarding the best therapeutic approach. Such patients may reasonably be entered into randomized trials of one or another therapeutic strategy. A series of such trials have been conducted over the last several years to compare the long-term outcomes of PTCR with medical management or with CABG. For the purpose of this review, data from these trials provide the best available insights into the long-term outcome of PTCR.

All these trials highlight the principal drawback to the long-term success of PTCR, restenosis. After balloon angioplasty, restenosis is encountered in at least 30% of patients with an initially successful dilatation. For certain coronary narrowings, stenting reduces but does not eliminate this

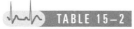 **TABLE 15–2**

Angioplasty Compared With Medical Therapy:
Single-Vessel Obstruction—6 Month Outcomes

Results	Medical Therapy (N = 107)	Angioplasty (N = 105)
Death	1	0
Myocardial infarction	1	0
Nonprotocol angioplasty	11	16
CABG*	0	7
Angina-free*	46%	64%
↑Exercise time*	+0.5 min	+2.1 min
↑QOL Score*	+2.0	+8.6

CABG, coronary artery bypass graft; QOL, quality of life.
*Difference is statistically significant.
Adapted from Parisi AF, Folland ED, Hartigan P: The Veterans Affairs ACE Investigators: A comparison of angioplasty with medical therapy in the treatment of single-vessel coronary artery disease. *N Engl J Med* 326:10, 1992.

problem.[14,15] The pathogenesis of restenosis and the efforts being directed at its prevention have been reviewed earlier in this text. Until the incidence of restenosis can be markedly reduced, the full potential for PTCR to benefit patients cannot be realized.

Because all these trials were designed, conducted, and reported, PTCR technology has leaped forward. In all trials, balloon angioplasty was considered the standard of care. In only a few of the most recent trials were stents used. Thus, the trials reviewed in the following paragraphs do not represent the state-of-the-art PTCR as described in the preceding chapters.

PTCR COMPARED WITH MEDICAL THERAPY

One randomized trial of PTCR compared with medical treatment for patients with stable coronary disease (stable angina, exercise-induced ischemia, or prior myocardial infarction) is available.[16,17] For these patients, their physicians agreed that either therapeutic approach was acceptable at the time the study was initiated. Those randomized to PTCR were treated with balloon angioplasty. Angiographic success in patients with single-vessel obstruction was 82%, and clinical success was 80%. (It should be recalled that these results are substantially inferior to current standards.)

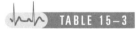 **TABLE 15-3**

Angioplasty Compared With Coronary Artery Bypass Graft (CABG) Meta-Analysis of 8 Trials at 1-Year Follow-Up

	Angioplasty (N = 1710)	CABG (N = 1661)
Death	2.9%	2.3%
Death + MI	7.9%	7.6%
Nonprotocol CABG*	17.8%	1.0%
CABG or angioplasty*	33.7%	3.3%
Angina grade ≥2	28.3%	10.8%

MI, myocardial infarction.
*Difference is statistically significant.
Adapted from Pocock SJ, Henderson RA, Rickards AF, et al: Meta-analysis of randomized trials comparing coronary angioplasty with bypass surgery. *Lancet* 346:1184, 1995.

Patients with single-vessel disease treated with angioplasty enjoyed improved exercise capacity, fewer symptoms, and improved quality of life compared with those randomized to medical treatment (Table 15-2).[16] In patients with multivessel obstruction, no statistically significant advantage was evident for either form of treatment.[17] Death and nonfatal myocardial infarction occurred equally as frequently in angioplasty and medically managed cohorts. Those assigned to angioplasty more often required CABG or repeat PTCR in the 6-month follow-up period.

Based on the latter data, it can be concluded that PTCR offers improved symptoms and quality of life compared with medical management, but patients who undergo PTCR more often require additional revascularization procedures, largely because of restenosis. An even greater advantage to PTCR might be apparent if the study were repeated with stenting to reduce restenosis.[14,15]

PTCR COMPARED WITH SURGICAL REVASCULARIZATION

At least nine recent trials report randomization to either CABG or PTCR of patients in whom revascularization was indicated because of symptoms. Such patients, frequently encountered in clinical practice, typically have disabling symptoms resistant to medical management, but no angiographic findings that dictate CABG. The results of all nine trials are remarkably consistent. Eight of the nine were recently subjected to a meta-analysis.[18] Based on this analysis, several statements can be made.

First, CABG offered no advantage in mortality or nonfatal myocardial infarction over PTCR for 3 to 5 years. However, 30% to 40% of patients randomized to PTCR required either CABG or repeated PTCR within the first year compared with only 5% to 10% of those assigned to CABG (Table 15-3). Again, this difference reflects the high restenosis rate that follows PTCR.

Second, those assigned to CABG reported less angina than those treated with PTCR at the end of the first year of follow-up. This finding may be explained by the combined effects of less complete initial revascularization and more restenosis with PTCR. It bears reemphasis that the rate of revascularization is strongly influenced by the restenosis rate after balloon angioplasty. More favorable outcomes would likely result if stenting were used.

Thus, two conclusions can be drawn to assist in choosing a therapeutic strategy for patients who may be treated with either revascularization strategy. First, CABG does not offer improved survival compared with PTCR. Second, the lesser morbidity associated with PTCR is offset by greater freedom from angina and from the need for repeat revascularization procedures when CABG is chosen.

♥ Summary

The previously cited data provide important information for the selection of treatment strategies for patients with coronary heart disease. PTCR, the most recent approach to therapy, offers a lower initial morbidity than CABG and is therefore the first choice of many patients. The price to be paid in the present state of the art is the frequent need for repeat revascularization in the first year after PTCR. On the other hand, the initial morbidity associated with PTCR is greater than that for medical therapy. However, patients may expect a greater improvement in symptoms and quality of life from that which occurs after PTCR. Thus, the therapeutic strategy must be individualized for each patient. The severity of their symptoms and their coronary atherosclerosis, taken together with their age and associated comorbid conditions, must be factored into the choice of treatment options.

As indicated in the opening paragraphs of this chapter, PTCR is a rapidly evolving technology. The ability of the cardiologist to treat stenoses using percutaneous approaches has improved dramatically. Apart from chronic total occlusions, few obstructions are unable to be successfully relieved.

The next few years are less likely to see a further reduction in restenosis beyond that presently resulting from the use of stents. Thus, the studies cited are not reflective of outcomes with current techniques and certainly do not reflect the increasing advantages of PTCR to be anticipated as the technology matures. Randomized clinical trials such as those reviewed are not very likely to be conducted in the future. They are expensive and difficult to conduct, particularly since physicians and patients are increasingly pleased with current PTCR results. Moreover, the pace of development of the technology is such that before a complicated trial can be designed and conducted, the equipment used has been rendered obsolete.

REFERENCES

1. Detre K, Holubkov R, Kelsey S, et al: The Co-Investigators of the NHLBI Percutaneous Coronary Angioplasty Registry. Percutaneous transluminal coronary angioplasty in 1985–86 and 1977–81. *N Engl J Med* 318:265, 1988.
2. Kuntz RE, Safian RD, Carrozza JP, et al: The importance of acute luminal diameter in determining restenosis after coronary atherectomy and stenting. *Circulation* 86:1827, 1992.

3. Lindsay J Jr, Pinnow EE, Reddy VM, Pichard AD: Discordance in the predictors of mortality vs. those of ischemic complications following transcatheter coronary intervention. *Cathet Cardiovasc Diagn* 32:312, 1994.

4. Lindsay J Jr, Pinnow EE, Pichard AD: New devices enhance hospital results of coronary angioplasty. *Cathet Cardiovasc Diagn* 43:1, 1998.

5. Ryan TJ, Faxon DP, Gunnar RM, et al: Guidelines for percutaneous transluminal coronary angioplasty. A report of the American College of Cardiology/American Heart Association Task Force on the assessment of diagnostic and therapeutic cardiovascular procedures. *J Am Coll Cardiol* 12:529, 1988.

6. Ellis SG, Roubin GS, King SB III, et al: In-hospital cardiac mortality after acute closure after coronary angioplasty: Analysis of risk factors from 8207 procedures. *J Am Coll Cardiol* 11:211, 1988.

7. Bergelson BA, Fishman RF, Tommaso CL: Abrupt vessel closure: Changing importance, management, and consequences. *Am Heart J* 134:362, 1997.

8. Mak K-H, Belli G, Ellis SG, Moliterno DJ: Subacute stent thrombosis: Evolving issues and current concepts. *J Am Coll Cardiol* 27:494, 1996.

9. Albiero R, Hall P, Itoh A, et al: Results of a consecutive series of patients receiving only antiplatelet therapy after optimized stent implantation. *Circulation* 95:1145, 1997.

10. Schomig A, Neumann FJ, Kastrati A, et al: A randomized comparison of antiplatelet and anticoagulant therapy after the placement of coronary-artery stents. *N Engl J Med* 334:1084, 1996.

11. Holmes DR Jr, Holubkov R, Vliestra RE, et al: The Co-Investigators of the National Heart, Lung, and Blood Institute Percutaneous Transluminal Coronary Angioplasty Registry: Comparison of the complications during percutaneous transluminal coronary angioplasty from 1977 to 1981 and from 1985 to 1986: The National Heart, Lung, and Blood Institute Percutaneous Transluminal Coronary Angioplasty Registry. *J Am Coll Cardiol* 12:1149, 1988.

12. Abdelmeguid AE, Topol EJ, Whitlow PL, et al: Significance of mild transient release of creatine kinase-MB fraction after percutaneous coronary interventions. *Circulation* 94:1528, 1996.

13. Altman DB, Racz M, Battleman DS, et al: Reduction in angioplasty complications after introduction of coronary stents: Results from a consecutive series of 2242 patients. *Am Heart J* 132:503, 1996.

14. Serruys PW, de Jaegere P, Kiemeneij F, et al: A comparison of balloon-expandable-stent implantation with balloon angioplasty in patients with coronary artery disease. *N Engl J Med* 331:489, 1994.

15. Fischman DL, Leon MB, Baim DS, et al: The Stent Restenosis Study Investigators: A randomized comparison of coronary-stent placement and balloon angioplasty in the treatment of coronary artery disease. *N Engl J Med* 331:496, 1994.

16. Parisi AF, Folland ED, Hartigan P: The Veterans Affairs ACE Investigators: A comparison of angioplasty with medical therapy in the treatment of single-vessel coronary artery disease. *N Engl J Med* 326:10, 1992.

17. Folland ED, Hartigan PM, Parisi AF: The Veterans Affairs ACE Investigators: Percutaneous transluminal coronary angioplasty versus medical therapy for stable angina pectoris. *J Am Coll Cardiol* 29:1505, 1997.

18. Pocock SJ, Henderson RA, Rickards AF, et al: Meta-analysis of randomized trials comparing coronary angioplasty with bypass surgery. *Lancet* 346:1184, 1995.

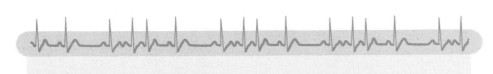

Index

Page numbers in *italics* denote figures; those followed by a t denote tables